Health and Educational Success - Recent Perspectives

Edited by Tebogo Maria Mothiba, Takalani Edith Mutshatshi and Thifhelimbilu Irene Ramavhoya

Published in London, United Kingdom

Health and Educational Success - Recent Perspectives
http://dx.doi.org/10.5772/intechopen.100697
Edited by Tebogo Maria Mothiba, Takalani Edith Mutshatshi and Thifhelimbilu Irene Ramavhoya

Contributors
Masenyani Oupa Mbombi, Mamare Adelaide Bopape, Livhuwani Muthelo, Moila Dimakatso Ophilia, Mabitsela Mphasha, Linda Skaal, Tebogo Maria Mothiba, Terry Jeremy Ellapen, Marine Burger, Yvonne Paul, Makwena Brink Ntjana, Lufuno Makhado, Angelina Maphula, Thendo Gertie Makhado, Ofhani Prudance Musekwa, Leepile Alfred Sehularo, Nombulelo Veronica Sepeng, Carol A. Cummings, Rosemary Reilly-Chammat, Ransford Kwaku Afeadie, Mary Naana-Essiaw, Susanna Adjei Arthur, Andrew Kweku Conduah, Dorothy Siaw-Marfo, Bridget Elikem Mensah, Hilary E. Fairbrother, Phillip B. Carpenter, Deena Khamees, Shane R. Cunha, Delelegn Emwodew Yehualashet, Binyam Tariku Seboka, Tizalegn Tesfaye Mamo, Mulugeta Namaro Yawo, Sheillah Hlamalani Mboweni, Petunia Tsheole, Aqsa Sohail, John Mamokhere, Netshidzivhani Mmbengeni Victor, Selepe Mose, Shannon Ramsey Jimenez

First published in London, United Kingdom, 2023 by IntechOpen
IntechOpen is the global imprint of INTECHOPEN LIMITED, registered in England and Wales, registration number: 11086078, 5 Princes Gate Court, London, SW7 2QJ, United Kingdom

British Library Cataloguing-in-Publication Data
A catalogue record for this book is available from the British Library

Additional hard and PDF copies can be obtained from orders@intechopen.com

Health and Educational Success - Recent Perspectives
Edited by Tebogo Maria Mothiba, Takalani Edith Mutshatshi and Thifhelimbilu Irene Ramavhoya
p. cm.
Print ISBN 978-1-80356-146-2
Online ISBN 978-1-80356-147-9
eBook (PDF) ISBN 978-1-80356-148-6

For EU product safety concerns:
IN TECH d.o.o., Prolaz Marije Krucifikse Kozulić 3, 51000 Rijeka, Croatia,
info@intechopen.com or visit our website at intechopen.com.

Meet the editors

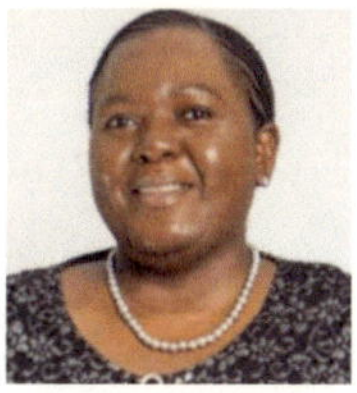

Tebogo Maria Mothiba is the Executive Dean of Faculty of Health Sciences, University of Limpopo, South Africa, where she was previously a research professor during 2018–2020. She is also a South African Research Foundation (NRF) C3-rated researcher. Her research interests are in health service management and non-communicable diseases such as diabetes mellitus and hypertension. She has been a co-principal investigator on projects such as the Scaling-up Packages of Interventions for Cardiovascular Disease Prevention in selected sites in Europe and the sub-Saharan Africa (SPICES) project at the University of Limpopo. She has participated in several funded research projects on strengthening health systems for maternal and child health as well as chronic diseases.

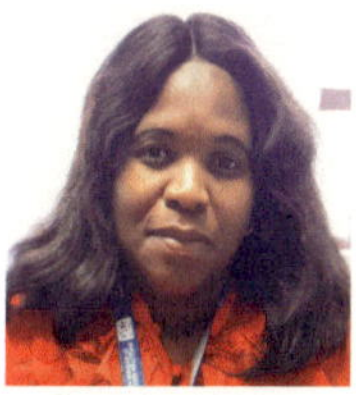

Thifhelimbilu I. Ramavhoya is a researcher, primary health care nurse specialist, and a midwifery lecturer in the Department of Nursing Science, University of Limpopo. She is an associate professor at the University of Limpopo, South Africa. She worked for 17 years as a clinical nurse practitioner and an acting operational manager in one of the primary healthcare facilities of Vhembe district. Her research interests include maternal and child health care, HIV and AIDS, and primary health care. She is a member of the Turfloop Research Ethics Committee at the University of Limpopo and a chairperson of community engagement. She is a journal reviewer and has published numerous articles of her own in accredited research journals.

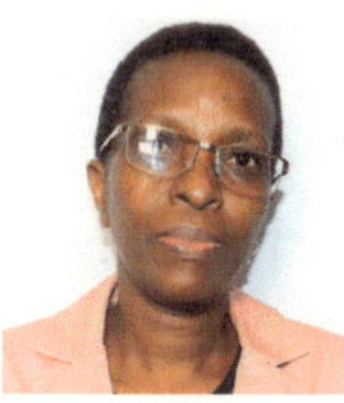

Takalani Edith Mutshatshi is an associate professor in the Department of Nursing Science, School of Health Care Sciences, Faculty of Health Sciences, University of Limpopo, South Africa. She worked as a child nurse specialist for nine years at Donald Fraser Hospital, South Africa, where she introduced Outpatient Child Health Services. She lectured at Limpopo College of Nursing for seven years. She has published articles in national and international peer-reviewed journals. She is a research coordinator in the Department of Nursing Science and serves on the School Research Ethics Committee at the University of Limpopo. She has supervised master's and doctoral student's research. She has won various research presentation awards at conferences. Her research interests are in health service management, child health, and occupational health.

Contents

Preface

The book originates from collaborative research attempts to reflect current perspectives on health and educational success. The authors are from diverse disciplines, pursuing interdisciplinary research activities focusing on health and educational successes from current perspectives. Collaborations are inclusive of medical practitioners, nurses, school-based educators, and other experts within the education and health sectors, all of whom were consulted to validate the information.

This book presents a scholarly discussion on various topics from current perspectives. It includes well-researched information on teachers', nurses', and doctors' views on success in health and education. Most of the book chapters present findings from original research that was conducted for master's and Ph.D. theses and articles. These chapters represent a significant reworking of the unpublished theses and thus the most recent information has been added along with accompanying citations. The book was also independently peer-reviewed by external experts in the field.

In this book, readers will learn about health and educational success from academics as well as established and novice researchers in the following chapters:

Chapter 1: "Perspective Chapter: Communication – Overcoming Generational Difference"

Chapter 2: "Perspective Chapter: Practical Approaches to Enhance Successful Lives among People Living with Epilepsy"

Chapter 3: "Innovations in Active Education Techniques: Team Based Learning, Flipping the Classroom, and Think-Pair-Share"

Chapter 4: "Knowledge of Sugar in Sugar-Sweetened Beverages in South Africa: A Survey of Postgraduate Students"

Chapter 5: "Perspective Chapter: Evidence-Based Medicine – A New Approach for Medical Education and Practice"

Chapter 6: "Awareness and Prevalence of Hepatitis B and C in Rural Areas of Lahore, Pakistan"

Chapter 7: "Perspective Chapter: Integrating Follow-up Care Management for Assessment and Management of Rape Survivors Diagnosed with PTSD and Depression in Primary Health Care Settings"

Chapter 8: "Perspective Chapter: Perspectives toward Overcoming Depression and Anxiety to Enhance Educational Success among Students in a Rural University Context"

Chapter 9: “Nurses’ Coping Strategies When Caring for Mental Health Care Users Diagnosed with Substance Use Disorders”

Chapter 10: “Patient Feedback to Enhance Residents’ Learning: A Patient and a Resident Perspective”

Chapter 11: “Perspective Chapter: Strengthening and Empowering Professional Health Educators’ Capacity and Practice”

Chapter 12: “Obstacles in the Nursing Training Programs”

Chapter 13: “Baseline Analysis for Effective Diabetes Intervention”

Chapter 14: “Factors Contributing to the Academic Challenges Faced by South African Physiotherapy, Occupational Therapy and Biokinetics Students”

Chapter 15: “In the Process of Being Left Behind: Rural-Urban Migration, Precarious Work Conditions, and the Health of Neglected Populations in Agbogbloshie, Accra, Ghana”

Chapter 16: “Perspective Chapter: Enhancing the Nurse-Initiated Management of Antiretroviral Therapy Training and Implementation - A Conceptual Framework”

Some of the chapters are perspective in nature and, as such, the authors use both narrative and integrative literature reviews to build on the known evidence-based practices. Some of the authors generated evidence-based information by using quantitative and qualitative research designs. The methodology used in this book can be transferred to other settings to generate new knowledge.

This book was designed to reach a wide audience with knowledge of the best practices used in various educational as well as clinical institutions, both private and public, to acquaint the individual communities both young and old and it can be applied in various settings.

Tebogo Maria Mothiba, Takalani Edith Mutshatshi and Thifhelimbilu Irene Ramavhoya
Office of the Executive Dean,
Faculty of Health Sciences and Department of Nursing Science,
University of Limpopo,
Polokwane, South Africa

Chapter 1

Perspective Chapter: Communication – Overcoming Generational Difference

Shannon Ramsey Jimenez

Abstract

Each generation has special characteristics brought out by the times in which they have lived, which has affected how they communicate in both reception and expression of information. This chapter examines key differences between the generations and discusses their application to medical education and patient care. Both older generations and younger generations will be discussed. This information was taken from industry, sales, and human resource literature and extrapolated to medical education. This review compares and contrasts the characteristics of the five unique working generations. Some of these characteristics include stoicism, altruism, idealism, and beneficence. The effects of these characteristics will be used to explain how generational differences affect communication specific to teaching, learning, and practicing medicine. This information is then used to show how to improve communication within those settings. In medical education, improved communication can facilitate better learning and more productive and pleasant experiences for the educator, the learner, and the patient.

Keywords: generation, communication, x, y, z, traditional, millennials, baby boomer

1. Introduction

Five generations are currently living together on the planet, and each generation is of the age to have formed their own opinions and expectations. The different generations include the Traditional Generation [>1945], the Baby Boomers [1945–1965~], then Generations X [1965–1980~], Generation Y- "Millennials" [1980–2000~], and Generation Z [2000–2010s~] [1]. Each generation has special characteristics brought out by the times in which they have lived, which in turn has affected the way they communicate in both reception and expression of information. The following chapter looks at key differences between the generations in the United States and discusses their application to medical education and patient engagement.

To better understand health professions students, educators need first to understand themselves. Everyone views the world through the lens of their own personal histories. Each generation will have a brief synopsis of characteristics followed by suggestions for health profession teachers and communication recommendations for learners. This chapter aims to improve communication between educators, learners, health professionals, and their patients. While this chapter focuses on generational differences in the United States, much of the content can be extrapolated to other parts of the world as well. People worldwide may experience history differently and, therefore, may have different characteristics. Using the information in this chapter, one can be mindful of the past and perceptions of the people around them and use that information to better relate and connect with others.

2. The traditional generation

The Traditional generation (aka Traditionals), those born before 1945, was shaped by the Great Depression and World War II, among other events. They have been described as "emotionally conservative," and this is one reason they are also called the "Silent Generation" [2]. They tend to be disciplined, more formal, and have a keen sense of duty. Traditionals like to follow the chain of command and prefer to make decisions based on what worked in the past, but they still seek out technological advances. They value respect, stability, privacy, integrity, order, consistency, practical communication skills, and paying your dues. Traditionals are loyal workers who are highly dedicated, risk-averse, and committed to teamwork and collaboration [2]. They want satisfying work opportunities that are stable, and they appreciate the personal touch such as handwritten notes [1].

2.1 For educators

Teachers from the Traditional Generation should try to understand that the formality and stoicism of their generation seem old-fashioned to younger generations. These characteristics mean less to younger generations than meaningful or genuine interactions [2]. Also, while paying your dues is important to Traditionals, younger generations believe if you are talented and work hard, you should be given a chance to prove yourself [2]. However, Traditionals, Millennials, and Generation Z do have a trait in common. It is their sense of duty [2]. While Traditionals' sense of duty is more targeted to their country or employer, Generation Z's sense of duty is more targeted at a cause. Younger and older generations are both proud of their work, but older generations are proud of the work product, and younger generations are prouder of the experience. All the generations mention wanting to contribute to the greater good as well [2].

2.2 For learners

When communicating with the Traditional Generation, learners should understand that a few well-chosen words of appreciation mean more to this generation. Showing respect is important to them. They expect students to work hard, not complain, and not look for a lot of recognition. However, when Traditionals praise someone, it is short but genuine and meaningful [2].

Learners should be relatively formal and direct but respectful when communicating with clinical teachers. Do not expect a lot of positive feedback, but when you get a few words, know it is meaningful. Appeal to their sense of duty. Be direct but polite. As they appreciate actions more than words, consider making a small card with a thank you. You may also consider doing something that saves them time, like gathering a patient's history or test results before they get in or while they are doing something else [3].

2.3 For healthcare providers

Patients from the traditional generation trust their physicians [4, 5]. They are more likely to do what their healthcare providers tell them to do without questioning it. They look to their physicians for education about their health nearly exclusively, and they expect to visit in person. Their physicians need to be explicit in recommendations as the traditional patient will tend to do precisely what you say [6]. While the recent pandemic has forced many to reach a certain comfort level with telehealth, they still prefer in-person visits when possible. They will sign up for a portal but will likely use it to review results only [7] (**Table 1**).

		General	Educators	Learners	Patients
Traditional >1945	Traits	Stoic, formal, risk-averse, dutiful, digital immigrants	Formal, rule follower, appreciates actions more than words		Implicit trust in their doctors
	Needs	Stability, a persona touch, personal satisfaction	Formal curriculum, know less formality is not disrespected to other generations.	Appreciate the few words of praise offered, be respectful, be direct but polite.	Explicit instructions, in-person interaction,
Baby Boomers 1945–1965	Traits	Optimistic, conflict avoidant, team- oriented, cause-oriented. "Show-me generation" strong sense of fairness	Actions mean more than words; nonconfrontational, love innovation, workaholic	Loves a cause, questions everything,	More likely to challenge physician's opinions
	Needs	To know they make a difference	Make a difference, be mindful of words as they can come out harsh	To be diplomatic, work hard, share ideas, appeal to a sense of fairness	Increase access to physicians through the portal to ask questions, personalized care
Generation X 1965–1980	Traits	"Latch-key kids," fiercely independent, pragmatic, creative, value actions, and accomplishment, cynical	Values hard work over intelligence, words can seem harsh	Results-driven, skeptical of authority, prefers a call	Skeptical of authority, fiercely independent, more likely to use the internet for information than the previous generations
	Needs	Structure and direction, work–life balance	Balance feedback to include positive reinforcement, be mindful of words	Be direct and practical, show independence	Provider to acknowledge internet info and prescribe good sites to find info

		General	Educators	Learners	Patients
Generation Y 1980—000	Traits	Confident, optimistic idealists, respect, dedication, meaning, words mean more than actions, good at teamwork	Actions mean more, dedicated	High expectations of authority, short attention span. Prefers text or e-mail to call.	Not likely to take physicians' advice. More likely to listen to advice online.
	Needs	Encouragement, coaching. To know they are making a positive difference in the world	Respect, positive contribution, be clear on what and how they are teaching, be encouraging	To be heard, balanced life, team activities, clear and organized material, rapid return of information, encouragement, validation be respectful	Acknowledgment, two-way digital communication, reputable sites to find information
Generation Z 2000–2010s	Traits	Still forming. Digital natives. Believe trust is earned, value meaning, social justice warriors. Values effectiveness over convenience		Prefer face-to-face communication. To be part of a greater good	The least likly to seek mental health treatment. Expects digital communication,
	Needs	Still forming		Frequent check ins/feedback. Use technology to communicate with students	Easy, instant/ convenient, digital communication with the healthcare system

Table 1.
Traits and needs of various generations pertaining to educators, learners, and patients. [the empty cells do not have enough in that category to characterize.]

3. The baby boomers

The Baby Boomer Generation are those born between 1945 and 1965, although the exact years vary slightly depending on who you are reading [1]. They witnessed and partook in the political and social turmoil of their time: the Vietnam War, the Civil Rights Movement, the John F. Kennedy (JFK) and Dr. Martin Luther King, Jr. (MLK) assassinations, Watergate, and the sexual revolution as well as Woodstock, and the freewheeling 1960s [2]. Baby Boomers grew up in an era of prosperity and optimism, bolstered by a sense that they are a unique generation capable of changing the world. They respect authority but do not always trust it. Many are accepting of diversity, optimistic, more politically liberal, conflict-avoidant, and relationship-oriented. They also thrive on the possibility of change and love a noble cause. They have a fierce sense of right and wrong. Baby Boomers have been described as the "Show Me Generation," which translates to words meaning little to them and actions meaning more [2].

3.1 For educators

The Baby Boomer Generation will tend to look on the bright side and hold back criticism due to their optimism and conflict avoidance [2]. However, because actions mean more to Baby Boomers than words, their verbal or written communication can seem insensitive and harsh to younger generations as the younger generation values words more. It is helpful to be mindful of their words and avoid "You" terms that can be interpreted as a personal attack. If they must give negative feedback, addressing the action and not the person is interpreted less harshly [3].

3.2 For learners

When communicating with the Baby Boomer generation, one should be diplomatic to avoid seeming confrontational. Confrontation can be interpreted as disrespect, which is something this generation will not tolerate well. Since they value actions, students should work hard and point out what their actions mean [3]. Speak up if you have ideas as Boomers enjoy innovation [2]. Keep a higher ground stance and appeal to their sense of right and wrong.

3.3 For healthcare providers

Baby boomers tend to see their physicians more often due to increasing health needs coupled with the desire to have some control over their health [6].

In part, because they are the "Show-me Generation," Boomers will tend to ask new and follow-up questions in the office and *via* a portal. They also expect high-quality, individualized healthcare [6]. Patients in their 1960s are just as likely as younger patients to register for their patient portal and will use it to ask questions and review results [6, 8]. Patients in this age range will use telehealth services but prefer to use them more for acute issues, and they like it due to convenience and affordability [7].

4. Generation X

Generation X (Xers, as they are known in short) are those born between approximately 1965 and 1980. Gen Xers grew up in a period of financial, familial, and societal insecurity associated with a significant recession. They witnessed their parents being laid off along with the decline of the American global power. Also, Xers grew up with a stagnant job market, corporate downsizing with limited wage mobility, and are the first individuals predicted to earn less than their parents did [2]. They have grown up in homes where both parents worked. This created a "latch-key kid" generation, where they were obligated to fend for themselves. They were influenced by music television (MTV), the HIV/AIDS epidemic, the fall of the Berlin Wall, and their mantra in high school was "question authority" because they felt authority had let them down [9].

Due to their economic hardships, Xers started to walk away from the workaholic lifestyle of the previous generation. They value a balance between work and life and are fiercely independent, entrepreneurial, pragmatic, and creative. They value actions more than words and accomplishment more than money [2].

4.1 For educators

Much like the Boomers, Xer's words may sometimes sound harsh to younger generations. They tend to be straight to the point and less formal [9]. They will notice when a student is trying their best or putting in more hours and be more likely to acknowledge hard work over intelligence. Being mindful of these personal tendencies will hopefully help mitigate them. Learning to give impersonal, balanced feedback can make interactions more meaningful. Making sure to include positive reinforcement and not just point out what a student does wrong is also helpful [3].

4.2 For learners

When communicating with the Gen X generation, be direct and practical. Do not be afraid to share ideas. As mentioned previously, Xers appreciate innovation. Learners should show independence and initiative, like looking things up before they are told or finding a patient's test results that they know the preceptor is waiting for. Asking thoughtful questions also shows that learners are listening and trying to learn, not just going through the motions or biding time until they can leave. Teachers can tell who is really trying and who is not [3].

4.3 For healthcare providers

Since the average age of practicing physicians is 53.8 [10], Gen X healthcare providers are more likely to be the same age or younger than most of the patients they see. This may create some sense of distrust that must be overcome by exhibiting confidence and excellence and educating patients thoroughly on your proposed diagnosis and recommendations.

Surprisingly, Xers are most likely to conduct independent research on conditions and medications – even more than Generation Y or Z. They are less likely to heed all of the physician's advice than the older generations (38%) but also less likely than Generation Z (43%) [5]. This is likely due to the aforementioned insecurity and independence they grew up with. Since so many patients investigate medical issues on the internet, the decision-making process may improve if efforts are made to share the burden of responsibility for knowledge. Further benefits may arise from physicians who assist patients in the information-gathering process [10]. To combat online misinformation, healthcare providers must positively influence patient selection of online materials [10]. This means that physicians should have some idea of certain websites they could recommend to their patients that are accurate and up to date.

5. Generation Y, aka millennials

Millennials are those born between 1980 and 2000, depending on who you listen to. Millennials are now the largest generation since the Baby Boomers' population is shrinking. They are also estimated to make up 75% of the workforce by 2025 [1]. This generation has been shaped by parental excesses, computers, dramatic technological advances, and relative peace. They were raised with close parental involvement (the so-called "helicopter parents"). As children, they were showered with constant praise and therefore may be overly confident [11]. As a result, Millennials are "optimistic idealists." They value respect, being heard, and dedication, and they want leaders who display these qualities. Millennials hold steadfast to ideas or causes but not as much to people or employers. They value meaning and validation and wish to contribute positively to the world [2].

Due to having increased interaction with technology and less with people, words mean more to this group, and they are more idealistic than their predecessors [2]. Millennials desire a more balanced life than the Xers. They have been characterized as "demanding" because they have a high expectation of those in authority [2].

5.1 For educators

Millennials have grown up in an increasingly multicultural society and appreciate diversity. They grew up with technology, change, and political turmoil, so they are adept at going with the flow [1]. This makes them good at teamwork so that they may be more comfortable or adept at interprofessional education activities [11]. Because of significant digital communication, Millennials have grown up with, they have a short attention span [11], are used to things being clear and categorized, and prefer it that way. For example, an educator may be teaching a millennial something all day, but if the educator does not say, "I am going to be teaching you now," it could be possible that the point is missed entirely by the millennial since they may not realize what is happening. Using specific words to relay what is happening or what needs to be observed by the student allows for better understanding since it is made clear to the learner from the beginning [3].

Millennials tend to expect a quick return of information. For example, if a millennial sends a presentation to an educator via e-mail, they will expect an acknowledgment of receipt. They prefer digital communication rather than phone calls by far. Millennials can get anxious with calls as they interrupt their day. Communication via phone may be more reactive and does not allow for well-thought-out ideas. They are likely to return e-mails on the weekend or at night. They perceive e-mails as less urgent than texts [12]. Millennials also tend to be less formal in their communication and seek connectivity with their coworkers and boss outside work. This may be more difficult for older educators or teaching physicians since they were trained to keep professional boundaries, and social interaction may be seen as taboo. It is acceptable to continue to lay firm boundaries but be sure to make the reasoning clear with positive communication [3]. Millennials are accustomed to "coaching" or "parenting" styles of feedback along with a lot of encouragement [11]. As mentioned previously, they appreciate validation and knowing they are contributing to the betterment of the world. Therefore, their contributions should be openly acknowledged if they cannot see them for themselves. Also, feedback, especially negative, should be framed as helping to improve them for their future patients and the greater good [13].

5.2 For learners

It is essential for learners in this generation to consider the adage "know thyself." It is also important to understand where your educators are coming from. While Generation Y is likely to be more technologically advanced than their teachers due to exposure, they should understand that the generations before them did a lot more with a lot less of the technological advances that they had the opportunity to know. Millennials should try to respect the contribution of the older generations, just like they want them to respect theirs. If their teacher or clinical educator does not e-mail or text them back right away or accept an invitation to something after work, it does not mean they are ignoring them. Older generations are more comfortable with a more distinct set of boundaries. However, if they do reach out to a millennial student by e-mail, text, or phone, they must think it is important, so the student should respond as soon as reasonable [3].

5.3 For healthcare providers

Perhaps because they are more technological-oriented and less people-oriented [2], they are the generation who is most likely NOT to heed their physician's advice [5]. However, they outspend baby boomers 2:1 on self-care [14]. Millennials are twice as likely as older generations to act on health advice they find online, believing that what they find online is as good as advice from a physician [15]. They expect to be able to communicate via technology for appointments, results, and consultations. Hence, they are unlikely to frequent an office that does not offer these [15]. Therefore, a provider should try to use these to communicate as well. Due to their exposure to technology, they tend to have short attention spans, so communication with them needs to be succinct and preferably dynamic [16]. It may also help to provide them with reputable websites so they can confirm or elaborate on the conversation with their provider.

6. Generation Z

Generation Z or Gen Z are people born around 1995 to 2010 [1]. They are just now entering the job market, so their characteristics are not fully known yet. They are called "digital natives" because they have known technology since birth [17]. Thus, they are deeply attached to technology and expect employers and schools to embrace it. Due to witnessing turbulent times and political turmoil, Gen Z has less trust for authority and believes respect is earned – more like Traditionals [17]. They value meaning and are motivated to contribute positively to the world. Gen Z members are technological idealists and social justice warriors [17].

Their generation is the most racially and ethnically diverse in history [18, 19] They embrace diversity and expect their leaders to do the same. They perceive that the world is smaller because of technology and use technology for communication more than any other generation. However, 72% of Gen Z workers prefer face-to-face communication at work, while 11% prefer texts, and 9% prefer e-mail [20]. Another study found that Gen Z respondents were more likely than technology-obsessed Millennials to value face-to-face communication, emphasizing effectiveness over convenience [21].

6.1 For educators

A study by The Center for Generational Kinetics found that 60% of Gen Z members prefer multiple check-ins with the boss during the week, and 40% of those workers would prefer that those check-ins happen at least daily [20]. According to the study, if these check-ins and interactions do not occur regularly, a Gen Z worker/student is likely to think they have done something wrong [22]. Therefore, didactic and clinical educators should understand that this generation will request frequent and instant feedback. However, it does not have to be lengthy. A few words of affirmation or correction will do much of the time. It may be beneficial to carve out a set time at the beginning or end of the day to give a little more formal feedback on whatever they are working on. Appeal to their beneficence and point out how they are contributing to the good of their patient or the community [3].

6.2 For learners

Try not to stereotype your teachers as "less connected" or in tune with tech, even though they may be. Generation Z's characteristics are much more like the Xer's than one may think in that you both like direct face-to-face communication and value innovative ideas. Healthcare Educators, particularly those in clinical practice, tend to be very busy. If they cannot give their students the feedback or attention that the students feel is needed immediately, they should be patient. Perhaps ask for a few minutes to discuss something at the end of the day or after the student has had a chance to look up the topic. The learner should offer to look up new research or guidelines and share them with their clinical educator so you can be a value-added resource as well. Learners should try to ask well-thought-out questions. They should also look things up while waiting but not in the room with the patient or while someone is talking to them. That can be perceived as disrespectful. The educator may think they are looking at social media instead of medical research [3]. Chances are that educators are going to be older than learners. Therefore, the learners should read the previous sections on the older generations to learn the best way to communicate with their educators.

6.3 For healthcare providers

Generation Z is the least comfortable visiting a physician [5]. Gen Z members are also 1.6 to 1.8 times more likely to report not seeking treatment for a behavioral health condition than millennials [16]. Because they are digital natives, they are more likely to go to social media for advice from other young people or follow mental health social media personalities to manage their behavioral health challenges. They are also more likely to use emergency rooms and crisis services. Gen Z is increasingly dissatisfied with the traditional healthcare model, and 45% do not have a primary care provider (PCP). They are turning to holistic and preventative care, seeking a convenient experience where they can have full autonomy over their health [23]. To improve communication with Generation Z, healthcare providers must embrace technology. They should offer patient portals and telehealth visits. They should also maintain a social media presence and try to post articles that may benefit various generations. Given the looming mental health crisis among Gen Z, [24], it is imperative that healthcare professionals find ways to improve Gen Z's comfort with and likelihood of accessing general and mental health services.

7. Conclusions

While this information in this chapter is focused on the differences between the generations, it is worthwhile to point out some similarities as well. Notably, several generations have similar descriptors. However, the magnitude of how much that descriptor applies is what changes over time. For example, Traditionals, Boomers, and Xers all value action more than words, but that characteristic became less prominent over time. While Millennials and Gen Z both value words more than actions, it seems more apparent in Z so far. It is also notable that beneficence is a common thread throughout the generations. It seems wanting to know that we are contributing to the greater good is a universal attribute.

Since empathy comes from being able to put oneself into another person's shoes, understanding each other's backgrounds that contribute to our personality traits will also contribute to our empathy. This, in turn, hopefully, will improve our communication and, therefore, our teaching results. Knowledge of generational differences can also be used by students and preceptors in their communication with patients.

This chapter has outlined many characteristics of various generations and communication strategies to use with them. Of course, these are broad generalizations, and other factors like personality type, cultural background, and personal history may keep some people from being stereotypically like the rest of their generation. That is why getting to know your learners by asking them about themselves and their goals is important for the teacher and the learner. Keeping these typical characteristics in mind when interacting with members of these generations can improve communication both ways. In medical education, improved communication can facilitate better learning and more productive and pleasant experiences for the teacher, the learner, and the patient.

Author details

Shannon Ramsey Jimenez
Arkansas College of Osteopathic Medicine, USA

*Address all correspondence to: shannon.jimenez@achehealth.edu

References

[1] Generational differences in the workplace [Infographic]. Purdue Global. Available from: https://www.purdueglobal.edu/education-partnerships/generational-workforce-differences-infographic/. Published 2021. [Accessed June 7, 2021]

[2] Tolbize A. Generational differences in the workplace. Rtc.umn.edu. Available from: https://rtc.umn.edu/docs/2_18_Gen_diff_workplace.pdf. Published 2008. [Accessed June 7, 2021]

[3] Jimenez S, Ford-Wilcox H. Generational differences in communication and translation to medical education. Osteopathic Family Physician. 2022;**14**(2):1-4. DOI: 10.33181/13068

[4] Medscape E. How generational factors impact patient engagement. Integrated healthcare executive. Available from: https://www.hmpgloballearningnetwork.com/site/ihe/article/how-generational-factors-impact-patient-engagement. Published 2022. [Accessed August 14, 2022]

[5] Katie A. Older generations place more trust in physicians than younger ones, study says. Beckershospitalreview.com. 2021. Available from: https://www.beckershospitalreview.com/digital-marketing/older-generations-place-more-trust-in-physicians-than-younger-ones-study-says.html. [Accessed 19 Aug 2022]

[6] Heath S. Understanding generational differences in patient engagement. Patient engagement HIT. Available from: https://patientengagementhit.com/news/understanding-generational-differences-in-patient-engagement. Published 2016. [Accessed August 14, 2022]

[7] Sathyanarayanan D et al. Telehealth use in geriatrics care during the COVID-19 pandemic—A scoping review and evidence synthesis. International Journal of Environmental Research and Public Health. 2021;**18**(4):1755. MDPI AG. DOI: 10.3390/ijerph18041755 [Accessed 15 Aug 2022]

[8] Heath S. Adoption of patient portals growing in older populations. EHR intelligence. Available from: https://ehrintelligence.com/news/adoption-of-patient-portals-growing-in-older-populations. Published 2016. [Accessed August 16, 2022]

[9] Gerber Ben S, Eiser AR. The patient-physician relationship in the internet age: Future prospects and the research agenda. Journal of Medical Internet Research. 2001;**3**(2):e15. JMIR Publications Inc. DOI: 10.2196/jmir.3.2.e15 [Accessed 19 Aug 2022]

[10] Newitt P. Physicians' average age by specialty. Beckersasc.com. Available from: https://www.beckersasc.com/asc-news/physicians-average-age-by-specialty.html#:~:text=The%20average%20age%20of%20a,to%20data%20firm%20Definitive%20Healthcare. Published 2022. [Accessed August 19, 2022]

[11] Levenberg P, Aaron M. The millennials in medicine: Tips for teaching the next generation of physicians. Journal of Academic Ophthalmology. 2014;**07**(01):e017-e020. DOI: 10.1055/s-0034-1396088

[12] 4-Fein K. What's left of generation X. Dissent Magazine. Available from: https://www.dissentmagazine.org/article/whats-left-of-generation-x. Published 2019. [Accessed June 7, 2021]

[13] Anderson E, Buchko AA, Buchko KJ. Giving negative feedback to millennials. Management Research Review. 2016;**39**(6):692-705. DOI: 10.1108/mrr-05-2015-0118

[14] Sherber N. The millennial Mindset. Journal of Drugs in Dermatology: JDD. 2018;**17**(12):1340-1342

[15] Goodwin J. Understanding the "Why" for gen Y: What millennials are looking for in healthcare practices. Mgma.Com. 2022. Available from: https://www.mgma.com/resources/quality-patient-experience/understanding-the-why%E2%80%9D-for-gen-y-what-millennials. [Accessed 19 Aug 2022]

[16] Gooch K. 6 Ways Gen Z interacts differently with the healthcare system. Beckershospitalreview.com. 2022. Available from: https://www.beckershospitalreview.com/strategy/6-ways-gen-z-interacts-differently-with-the-healthcare-system.html. [Accessed 19 Aug 2022]

[17] Frances T, Hoefel F. 'True Gen': Generation Z and its implications for companies. McKinsey.com. Available from: https://www.mckinsey.com/industries/consumer-packaged-goods/our-insights/true-gen-generation-z-and-its-implications-for-companies?cid=eml-web. Published 2018. [Accessed June 7, 2021]

[18] Who is Gen Z and how will they impact the workplace. Western Governors University. Available from: https://www.wgu.edu/blog/who-is-gen-z-how-they-impact-workplace1906.html. Published 2019. [Accessed June 7, 2021]

[19] Parker K, Graf N, Igielnik R. Generation Z looks a lot like millennials on key social and political issues. Pew research center's social & demographic trends project. Available from: https://www.pewsocialtrends.org/2019/01/17/generation-z-looks-a-lot-like-millennials-on-key-social-and-political-issues. Published 2019. [Accessed June 7, 2021]

[20] Campiere A. How generation Z communicates at work: Ryan Jenkins, Others Weigh IN. PCMA. Available from: https://www.pcma.org/how-generation-z-communicates-work/. Published 2019. [Accessed June 7, 2021]

[21] Yozell Associates. Generation Z Values Face-To-Face Business Communication. Yozell Associates; Employee Benefits Newsletter. Available from: http://yozell.com/blog/generation-z-values-face-face-business-communication. Published 2017. [Accessed June 7, 2021]

[22] Denison E. Generation Z Research – State of Gen Z™ 2018 – The Center for Generational Kinetics. The Center for Generational Kinetics. Available from: https://genhq.com/generation-z-research-2018. Published 2018. [Accessed June 7, 2021]

[23] Sing Sonia IM, Christina IM. The rise of digital natives: How millennials and Gen Z are transforming healthcare - AVIA. AVIA. 2021. Available from: https://aviahealth.com/insights/the-rise-of-digital-natives-how-millennials-and-gen-z-are-transforming-healthcare/#:~:text=Gen%20Z%20is%20increasingly%20dissatisfied,full%20autonomy%20over%20their%20health. [Accessed 19 Aug 2022]

[24] Benton TD, Boyd RC, Njoroge WF. Addressing the global crisis of child and adolescent mental health. JAMA Pediatrics. 2021;**175**(11):1108-1110. DOI: 10.1001/jamapediatrics.2021.2479

Chapter 2

Perspective Chapter: Practical Approaches to Enhance Successful Lives among People Living with Epilepsy

Lufuno Makhado, Angelina Maphula, Thendo Gertie Makhado and Ofhani Prudance Musekwa

Abstract

Epilepsy is a neglected noncommunicable condition in this era. Therefore, it is imperative that practical approaches to enhance the management of epilepsy for the success of people living with epilepsy (PLWE) be analyzed and described. The chapter will encompass the challenges faced by people living with epilepsy, their needs, the PLWE resilience and coping strategies, epileptic seizure first-aid management, and support for people living with epilepsy. The issues aforementioned can potentially shape the future of the people living with epilepsy if attended to effectively. It is high time that epilepsy and people living with epilepsy are given the attention they require to reduce the stigma attached, misconceptions, maltreatment, mismanagement, and negative cultural and religious beliefs, as this will encourage the people living with epilepsy to accept themselves and partake in the family, community, school, and societal engagements without any fear.

Keywords: management, people living with epilepsy, seizures, resilience, support

1. Introduction

Epilepsy is a condition characterized by experiences of unprovoked seizures caused by synchronous or excessive neural activity [1]. An enduring predisposition characterizes it to seizures and results in neurobiological, cognitive, psychological, and social consequences. People living with epilepsy (PLWE) experience altered sensations, behavior, and consciousness due to a discharge of nerve tissue on muscles. The misconceptions and ill understanding of epilepsy constitute the prevalence of epilepsy. The World Health Organization [2] shows that 70% of people living with epilepsy could live free of seizures due to effective scientific medication attained at a low cost. However, this is not so due to a lack of knowledge of the disorder. According to the World Health Organization [2], epilepsy does not get as much attention as it deserves from health practitioners and policymakers. There is a noticeable gap in knowledge of epilepsy between African countries, European countries, Asian countries, and America. In the United Kingdom, a national survey collected shows very low stigma and knowledge satisfaction [3]. In Asia, although Karimi and Akbarian [4] show that PLWE have somewhat adequate knowledge about the disease, Thapa et al. [5] show inadequate knowledge in the general public. General awareness of the disease is not certain in Asia, especially because some believe sleep deprivation and certain drinks and foods trigger seizures [4].

In rural sub-Saharan African countries, there is a persistent prevalence of epileptic misconceptions [6], and this is supported by Kaddumukasa et al. [7] who reported among other things that epilepsy is considered a curse from God and is caused by witchcraft that PLWE are considered to be insane and should be isolated. A couple of studies done in African countries show how knowledgeable people in Africa are about epilepsy. Armah-Ansah et al. [8] state that although about 97.5% of people said to have heard about epilepsy, they still share negative attitudes toward it, resulting in isolation and stigma. In Ethiopia, 97% have never heard about epilepsy, 85.6% proved not knowledgeable about epilepsy, and 86.8% expressed a generally negative attitude toward epilepsy and PLWE [9]. These statistics are incomparable to the 5.9% who had never heard of epilepsy in Asia [5]. Kaddumukasa et al. [7] show that perceptions, stigma, and misconceptions about epilepsy are based on culture and wrong information taught. Besides an increased mortality rate, the ill information and knowledge on epilepsy bear fruit to several challenges experienced by PLWE, their families/caregivers, and those in close relationship with them.

In most cases, it is found that PLWE are excluded due to negative beliefs held by the general public. According to Kaddumukasa et al. [7], PLWE are excluded from community involvement. They are not allowed to play with other people as epilepsy is believed to be contagious, which adds to their isolation and segregation. This shows that PLWE, along with their families, are marginalized. In their study, Henok and Lamaro [9] show that 30% of their study's sample believe that PLWE should be isolated from society, and 40% said they are associated with PLWE and have their children isolated from any known person with epilepsy. As a means of precaution, their families put measures that isolate them. Along with forced social exclusion, PLWE isolates themselves because they feel ashamed and rejected.

A study revealed that people without the disease refuse to marry PLWE [7]. This results in a negative outlook on marriage from PLWE. How others view epilepsy and their attitude toward it causes great distress for PLWE. This results in interpersonal challenges, and they become impatient with other people expressing consistent general agitation [10]. Furthermore, the literature reveals that PLWE often experiences shame, which evokes guilt, grief, and anger [10–12]. Guilt often comes from the feelings of burdening others. For most, epilepsy leads to fear and anxiety [12].

In addition, PLWE generally experiences anxiety disorders and mood disorders. The weight of stigma, discrimination, and social limitation often leads to low self-esteem and depression, contributing to suicide. PLWE may not be able to perform day-to-day tasks, and they may also have physical injuries [13]. In addition, epilepsy can impact speech and add to language difficulties [14].

As a global crisis that affects over 50 million people and increasing due to new births, epilepsy implores intensive research, especially in low-middle-income countries. Countries in Africa show insufficient levels of knowledge mostly influenced by their traditional African culture and background compared to other countries, such as Europe and the United States of America, which do noy share the same beliefs [15]. It is evident that the level of knowledge that one has on epilepsy ultimately influences their ideas about epilepsy, which contributes to their attitudes and behavior toward epilepsy and PLWE. In most cases, these attitudes and behaviors result in negative impacts as they result from ignorance and prejudice.

PLWE generally experience a low quality of life and are burdened with the effects the disorder has on their lives and the lives of those close to them. The root of this is insufficient fallacious knowledge and understanding of epilepsy. Misconceptions about epilepsy, stigma, and ill social coping mechanisms of PLWE may be due to a lack of accurate knowledge about epilepsy. PLWE experience social exclusion, anxiety, guilt, and embarrassment because of epilepsy. The lack of education and precise knowledge on epilepsy prolongs such psychological and social distress. In addition to these, misconceptions hinder prompt diagnosis and appropriate treatment [16]. Misconceptions may be because community members are not open to talking about epilepsy. Epilepsy South Africa [17] shows that by the age of 20 years, 75% have already experienced their first seizure. This means that most people have their first seizure during their childhood. Murugupillai et al. [18] show that parents avoid talking about epilepsy with their children. This then promotes the misconceptions as they grow up believing in all that they come across in their life span.

Consequently, this is the start of stigma, and the spread of misconceptions about epilepsy as ideas about epilepsy are spontaneously made up upon experiencing the seizure or witnessing another young person having an epileptic seizure. Hence, this chapter aims to provide the challenges faced by PLWE, their needs, the immediate management of seizures, care, and support of PLWE to widen the understanding and provide practical approaches to promote a conducive environment for PLWE.

2. Challenges faced by PLWE

To improve the everyday living of PLWE and enhance their quality of life, it is important to ask the questions: "what is the impact of epilepsy?" and "How is it like LWE?". By answering these questions, we can begin to understand the challenges PLWE has and ultimately achieve the goal. This section will highlight the challenges experienced by PLWE, the physical, psychosocial, economic, and existential challenges.

2.1 Physical challenges

In the occurrences of seizures, more often than not, patients experience uncontrolled physical challenges, e.g. urinal excretion. Some patients sustain physical injuries in the least end; they are nonfatal; however, in the end, death may result. A study done evaluating injuries among PLWE found that 85.5% have sustained an injury during a seizure [19]. On the other hand, Bifftu et al. [20] reported 27.8% of physical injuries. Some of these injuries include as follows:

- Soft tissue injury [19, 21]
- Dental and tongue injury [19–22]
- Head and/or brain injury [19, 20, 22, 23]

- Burns [19–23]
- Fractures [20–24]
- Memory and concentration problems [25, 26]
- Treatment challenges in terms of experiencing a high number of adverse side effects [25–28]

Some physical challenges result from seizure aftermath and may only apply to PLWE who experience generalized or focal motor seizures. Regardless of the type of epilepsy, physical challenges (living with injuries and those that are a direct result of seizure occurrence) can negatively impact the quality of life. An epileptic experiencing mood and behavioral side effects are just as challenged as a person with a visible injury, e.g. a person with a burn or dental injury may encounter frequent stares that leave them feeling embarrassed. In essence, many physical challenges experienced are much connected with psychosocial challenges.

2.2 Psychosocial challenges

Generally, psychosocial challenges vary across ages [27–29]. PLWE are often stigmatized, prejudiced, and segregated because they are LWE. PLWE are also often excluded from educational opportunities [30]. These challenges often result in comorbidities such as depressive disorders, anxiety disorders, and stress disorders. In addition to these issues, PLWE have suicidal thoughts, they fear being alone, fear being in social spaces, suffer continuous embarrassment, and lose relationships due to this disease, and this often leads to isolation [28–32]. In most cases, epilepsy's psychosocial consequences are not directly caused by the disorder; instead, they result from external factors such as behaviors and attitudes about epilepsy and PLWE.

2.3 Economic challenges

Epilepsy poses financial challenges for PLWE as well as their caregivers/families. The WHO [30] shows that "out-of-pocket costs" become burdensome. These costs are used to purchase treatment, travel to health care facilities, and pay for therapies. In some instances, young people drop out of school (and essentially become unemployed) due to the disease burden. In one study, experiences of epileptic seizures at a workplace resulted in resignation from their work [33]. Consequently, on a personal and household level, PLWE experience or contribute to a financial burden.

2.4 Treatment challenges

This challenge contributes to physical, lifestyle/social, and economic challenges. Patients on anti-epileptic drugs (AEDs) may experience tiredness, dizziness, headaches, memory loss, and issues with attention [25, 32]. Social side effects of treatment may include altering eating schedules and what they eat and monetary challenges because of treatment costs. In their findings, Fazekas et al. [34] report that epilepsy treatment side effects are often unbearable to PLWE. In addition to the hostile experience of treatment, about 7–20% of children and 30–40% of adults living with epilepsy are said to be drug-resistant [35]. In addition, convenience, drug side effects, and unavailability of treatment result in the growing dependence on traditional treatment from traditional healers of epilepsy [36].

Treatment challenges are often experienced in low-middle-income countries where we find low-quality health facilities, access to health care services, short medicine supply, and cost of purchased medication. According to WHO [30], about three-quarters of PLWE may not receive proper medication, and there is a treatment gap within the low-middle-income countries. It is reported that less than 50% of PLWE have access to anti-epileptic medication.

Epilepsy is a disease that may be cured. However, in most instances, it can only be managed. In this regard, it is possible that PLWE may experience lifelong challenges if there is no intentional intervention to mitigate the effects of the factors deemed to be challenging and meet their needs.

3. Needs of PLWE

Reflecting on the previous section, the needs of PLWE are pivotal to increasing the quality of life, especially because their challenges influence areas where they need support. There is a need for easier access to care and treatment, especially in low-middle-income countries. What's more, PLWE needs financial support/access to more medication options, eliminating generalized diagnosis and prescription of medication.

WHO [30] suggests that to increase PLWE's quality of life, there needs to be a change in the legislature and an increase in the international standard of the law to be inclusive and considerate of PLWE. This may help protect PLWE in schools and workplaces and give them equal opportunities to attain a future and profession. PLWE who reside in underserved populations generally have low self-management because of a lack of education and equipment [37]. Musekwa et al. [12] and Yeni et al. [38] show that education (educating the public, PLWE, and caregivers about epilepsy) has become a need and a way to increase the quality of life and PLWE.

Fazekas et al. [34] reflect that the greater need is to relieve their psychosocial challenges, what's more, there is a need for therapy and social support for PLWE. Yeni et al. [38] add a close correlation between mental health and the quality of life for PLWE. Focusing on fulfilling this need will help in decreasing psychosis comorbidities, attaining positive mental health, strengthening coping mechanisms, and building resilience.

4. PLWE resilience and coping strategies

The ability to cope and function while living with epilepsy daily may be challenging. This section provides the strategies that can enhance and strengthen PLWE's resilience and coping with the condition.

4.1 Making connections

The importance of good relationships with close family members, friends, and others cannot be overemphasized [39–41]. This can be achieved by accepting help and support from those who care about PLWE and are willing to listen to them, strengthening resilience. Some people find that being active in civic groups, faith-based organizations, or other local groups provides social support and can help reclaim hope [42–47]. As much as PLWE are making connections with the significant others, reciprocal attention must be provided from the significant others. It has been noted that assisting others in their time of need can also benefit the assister [48]. As a result, this puts PLWE in the position to help those in need, as it is likely to offer assistance in a crisis.

4.2 Looking beyond the crises

You cannot change the fact that highly stressful events happen, but you can change how you interpret and respond to these events. The psychosis of epilepsy can be overwhelming, and its neurobiological basis remains unclear [49]. The misconceptions, stigma, and myths attached to epilepsy arise due to a lack of understanding regarding epilepsy among populations. As a result, PLWE needs to look beyond the present to see how future circumstances may be better. In dealing with difficult situations, PLWE must be able to notice subtle ways in which they might feel a bit better.

4.3 Accept that change is a part of living

People with epilepsy often experience changes in their quality of life, such as reduced mobility and having difficulties learning, attending school, working, and interacting with others [50–52]. Most PLWE live a full, active life that includes school, friends, sports, and other relevant activities most people living without epilepsy engage in. The extent to which epilepsy interrupts a PLWE's life depends on the type of epilepsy, the effectiveness of treatment, and many other factors. To help PLWE become more independent, ensure they receive appropriate care and support throughout their transition in life. The vast majority of people with epilepsy can drive, go to college, get a job, get married, and raise a family [53–55]. Learning about epilepsy, your rights and responsibilities, and where to find support and resources will help you live a happy and fulfilling life [56]. As a result of epileptic adverse situations, some goals may no longer be achievable. However, PLWE can surpass this by accepting circumstances that cannot be changed to help them focus on changeable circumstances.

4.4 PLWE to take decisive action to achieve their goals

We all have goals in life, and PLWE are not excluded. Therefore, it is also essential for PLWE to develop realistic goals. These may be short- or long-term goals, but they provide a reason to carry on living and striving for a better tomorrow. PLWE should engage in regular activities no matter how small they may seem; small accomplishments will enable them to move forward toward their goals [46]. Focus on what you can accomplish today rather than on impossible tasks. Take action as much as possible when faced with adverse circumstances. It is better to take action than to avoid problems and stress by wishing that they would go away [46].

4.5 Look for opportunities for self-discovery and nurture a positive self-view

As a result of epilepsy, PLWE may learn something about themselves and find that they have grown somehow. Through the experience of the epileptic condition, epilepsy-related tragedies and hardship, most PLWE reported improved relationships, a greater sense of strength even when feeling vulnerable, an enhanced sense of self-worth, and a more developed spirituality [57]. Resilience can be built by PLWE trusting their instincts and developing confidence in their ability to solve problems.

4.6 Take care of yourself by maintaining a hopeful outlook

People living with epilepsy should be attentive to their own needs and feelings. They should engage themselves in activities that they enjoy and find relaxing. Regular physical activities and exercises are highly recommended. Self-care helps PLWE keep their minds and bodies primed to deal with any situation requiring resilience. An optimistic outlook enables you to expect that good thing will happen in your life. Thus, PLWE needs to attempt to visualize what they want rather than worry about their fear. PLWE must identify ways that are likely to work well for them as part of their strategy for nurturing resilience.

5. Management of epileptic seizures first aid

This section intends to provide the first-aid quick guide for seizures, and the guide is particularly relevant for tonic–clonic seizures as the person fits, shakes, or jerks. Before the first aid, a brief description of the seizures is described. According Centers for Disease Control and Prevention seizures are classified into two groups [58], thus general and focal seizures.

Both absence and tonic–clonic seizures are generalized seizures that affect both sides of the brain. There can be rapid blinking or a few seconds of staring into space during absence seizures, which are sometimes called petit mal seizures. The effects of tonic–clonic seizures, also called grand mal seizures, can include crying out, losing consciousness, falling to the ground, having muscle jerks or spasms, and feeling fatigued afterward. As opposed to focal seizures, partial seizures occur only in one part of the brain. Depending on their complexity, they can be classified as simple focal, complex focal, or secondary generalized seizures. Simple focal seizures affect a small area of the brain and can cause twitching or unusual sensations. The other type of seizure is complex focal seizures, which can leave a person with epilepsy confused or bewildered. As a result, the person may be unable to react to queries or directions for a few minutes. Finally, a secondary generalized seizures originates in one section of the brain but extend to both sides. In other words, the individual has a focused seizure initially, followed by a generalized seizure [59].

Although seizures can be terrifying to witness, they are not always a medical emergency. Habitually, once the seizure stops, the person recovers, and their breathing goes back to normal. Now it is important to know what to do in case of a seizure, and the following guide [59] provides a step-by-step directive of how to attend to the person:

- Try to stay calm.
- Look around—is the person in a dangerous place? If not, do not move them. Move objects around the person like furniture, away from them.
- Note the time the seizure starts.

- Cushion their head with something soft if they have collapsed to the ground.
- Look for medical jewelry or an ID card for information about what to do.
- Do not hold them down.
- Do not put anything in their mouth.
- Try to stop other people crowding around.
- After the seizure has stopped, gently put them into the recovery position and check that their breathing is returning to normal. Gently check their mouth to see that nothing is blocking their airways, such as food or false teeth. If their breathing sounds difficult after the seizure has stopped, call for an ambulance.
- Try to minimize any embarrassment. If they have wet themselves, deal with this as privately as possible.
- Stay with the person until the seizure ends and they are fully awake. After it ends, help the person sit in a safe place. Once they are alert and able to communicate, tell them what happened in straightforward terms. They may need gentle reassurance.
- Do not give them anything to eat or drink until they are fully recovered.
- When to call for medical assistance

Usually, when a person has an epileptic seizure, there is no need to call an ambulance. However, always call for emergency assistance in case any of the following apply:

- you know it is the person's first seizure;
- they have injured themselves badly;
- they have trouble breathing after the seizure has stopped;
- one seizure immediately follows another with no recovery in between;
- the seizure lasts 2 minutes longer than is usual for them; or
- you do not know how long their seizures last.
- Suppose you need to call the emergency services on an Android or iPhone device. In that case, there are ways to send your GPS location to the emergency services simultaneously automatically.

Some people recover quickly from a tonic–clonic seizure, but they will often be exhausted, want to sleep, and may not feel back to normal for several hours or days [60].

6. Supporting people living with epilepsy

Caring for people living with epilepsy can involve several skills, including technical tasks such as dealing with medical equipment, emotional support, being able to adapt if needs change, or working with health care professionals involved in the person's health or care. These roles may be in addition to other demands in terms of parents or caregivers such as their family, other relationships, work, home, financial constraints, social life, their own health, and hopes and wishes. Parents or caregivers may cope well with multitasking, or they may find it difficult to cope as some areas of their lives are being neglected. As a teacher in a school setting, it may be hard to merely focus on PLWE while having a class with multiple learners with different care needs that also seek their attention, let alone their teaching role. However, according to the Epilepsy Society (UK) [61], it is essential that parents, caregivers, and teachers who are caring for someone with epilepsy, the following are the aspects or activities they should do to support PLWE:

- keeping them safe during and after a seizure,
- calling for medical help, or giving first aid or emergency medication,
- staying with them or seeing them home safely after a seizure,
- noting any pattern or trigger to their seizures, which may help if they do not recall their seizures,
- helping them with their routine of taking anti-epileptic drugs (AEDs),
- going with them to appointments, helping to take notes, or providing descriptions of seizures to the person with epilepsy and their health care providers,
- acting as a representative or advocate for the person, with their health care providers involved in their care
- joining in with leisure activities that might pose a safety risk if they were to have a seizure, such as swimming, etc.
- providing transport if necessary
- helping them to adapt their home or lifestyle to provide a safe living environment.

The activities aforementioned are critical to the care of someone with epilepsy and may present a lot of responsibility to the parent, caregiver, or teacher. It should also be noted that these activities are very vital and valuable to PLWE. Apart from attending to the presented activities, it should be noted that co-morbid exist as well. Thus, PLWE may also have other conditions that require extra care needs. Given the need for social welfare's support for PLWE, sometimes this becomes a turmoil as seizures may be infrequent or unwitnessed by others. Thus, other people may not see the need for care; hence, some social services do not always distinguish epilepsy as a condition with particular care needs.

Caring and supporting PLWE carries physical attention and psychological and emotional attention needs. Thus, living with epilepsy can have a psychological impact which may also affect parents, caregivers, or teachers as their caregivers. This could include stress, depression, or mood changes. In addition, as epilepsy is an individual condition, it can change over time [61]. The amount of care that is needed may increase or decrease. The situation of the parent, caregiver, or teacher could change. They may become physically unable or have now focused on their own health needs as well as the need to regain their independence. It may also be that those providing care are even caring for more than one person, increasing the caregiver's strain. This is some of the baggage that comes with caring for people living with epilepsy, and there is a need to find ways to cope and maintain the caring role. In contrast, some people may expect that the caregiver can continue to manage regardless of their own needs or strains just because they always have done before.

7. Conclusions

The chapter provided the challenges faced by PLWE as well as their needs. We further provided approaches to promote resilience and coping among the PLWE, the immediate management of seizures, and care and support of PLWE. The issues aforementioned can potentially shape the future of the PLWE if attended effectively. It is high time that epilepsy and PLWE are given the attention they require to reduce the stigma attached, misconceptions, maltreatment, mismanagement, and negative cultural and religious beliefs, as this will encourage the PLWE to accept themselves and partake in the family, community, school, and societal engagements without any fear.

Acknowledgements

The author acknowledges the GladAfrica Epilepsy Foundation Trust and the GladAfrica Epilepsy Research Project to stimulate this chapter's conceptualization.

Conflict of interest

The authors declare no conflict of interest.

Author details

Lufuno Makhado*, Angelina Maphula, Thendo Gertie Makhado
and Ofhani Prudance Musekwa
University of Venda, Thohoyandou, South Africa

*Address all correspondence to: lufuno.makhado@univen.ac.za

References

[1] England MJ, Austin JK, Beck V, Escoffery C, Hesdorffer DC. Erasing epilepsy stigma: Eight key messages. Health Promotion Practice. 2014;**15**(3):313-318

[2] World Health Organization. Epilepsy: A Public Health Imperative: Summary. Geneva, Switzerland: World Health Organization; 2019

[3] Holmes E, Bourke S, Plumpton C. Attitudes towards epilepsy in the UK population: Results from a 2018 national survey. Seizure. 2019;**65**:12-19

[4] Karimi N, Akbarian SA. Knowledge and attitude toward epilepsy of close family members of people with epilepsy in North of Iran. Advances in Medicine. 2016. 6 p. Available from: https://downloads.hindawi.com/journals/amed/2016/8672853.pdf

[5] Thapa L, Bhandari TR, Shrestha S, Poudel RS. Knowledge, beliefs, and practices on epilepsy among high school students of Central Nepal. Epilepsy Research and Treatment. 2017;**1187**:7

[6] Mbelesso P, Luna J, Yangatimbi E, Mboukou C, Preux PM. Sociocultural representations of epilepsy in the Central African Republic: A door-to-door survey. Seizure. 2019;**67**:23-26

[7] Epilepsy South Africa. Epilepsy South Africa Services + programmes. 2017. Available from: https://epilepsy.org.za/new/uploads/files/Epilepsyinformation2017/2017%20Activity%20Booklet%20for%20Children.pdf

[8] Kaddumukasa M, Kaddumukasa MN, Buwembo W, Munabi IG, Blixen C, Lhatoo S, et al. Epilepsy misconceptions and stigma reduction interventions in sub-Saharan Africa, a systematic review. Epilepsy and Behavior. 2018;**85**:21-27

[9] Armah-Ansah EK, Oteng KF, Affum JB. Population and health students knowledge, attitude and perception towards epilepsy patients. Epilepsy Journal. 2018;**4**(132):2472-2895

[10] Henok A, Lamaro T. Knowledge about and attitude towards epilepsy among menit community, Southwest Ethiopia. Ethiopian Journal of Health Sciences. 2017;**27**(1):47-58

[11] Siriba RM. The experiences of people living with epilepsy in Nzhelele, Limpopo Province. A thesis submitted in partial fulfilment of the requirements for the degree of Master of Psychology in the Faculty of Humanities at the University of Limpopo. South Africa. 2014

[12] National Center for Chronic Disease Prevention and Health Promotion, Division of Population Health. Epilepsy, information for specific groups: Training for professionals. 2018. Available from: https://www.cdc.gov/epilepsy/groups/professionals.htm

[13] Musekwa OP, Makhado L, Maphula A, Mabunda JT. How much do we know? assessing public knowledge, awareness, impact, and awareness guidelines for epilepsy: A systematic review. The Open Public Health Journal. 2020;**13**(1)

[14] Keikelame MJ, Swartz L. It is always HIV/AIDS and TB: Home-based carers' perspectives on epilepsy in Cape Town, South Africa. International Journal of Qualitative Studies on Health and Well-being. 2016;**11**(1):30213

[15] Mula M, Sander JW. Psychosocial aspects of epilepsy: A wider approach. BJPsych Open. 2016;**2**(4):270-274

[16] Ekeh BC, Akpan EE, Ekrikpo UE. The knowledge, attitude and perception towards epilepsy amongst health workers in a tertiary hospital in Uyo, Southern Nigeria. Journal of Advances in Medicine and Medical Research. 2016:1

[17] Makhado L, Makhado TG, Lebese RT, Maphula A, Maputle MS, Mabunda JT, et al. GladAfrica epilepsy research project (GERP): Initiation, launch and community interest report. Africa Journal of Nursing and Midwifery. 2020;**22**(2):5

[18] Murugupillai R, Wanigasinghe J, Muniyandi R, Arambepola C. Parental concerns towards children and adolescents with epilepsy in Sri Lanka–Qualitative study. Seizure. 2016;**34**:6-11

[19] Mollaoğlu M, Bolayir E. Injuries in patients with epilepsy and some factors associated with injury. Nöro Psikiyatri Arşivi. 2013;**50**(3):269

[20] Bifftu BB, Tadesse Tiruneh B, Mekonnen Kelkay M, Bayu NH, Tewolde AW, Takele WW, et al. Seizure-Related Injuries Among People with Epilepsy at the Outpatient Department of the University of Gondar Hospital. Northwest Ethiopia: Cross-sectional institutional-based study. Neurology Research International; 2017. p. 2017

[21] Nguyen R, Tellez-Zenteno J. Injuries in epilepsy: A review of its prevalence, risk factors, type of injuries and prevention. Neurology International. 2009;**1**(1):72-78

[22] International League Against Epilepsy. Seizure-related injuries common: Head wounds and drowning risk top list of dangers. Epigraph. 2019. Available from: https://www.ilae.org/journals/epigraph/epigraph-vol-21-issue-1-winter-2019/seizure-related-injuries-common-head-wounds-and-drowning-risk-top-list-of-dangers

[23] Willems LM, Watermann N, Richter S, Kay L, Hermsen AM, Knake S, et al. Incidence, risk factors and consequences of epilepsy-related injuries and accidents: A retrospective, single center study. Frontiers in Neurology. 2018;**9**:414

[24] Sirven JI, Shafer PO, Schachter S. Types of injuries from seizures [Internet]. 2013 [Cited 27 April 2022]. Available from: https://www.epilepsy.com/preparedness-safety/staying-safe/types-injuries

[25] Henning O, Landmark CJ, Henning D, Nakken KO, Lossius MI. Challenges in epilepsy–The perspective of Norwegian epilepsy patients. Acta Neurologica Scandinavica. 2019;**140**(1):40-47

[26] Epilepsy foundation. Thinking and Memory [Internet]. 2022 [Cited 27 April 2022]. Available from: https://www.epilepsy.com/complications-risks/thinking-and-memory

[27] Stafstrom CE. Using artwork to understand and address the psychosocial challenges facing children and adolescents with epilepsy. Epilepsy & Behavior. 2019;**101**:106572

[28] Sen A, Jette N, Husain M, Sander JW. Epilepsy in older people. The Lancet. 2020;**395**(10225):735-748

[29] Batchelor R, Taylor MD. Young adults with epilepsy: Relationships between psychosocial variables and anxiety, depression, and suicidality. Epilepsy & Behavior. 2021;**118**:107911

[30] World Health Organization (WHO). Epilepsy. Fact Sheets. World Health Organization; 2022. Accessed from:

https://www.who.int/news-room/fact-sheets/detail/epilepsy

[31] Mühlenfeld N, Störmann P, Marzi I, Rosenow F, Strzelczyk A, Verboket RD, Willems LM. Seizure related injuries-frequent injury patterns, hospitalization and therapeutic aspects. 2021. Accessed from: https://www.sciencedirect.com/science/article/pii/S1008127521001619

[32] Tsvere M, Chiweshe MK, Mutanana N. General side effects and challenges associated with anti-epilepsy medication: A review of related literature. African Journal of Primary Health Care and Family Medicine. 2020;**12**(1):1-5

[33] Nishida T, Terada K, Ikeda H, Inoue Y. Seizures, accidental injuries at work, and reasons for resignation in people with epilepsy. Epilepsy & Behavior. 2020;111:107237. WHO. Epilepsy [Internet]. 2022. [Cited 27 April 2022]. Available from: https://www.who.int/newsroom/factsheets/detail/epilepsy#:~:text=People%20with%20epilepsy%20tend%20to,conditions%2C%20including%20anxiety%20and%20depression

[34] Fazekas B, Megaw B, Eade D, Kronfeld N. Insights into the real-life experiences of people living with epilepsy: A qualitative netnographic study. Epilepsy & Behavior. 2021;**116**:107729

[35] Xue-Ping W, Hai-Jiao W, Li-Na Z, Xu D, Ling L. Risk factors for drug-resistant Epilepsy: A systematic review and meta-analysis. Medicine. 2019;**98**(30):e16402.

[36] Auditeau E, Chassagne F, Bourdy G, Bounlu M, Jost J, Luna J, et al. Herbal medicine for epilepsy seizures in Asia, Africa and Latin America: A systematic review. Journal of Ethnopharmacology 2019;234:119-153.

[37] Pandey DK, Levy J, Serafini A, Habibi M, Song W, Shafer PO, et al. Self-management skills and behaviors, self-efficacy, and quality of life in people with epilepsy from underserved populations. Epilepsy & Behavior. 2019;**98**:258-265

[38] Yeni K, Tulek Z, Simsek OF, Bebek N. Relationships between knowledge, attitudes, stigma, anxiety and depression, and quality of life in epilepsy: A structural equation modeling. Epilepsy & Behavior. 2018;**85**:212-217

[39] Adu J, Oudshoorn A, Anderson K, Marshall CA, Stuart H, Stanley M. Policies and interventions to reduce familial mental illness stigma: A scoping review of empirical literature. Issues in Mental Health Nursing. 2021:1-5

[40] Adu J, Oudshoorn A. The deinstitutionalisation of psychiatric hospitals in Ghana: An application of Bronfenbrenner's social-ecological model. Issues in Mental Health Nursing. 2020;**41**(4):306-314

[41] Smallwood E, Legari S, Sheldon S. Group art therapy for the psychosocial dimension of epilepsy: A perspective and a preliminary mixed-methods study. Canadian Journal of Counselling and Psychotherapy/Revue Canadienne de Counseling et de Psychothérapie. 2020;**54**(3):286-323

[42] Hathaway DB, Dawes M. Addiction and Twelve-Step Spirituality. In: Peteet JR, Moffic HS, Hankir A, Koenig HG, editors. Christianity and Psychiatry. Springer; 2021 Sep 2; 147-162. https://doi.org/10.1007/978-3-030-80854-9_11

[43] Yabanci B. Work for the nation, obey the state, praise the ummah: Turkey's government-oriented youth organisations in cultivating a new nation. Ethnopolitics. 2021;**20**(4):467-499

[44] Clements TP, Clements AD. Community is the vehicle to recovery. From The front lines of the Appalachian addiction crisis: Healthcare providers discuss opioids. Meth and Recovery. McFarland & Company, Inc. 2020: 135-155

[45] Ventevogel P. Interventions for mental health and psychosocial support in complex humanitarian emergencies: Moving towards consensus in policy and action? In: Mental Health of Refugee and Conflict-Affected Populations. 2018. pp. 155-180

[46] Epilepsy Ontario. Living with epilepsy. 2018. Retrieved from: https://epilepsyontario.org/living-with-epilepsy/life-fulfillment/10-ways-to-build-resilience/

[47] de Wolf F. Religion, spirituality and psychosocial support activities to people affected by a humanitarian crisis: The role of faith-based organisations (Doctoral dissertation). 2018

[48] World Health Organization. Mental Health and Psychosocial Considerations During the COVID-19 Outbreak. 2020. Geneva, Switzerland: World Health Organization; 2020

[49] Allebone J, Kanaan RA, Maller JJ, O'Brien T, Mullen S, Cook M, et al. Enlarged hippocampal fissure in psychosis of epilepsy. Epilepsy & Behavior. 2020;**111**:107290

[50] Min A, Miller W, Rocha L, Börner K, Brattig Correia R, Shih PC. Just in time: Challenges and opportunities of first aid care information sharing for supporting epileptic seizure response. Proceedings of the ACM on Human-Computer Interaction. 2021;**5**(CSCW1):1-24

[51] Shih P, Francis-Auton E, Nikpour A, Herkes G, Bleasel A, Rapport F. Enhancing quality of life among epilepsy surgery patients: Interlinking multiple social and relational determinants. Epilepsy & Behavior. 2020;**102**:106721

[52] Lindsay S, Thiyagarajah K. The impact of service dogs on children, youth and their families: A systematic review. Disability and Health Journal. 2021;**14**(3):101012

[53] Michaelis R, Niedermann C, Reuber M, Kuthe M, Berger B. Seizures have become a means of somehow learning things about myself–A qualitative study of the development of self-efficacy and mastery during a psychotherapeutic intervention for people with epilepsy. Epilepsy & Behavior. 2018;**84**:152-161

[54] Algahtani H, Shirah B, Alzahrani A, Shaheen M. Perception and attitude of the general population towards epilepsy in Jeddah, Saudi Arabia. Journal of Epilepsy Research. 2019;**9**(1):42

[55] Mann C, Süß A, von Podewils F, Zahnert F, Langenbruch L, Bierhansl L, et al. Gender differences in concerns about planning to have children and child-rearing among patients with epilepsy: A prospective, multicenter study with 477 patients from Germany. Epilepsy & Behavior. 2022;**129**:108650

[56] Moser E, Chan F, Berven NL, Bezyak J, Iwanaga K, Umucu E. Resilience and life satisfaction in young adults with epilepsy: The role of person-environment contextual factors. Journal of Vocational Rehabilitation. 2020;**52**(2):157-171

[57] Potage JN. A sense of hope: Parents treating their epileptic child with cannabidiol (Doctoral dissertation, Walden University)

[58] CDC. Epilepsy: Types of seizures. 2022. Retrieved from: https://www.cdc.

gov/epilepsy/about/types-of-seizures.htm#:~:text=Tonic%3A%20Muscles%20in%20the%20body,jerking%20parts%20on%20the%20body

[59] National Centre for Chronic Disease Prevention and Health Promotion, Division of Population Health. Types of seizures. [Internet]. 2020 [Cited 27 April 2022]. Available from: https://www.cdc.gov/epilepsy/about/types-of-seizures.htm

[60] CDC. Epilepsy: Seizure first aid. 2022. Retrieved from: https://www.cdc.gov/epilepsy/about/first-aid.htm

[61] Epilepsy Society UK. Caring for someone with epilepsy. 2020. Retrieved from: https://epilepsysociety.org.uk/about-epilepsy/information-carers/caring-someone-epilepsy

Chapter 3

Innovations in Active Education Techniques: Team Based Learning, Flipping the Classroom, and Think-Pair-Share

Hilary E. Fairbrother, Phillip B. Carpenter, Shane R. Cunha and Deena Khamees

Abstract

Team-based learning, flipped classroom, and think-pair-share are active learning pedagogies used commonly in undergraduate medical education today. They are based on constructivist learning theory and are effective to use to actively teach foundational knowledge to medical students. They also help students work on team dynamics, critical thinking, and clinical knowledge application. These techniques can be employed without expensive technology or special training. Medical education was grossly affected by the COVID-19 pandemic and the inability to assemble in person. These educational techniques all allow for enhanced and active remote learning. With the amplification of remote education delivery during the pandemic, it is easy to see how we can use these techniques to spread foundational medical education more equitably across the globe.

Keywords: undergraduate medical education, active learning, team-based learning, flipped classroom, think-pair-share

1. Introduction

Medical students have become increasingly apathetic to traditional lecture-based teaching methods, particularly as they fail to engage the attention of the learners and have been described as an inferior pedagogy with respect to the development of critical thinking skills [1–3]. Indeed, student concentration is well known to shortly dissipate during lecture time [4]. As a result, non-compulsory lecture-based curricula receive poor classroom attendance and overreliance on third-party educational or other external resources. Further, as compelling evidence with respect to important factors such as failure rates has been put forward, the inferior nature of lecture-based teaching pedagogies in the science, technology, engineering, and math (STEM) fields of study relative to active learning pedagogies has been revealed [5, 6]. Active learning methods emphasize the application of information during class time. Such problem-solving skills promote higher-order thinking in the Bloom's taxonomy. In fact, evidence show that lecture-based delivery of information is outdated and inefficient. Active learning is a superior method for delivering content in the STEM fields [5]. Further, it may no longer be appropriate to use lecture-based teaching as the comparative standard for teaching efficacy, but rather that different active learning modalities should be compared to each other [6].

Active learning models such as cooperative, team-based learning (TBL), and flipped classroom (FC) pedagogies have been developed to address the inadequacies of lecture-based teaching as they strive to eliminate the ineffectiveness of passive learning [7, 8]. Indeed, many medical schools have revised their curriculum to emphasize active learning pedagogies [9, 10]. TBL is a small group format that highlights knowledge application. FC settings reverse the traditional lecture-homework learning model that has dominated education for years and promotes student engagement and learning [11, 12].

Cooperative learning is an active strategy that has been shown to promote student engagement and learner satisfaction [8, 13, 14]. Its successful implementation requires strong interpersonal skills and peer teaching. One type of cooperative learning pedagogy called think-pair-share (TPS) was developed by Lyman and colleagues [15] and has been successfully implemented in healthcare education [16]. TPS is a 3-pronged approach that promotes individual, cooperative, and full class input.

Although these active learning platforms represent promising teaching pedagogies for increasing medical student engagement and acquisition of higher order learning skills some challenges remain. This includes variations in the degrees of improvement of learning outcomes relative to traditional lectures as well as continued student engagement and in-person attendance [10, 17–19]. Thus, in and by itself, the active learning is not necessarily sufficient to address issues such as engagement and attendance.

This chapter will discuss and describe TBL, FC, and TPS as active and progressive educational pedagogies. Descriptions of practical application of each of these strategies will be followed by specific pandemic-stimulated remote learning lessons learned. The technology required to use these techniques will be discussed and specific challenges of special populations and unique education delivery challenges will be reviewed and examined.

2. Educational pedagogies used to activate learning in medical school

2.1 Team-based learning (TBL)

2.1.1 Literature review and learning theory

TBL is a small group format that highlights knowledge application. TBL follows the principles of constructivist educational theory [20]. Constructivist theory was developed from cognitive learning theory and postulates the following four main concepts. Firstly, the teacher is a guide to the educational content and a facilitator for the students. Secondly, learning is active and should employ small group formats. Thirdly, teachers are expected to highlight and explain the inconsistencies between students' foundational knowledge and future experiences. Finally, students should have time to reflect on their learning experiences [21].

In TBL, students are expected to prepare for the application exercise independently and this initial knowledge is tested at the start of the TBL session through an Individual Readiness Assurance Test (IRAT). Students are then broken up into assigned small groups and the same knowledge is tested in the Group Readiness Assurance Test (GRAT). Students are then brought back together for a review of the assurance test material before they are again sent into their assigned groups to complete the Application Exercise (AE). After the application exercise is complete, the large group is brought back together to review the AE. TBL is favorably reviewed by most students and faculty and multiple studies have noted that it has equivalent teaching efficacy to lecture and helps increase test grades of lower performing students [22].

The practice of medicine involves complex knowledge processing, application, and integration. Simple regurgitation of facts will not lead to the necessary skills that students must learn to practice clinical medicine. These critical thinking skills are not easily taught in passive, lecture-based formats. Classically, medical schools have used passive techniques to assist students' obtainment of foundational knowledge during the initial phase of school followed by a precepting environment during latter phases of medical school when students join the healthcare team to deliver patient care. In this way, students both observe the clinical reasoning and knowledge application and begin to practice this skill themselves. TBL allows educators to introduce concept integration and critical thinking skills in a small group format [23]. TBL can be used with an in-person or remote design; synchronously or asynchronously. A single professor or a small group of educators can efficiently teach a very large number of students using TBL making this pedagogy one of the easiest to access regarding limited resource settings. There is no specific technology that is required to run a complete and successful TBL session, though this chapter will address how TBL can use technology to facilitate active learning in a remote setting.

2.1.2 Practical application and examples

TBL is used in our school's curriculum longitudinally throughout the first semester of the first year of medical school. 18 separate sessions are held over the course of almost 5 months with the goal of applying foundational medical knowledge clinically. At the start of each week, our students have an introduction to the clinical subject matter. Throughout the week students have a variety of lectures and active learning covering the foundational knowledge that supports the clinical case. On the last day of the week, the students go through the TBL session.

A best practices specific example would progress as follows:

- ***Monday***: A 30-minute introduction to cystic fibrosis (CF) delivered jointly by a physician and PhD scientist followed by a 20-minute interview with a patient living with CF.
    - Learning objectives: cell membrane and channel biology, a clinical overview of CF, and a review of the genetics related to CF
- Foundational content (during the week):
    - Osmosis

- Carrier-mediated transport
- Cell structure, diffusion, and transport
- Genetic patterns of inheritance

- ***Friday:*** The two-hour TBL session is run by three to four educators including a clinical physician and the relevant PhD science content experts.
    - IRAT – students answer multiple choice content individually on the week's content
    - GRAT – immediately after the IRAT in a group of 6–8, students answer identical questions, receiving real-time feedback when they give the correct answer
    - Debrief – the educators go over any questions that had a low number of correct answers once students were in their small group
    - AE – students work through a clinical case, answering a variety of multiple choice and short answer questions as they follow a case of a patient with cystic fibrosis.
    - Final debrief – educators go through each question of the AE to verify that students have accurate learning and application of clinical concepts.

2.1.3 Covid-19 pandemic effects and remote learning and technology usage

The COVID-19 pandemic grossly affected the delivery of undergraduate medical education in the United States (US). Overnight classes were canceled, and all foundational curriculum delivery was made remote for a year. One of the excellent aspects of TBL is the ability to implement this pedagogy remotely. TBL is incredibly flexible, and with a modicum of technology use can be used in a robust fashion without student/faculty physical proximity.

To deliver a TBL AE remotely, there must be a way for students to answer questions and for faculty to review answers contemporaneously. There also needs to be a way for students to communicate (ideally video-enabled) in a small group, and with the entire class. In our experience, we found that we used a content delivery and a video communication platform concurrently. There exist online platforms specifically for TBL, and our institution used InteDashboard™. The downside of commercial products such as this is the monetary expense. The upside is that they are designed to facilitate the educator in both designing and delivering an AE. Free platforms such as Google Forms could be used in low-resource settings. A concomitant video-enabled communication platform is then employed to allow for small group work and large group collective review with the instructors. Common products used are Zoom and Webex though free products exist such as Google Hangouts, Slack, and Skype.

2.1.4 Unique challenges of TBL

TBL can be a challenging pedagogy both for the faculty and the students. While it is usually rated higher than lecture-based teaching it can take students multiple sessions to be comfortable with this educational delivery format [24]. Faculty often need hours of training in TBL design and delivery before it can be performed satisfactorily. Creating original TBL cases can introduce a large burden on faculty, and this can be a barrier to using TBL repeatedly throughout a curriculum [25]. We suggest using open-access medical information such as MedEdPORTAL (https://www.mededportal.org/) to access pre-existing TBL cases significantly decreasing the initial time investment required when introducing TBL to a curriculum.

When done well, TBL will push students to stretch beyond memorization into critical thinking. Clinical cases also often introduce elements of ambiguity, ethics, and clinical uncertainty and this can make students uncomfortable, though we argue that this is exactly what medical students need to become competent physicians who lead teams of healthcare professionals.

2.2 The flipped classroom (FC)

2.2.1 Literature review and learning theory

The flipped classroom (FC) pedagogy involves a combination of pre-assigned, independent, asynchronous content and dependent, synchronous teaching [26]. The traditional lecture is often transformed or replaced by content that is expected to be reviewed prior to synchronous, interactive sessions where faculty may go over a case, model problem solving, and in general applying the concepts covered in the assigned pre-work. FC has been shown to increase student motivation and satisfaction with curriculum when compared to classic lecture, and it is at least as effective in teaching material when compared to more passive pedagogies [17]. FC, like TBL, is based on constructivist learning theory.

Flipped classroom settings reverse the traditional lecture-homework learning model that has dominated education for years. Rather, the flipped model involves pre-session learning (i.e. video or reading) followed by class, active learning (i.e. problem solving or case study). When combined with Audience Response Systems (ARS) such as Poll Everywhere® (PE), the flipped classroom has been shown to promote student engagement and learning [11, 12]. ARS allow teachers to synchronously question their students during education delivery and analyze these results. PE is a specific ARS that allows for the embedding of polls and questions into a PowerPoint lecture with immediate analysis. Although the flipped classroom model represents a promising teaching pedagogy for increasing medical student engagement and acquisition of higher order learning skills some challenges remain. This includes variations in the degrees of improvement of learning outcomes relative to traditional lectures as well as continued low attendance and student engagement [10, 17–19]. Thus, in of and by itself, the flipped model is not necessarily sufficient to address issues such as attendance and engagement.

2.2.2 Practical application and examples

The first step to creating an FC active learning session is to translate or replace the lecture material with content that can be studied by the learners prior to attending a synchronous session with the professor. This takes a different skill set than delivering a conventional lecture. In the addition, modern learners are often not satisfied with preparatory material being all reading from a book. This introduces multiple different challenges for educators. First, teaching a video is different from teaching to an audience. When teaching to an audience, student comprehension is readily apparent to the lecturers and additional opportunities to rephrase difficult concepts may be pursued. In addition, one may employ engaging with the students as a means of transitioning between concepts. Second, utilizing video editing software to make the video short and concise is critical. This software allows educators to remove unintended gaffes or poorly expressed concepts.

A best practice, specific example of the process of converting a 50-minute lecture on hemodynamics into short videos is discussed in next two paragraphs. First, the lecture comprised of 36 slides was subdivided into the main fundamental concepts such as resistance to flow, blood flow, and regulation of vessel compliance. Then, each slide was evaluated for [1] the placement or flow of information in the slide, [2] potential ambiguity in the written text, and [3] figure quality. This process led to the clarification of inexplicit text previously expounded upon during lecture and the inclusion of more informative and straightforward figures. A script was then created of the information to be discussed on each slide using concise phrases that were audibly rehearsed and reworked to better represent the lecturer's instinctive spoken word choice. While the initial purpose of using a script was to create a concise and effective video, an unintended benefit includes having a well-developed work product should the video require future additions or modifications. In addition, students greatly appreciate using the script as an additional study aide to facilitate comprehension of the video content.

When making the video, there are many software options, and our institution uses Panopto. While the explicit software used is not critical, look for intuitive platforms that are not overly complicated if creating content without professional assistance. First, to create high-quality audio, use a headset with a noise-canceling microphone to reduce ambient noise. Second, when interacting with the PowerPoint slide, use the laser pointer option to focus the viewer's attention on specific text or figures on the slide. Third, consider enabling the camera on your computer to video yourself discussing the slides. This option affords the students an opportunity to develop a personal connection with the lecturer even though it's not a live connection. Fourth, remember the editing process will help you achieve a high-quality, short video with accurate and concise descriptions. When making the video, if you misspeak, pause to create a time gap of 1–2 seconds, and then try again. During the editing process, the bloopers can be removed such that an hour-long unedited video may be pared down to a 5–10 minute polished video. Finally, utilize the pause function in your video software. Even using a script, it can be difficult to seamlessly describe many high-yield concepts on a slide. Alternatively, you can focus on one concept at a time by utilizing the pause function between concepts to reset your attention in the script and on the slide. These pauses are easily removed during the editing process.

Once the lecture content is converted to short videos to be previewed by students, the time allotted for the lecture can be utilized for an active learning session when the students can apply the knowledge learned from the videos. Our institution uses an ARS called Poll Everywhere that allows students to answer questions via a computer or cell phone. The goal of the ARS is to engage the audience, its greatest value is enabling the coalescence of instantaneous feedback from in-person and/or remote audience members. Using a video conferencing application combined with the FC pedagogy, a lecturer can facilitate an active learning session where students in their remote locations can respond to questions via an ARS. In the case of Poll Everywhere, this can be instantaneously revealed in the PowerPoint presentation. A productive and interactive learning experience no longer requires the students and facilitators to be in the same location.

2.2.3 Covid-19 pandemic effects and remote learning

During the COVID-19 pandemic, FC increased in popularity at our institution. Many faculty created videos at home, consolidating hours of lecture into videos. Some faculty also mapped content to third-party content resources and focused on knowledge curation and application rather than basic content delivery. Interactive FC sessions were easily held throughout the lockdown remotely using both ARS and video communication platforms. In fact, many professors felt that remote FC delivery was superior to in-person because the chat function of the communication platform decreased the barrier to student involvement. While many students may feel intimidated and scared to offer an answer verbally in front of a class of their peers, entering text into the chat on a video conference seemed to be less intimidating and there was a large amount of participation from a wider array of learners.

2.2.4 Technologies employed

Specific technologies employed at our institution would be Panopto to record audio narration to PowerPoint slides, Camtasia to allow for animation of PowerPoint slides, Poll Everywhere as an ARS that could be embedded within PowerPoint presentations, and Webex as a video conferencing platform. These are by no means the only technologies available, and there are multiple free options including such as Prezi for slide preparation and presentation and Slido, Kahoot!, MeetingPulse as ARS's.

2.2.5 Unique challenges of FC

Flipping even a single hour of lecture content can take an extraordinary amount of time. Even if the software and ARS are free, FC can involve a tremendous amount of faculty time which is one of the most expensive resources in healthcare education. One study found that the time required to prepare for a semester-long course increased by 127% when the sessions were all converted to an FC format [27].

When surveyed, there always exists a cohort of learners who do not rate FC highly, particularly in the context of video streaming of third-party resources. With the rise of competing, professionally sourced content made explicitly to align to national US standardized exams, there are students who see FC sessions as an inefficient way to learn. This indicates that multiple, blended teaching pedagogies (active and passive) may reflect the optimal delivery of content and grooming of critical thinking skills required for successful medical education.

2.3 Think-pair-share (TPS)

TPS is a 3-pronged approach that promotes individual, cooperative, and full class input. A question is first posed to students who are given time to think individually about what the answer might be. Students are then asked to confer with their peers (or they can be assigned to a specific peer) to discuss their answers in a pair or small group. Finally, several of the small groups share with the larger group what they think the answer to be. This is an active pedagogy based on social constructivist learning theory.

2.3.1 Practical application and examples

At our institution, we developed an instructional pedagogy that used FC and the TPS learning model. A series of traditional biochemical lectures that included material mapping to the USMLE Step 1 Exam Content Outline was streamlined and recorded. The videos were made available to students prior to the flipped session. During class, the students answered clinically-focused questions derived from this material via the ARS. First, the students were presented with a question that they answered using PE as individuals with no peer consultation. After the responses were recorded, the same question was posed to the class again, and after "thinking and pairing" with their peers, a second individual response was recorded. Afterward, the instructor revealed the individual (Pre or pretest) and post-collaborative (Post or posttest) responses and opened the question for full class discussion and annotation. The benefit of using an ARS is the availability of immediate poll results; where students see the correct answer and instructors can gauge knowledge gaps and address misconceptions. This type of Just-In-Time Teaching (JiTT) promotes effective use of class time [28]. JiTT involves students through active learning and instructors use teaching time to address areas of misunderstanding identified by the activities.

For TPS, an ideal question is one that displays significant improvement in performance after peer consultation because it represents a point in the session where collective, active learning has the greatest impact. When we studied this at our own institution, we found that the statistically significant questions were application-based questions that required higher-level thinking skills as per Bloom's taxonomy. We found that many of the statistically insignificant questions had high baseline pretest scores and could be labeled as first-order questions. (i.e. "easy" as they utilize lower levels on Bloom's Taxonomy). Collectively, our data showed that our flipped-TPS model led to improved assessment performance through collaborative learning. Further, our survey data revealed a preference for this pedagogy over the traditional lecture model, consistent with the average recorded attendance of 74% [29].

2.3.2 Unique challenges of TPS: how useful is the "share?"

Classically, during the sharing portion of TPS, educators would either ask learners to volunteer their answers or randomly call on a student. When professors allow students to volunteer, it is common practice that a few students may dominate the discussion. Also, in terms of bias, students with same gender identity and from similar cultural backgrounds are more likely to volunteer their answers [30]. When students know that they may be randomly called on, this can be an extraordinary source of stress for individual students and can decrease overall class attendance. Using an ARS rather than relying on an individual share outside of the context of the responses of the entire group diminishes many of these challenges. Finally, during the recent pandemic, when TPS sessions were made remote, students were noted to be more active in the chat than they were when the meetings were in person. It is due to this that the faculty requested that TPS sessions remain virtual and synchronous even as attendance restrictions from the pandemic were lifted.

3. International implications: a broader perspective galvanized by a pandemic

While there is incredible diversity in the final approach to and practice of medicine across the country and world, the foundational knowledge of medicine is rather universal. This allows educators to share their approaches, educational interventions, and adaptations with each other globally. Indeed, we saw this at a possibly unprecedented level during the COVID pandemic. With a need for virtual education, many well-resourced institutions made this pivot well to minimize disruption of education [31]. Yet others may face obstacles such as limitations in technology, relevantly skilled staff, and funding [32]. Foundational medical education transcends regional and cultural differences such that interventions developed may be shared in free, open access formats - greatly narrowing this gap. Outside of such pressing needs and at a more practical level, we may avoid duplication of efforts in the design and implementation of the same or near-identical educational interventions. Existing, accessible resources may be curated to satisfy the unique population and needs at hand. Accordingly, such efforts may be allocated toward growth and innovation, which are then shared again, further elevating medical educators. Perhaps more satisfying are benefits such as fostering a sense of collaboration in teaching and learning nationally and internationally. Both educators and learners may share their thoughts, views, successful strategies, frustrations, and more with others – creating a community and sense of connection, thereby broadening their views of the practice of medicine to an international stage. Furthermore, such a mindset may be extended into the future practices of today's learners, resulting in an ever richer and more robust professional experience for physicians and care for patients.

4. Remote learning – broader implications

The pandemic has brought us an unprecedented increase and the use of remote learning. While the subject matter itself may be well conveyed via such remote strategies, there are less tangible aspects of medical education that may be lost in the process. In-person learning allows more readily for student socializing, fostering a sense of community. Indeed, without it, we have seen a marked increase in student self-reports of isolation, anxiety, and depression [33]. Those students also report decreased satisfaction with their medical education [33]. In addition to these potentially devastating consequences, there may be evidence that a weak or nonexistent "classroom community" may harm students' preparedness and performance clinically [34]. This community can build students' communication and teamwork skills both formally via targeted educational programming and informally via the natural proceedings of classroom and group work interactions - what may often be referred to as the hidden curriculum [34, 35].

The students' community is not the only one at risk in remote learning, but also those connections between students and educators, which would normally allow for the less tangible benefits of education. Without this, students may find it difficult to establish a mentorship, which has been shown to be necessary for the ideal professional growth of medical professionals [34, 36]. Educators may lose the reward that is feeling the successful engagement of students during an educational session or witnessing the students' growth and graduation to more complex material and roles. Additionally, it may be difficult for faculty to role model appropriate attitudes and behaviors over remote learning modalities [37, 38].

5. Conclusions

In conclusion, TBL, FC, and TPS are active learning pedagogies based on constructivist educational theory. These are well-liked by students, and accessible and trusted techniques to introduce active learning into healthcare education. This chapter explained each of these pedagogies and then gave specific examples of how to take traditional lecture-based content and evolve it into one of these engaging educational formats. The technology recommended to employ these tactics was discussed, particularly through the lens of the recent Covid-19 pandemic which caused much of foundational graduate medical education to be delivered remotely. Finally, the international implications of being able to deliver content remotely and some of the consequences of remote learning were reviewed.

Acknowledgements

The authors would like to thank Peggy Hseih, Aaron Poliak, Allison Ownby, Litao Wang, The Department of Emergency Medicine at McGovern Medical School, and McGovern Medical School. There was no outside funding received for this project.

Conflict of interest

The authors declare no conflict of interest.

Author details

Hilary E. Fairbrother[1*], Phillip B. Carpenter[2], Shane R. Cunha[3] and Deena Khamees[4]

1 UTHealth Houston Department of Emergency Medicine, McGovern Medical School, Houston, United States

2 Department of Biochemistry and Molecular Biology, McGovern Medical School, Houston, United States

3 Department of Integrative Biology and Pharmacoogy, McGovern Medical School, Houston, United States

4 Texas Innovation and Education Research Lab, UTHealth Houston Department of Emergency Medicine, Houston, Texas, United States

*Address all correspondence to: hilary.e.fairbrother@uth.tmc.edu

References

[1] Mazur E. Education. Farewell, lecture? Science. 2009;**323**(5910):50-51

[2] Chan L. Teaching Anatomy: A Practical Guide. 1st ed. New York, NY: Springer International Publishing; 2015. pp. 61-72

[3] Steinert YSL. Strategies for increasing participation in large group presentations. Medical Teacher. 1999;**21**:37-42

[4] Stuart J, Rutherford RJ. Medical student concentration during lectures. Lancet. 1978;**2**(8088):514-516

[5] Freeman S, Eddy SL, McDonough M, Smith MK, Okoroafor N, Jordt H, et al. Active learning increases student performance in science, engineering, and mathematics. Proceedings of the National Academy of Sciences of the United States of America. 2014;**111**(23):8410-8415

[6] Wieman CE. Large-scale comparison of science teaching methods sends clear message. Proceedings of the National Academy of Sciences of the United States of America. 2014;**111**(23):8319-8320

[7] Abdel Meguid E, Collins M. Students' perceptions of lecturing approaches: Traditional versus interactive teaching. Advances in Medical Education and Practice. 2017;**8**:229-241

[8] Crouch CME. Peer instruction: Ten years of experience and results. American Journal of Physics. 2001;**69**:970-977

[9] Laird-Fick HS, Solomon DJ, Parker CJ, Wang L. Attendance, engagement and performance in a medical school curriculum: Early findings from competency-based progress testing in a new medical school curriculum. PeerJ. 2018;**6**:e5283

[10] White CMM, Bradley E, Roy P, Yoon M, Martindale J, Worden MK. Challenges to engaging medical students in a flipped classroom model. Medical Science Educator. 2015;**25**:219-222

[11] Gubbiyappa KS, Barua A, Das B, Vasudeva Murthy CR, Baloch HZ. Effectiveness of flipped classroom with poll everywhere as a teaching-learning method for pharmacy students. Indian Journal of Pharmacology. 2016;**48**(Suppl. 1):S41-SS6

[12] Graham KL, Cohen A, Reynolds EE, Huang GC. Effect of a flipped classroom on knowledge acquisition and retention in an internal medicine residency program. Journal of Graduate Medical Education. 2019;**11**(1):92-97

[13] Hanson MJ, Carpenter DR. Integrating cooperative learning into classroom testing: Implications for nursing education and practice. Nursing Education Perspectives. 2011;**32**(4):270-273

[14] Copp SL. Using cooperative learning strategies to teach implications of the Nurse Practice Act. Nurse Educator. 2002;**27**(5):236-241

[15] Lyman F. The responsive classroom discussion. In: Anderson AS, editor. Education UoMCo. College Park, MD: Mainstreaming Digest; 1981. pp. 109-113

[16] Fitzgerald D. Employing think-pair-share in associate degree nursing curriculum. Teaching and Learning in Nursing. 2013;**8**:88-90

[17] Chen F, Lui AM, Martinelli SM. A systematic review of the effectiveness of flipped classrooms in medical education. Medical Education. 2017;**51**(6):585-597

[18] Gillette C, Rudolph M, Kimble C, Rockich-Winston N, Smith L, Broedel-Zaugg K. A meta-analysis of outcomes comparing flipped classroom and lecture. American Journal of Pharmaceutical Education. 2018;**82**(5):6898

[19] White C, Bradley E, Martindale J, Roy P, Patel K, Yoon M, et al. Why are medical students 'checking out' of active learning in a new curriculum? Medical Education. 2014;**48**(3):315-324

[20] Hrynchak P, Batty H. The educational theory basis of team-based learning. Medical Teacher. 2012;**34**(10):796-801

[21] Kaufman DM. Applying educational theory in practice. British Medical Journal. 2003;**326**(7382):213-216

[22] Kang KA, Kim SJ, Oh J, Kim S, Lee MN. Effectiveness of simulation with team-based learning in newborn nursing care. Nursing & Health Sciences. 2016;**18**(2):262-269

[23] Michaelsen LPD, McMahon K, Levine R. Team-based Learning for Health Professions Education: A Guide to Using Small Groups to Improving Learning. Sterling, VA: Stylus Publishing, LLC; 2008

[24] Davidson LK. A 3-year experience implementing blended TBL: Active instructional methods can shift student attitudes to learning. Medical Teacher. 2011;**33**(9):750-753

[25] Brandler TC, Laser J, Williamson AK, Louie J, Esposito MJ. Team-based learning in a pathology residency training program. American Journal of Clinical Pathology. 2014;**142**(1):23-28

[26] Youhasan P, Chen Y, Lyndon M, Henning MA. Exploring the pedagogical design features of the flipped classroom in undergraduate nursing education: A systematic review. BMC Nursing. 2021;**20**(1):50

[27] McLaughlin JE, Roth MT, Glatt DM, Gharkholonarehe N, Davidson CA, Griffin LM, et al. The flipped classroom: A course redesign to foster learning and engagement in a health professions school. Academic Medicine. 2014;**89**(2):236-243

[28] Novak GM, Patterson ET, Gavrin AD, Christian W. Just-in Time Teaching: Blending Active Learning with Web Technology. New Jersey: Prentice-Hall; 1999

[29] Carpenter PB, Poliak A, Wang L, Ownby AR, Hsieh P. Improved performance in and preference for using think-pair-share in a flipped classroom. Medical Education. 2020;**54**(5):449-450

[30] Cooper KM, Schinske JN, Tanner KD. Reconsidering the share of a think-pair-share: Emerging limitations, alternatives, and opportunities for research. CBE Life Science Education. 2021;**20**(1):fe1

[31] Khamees D, Peterson W, Patricio M, Pawlikowska T, Commissaris C, Austin A, et al. Remote learning developments in postgraduate medical education in response to the COVID-19 pandemic - A BEME systematic review: BEME Guide No. 71. Medical Teacher. May 2022;**44**(5):466-485

[32] Dawidziuk A, Kawka M, Szyszka B, Wadunde I, Ghimire A. Global access to technology-enhanced medical education

during the COVID-19 pandemic: The role of students in narrowing the gap. Global Health: Science and Practice. 2021;**9**(1):10-14

[33] Chakladar J, Diomino A, Li WT, Tsai JC, Krishnan AR, Zou AE, et al. Medical student's perception of the COVID-19 pandemic effect on their education and well-being: A cross-sectional survey in the United States. BMC Medical Education. 2022;**22**(1):149

[34] Hafferty FW, Franks R. The hidden curriculum, ethics teaching, and the structure of medical education. Academic Medicine. 1994;**69**(11):861-871

[35] Azmand S, Ebrahimi S, Iman M, Asemani O. Learning professionalism through hidden curriculum: Iranian medical students' perspective. Journal of Medical Ethics and History of Medicine. 2018;**11**:10

[36] Bettin KA. the role of mentoring in the professional identity formation of medical students. The Orthopedic Clinics of North America. 2021;**52**(1):61-68

[37] Shrank WH, Reed VA, Jernstedt GC. Fostering professionalism in medical education: A call for improved assessment and meaningful incentives. Journal of General Internal Medicine. 2004;**19**(8):887-892

[38] Cruess SR, Cruess RL, Steinert Y. Role modelling–making the most of a powerful teaching strategy. British Medical Journal. 2008;**336**(7646):718-721

Chapter 4

Knowledge of Sugar in Sugar-Sweetened Beverages in South Africa: A Survey of Postgraduate Students

Netshidzivhani Mmbengeni Victor, Selepe Mosa and John Mamokhere

Abstract

This survey investigated the level of knowledge of sugar in sugar-sweetened beverages by postgraduate students enrolled at the University of Limpopo in the 2019 academic year. A survey questionnaire was sent to three hundred and fifty-nine (359) students as a target population, and two hundred and seventy-eighth (278) questionnaires were returned. The results are based on 77% of the target population. On average, the respondents correctly answered just over half of the items on added sugar in SSBs, with M = 56.02% and SD = 22.03%. There is sufficient evidence to say that the level of knowledge of added sugar between male and female University of Limpopo postgraduate students are different ($t (177) = 2.763$, $p = .011$), using the 5% level of significance. Knowledge and awareness of added sugar are not sufficient components to influence the use of nutrition labels. The findings conclude that there is a relationship between gender and knowledge of added sugar in sugar-sweetened beverages and found that no relationship exists between BMI and knowledge of added sugar in sugar-sweetened beverages. There is a need for user-friendly terminology on nutrition labels.

Keywords: knowledge, sugar tax, sugar-sweetened beverages, postgraduate students, South Africa

1. Introduction

Sugar consumption has increased globally from 130 to 178 million tonnes (World Cancer Research Fund, 2015), and the general consumption of sugar was noted to exceed the WHO guidelines in many countries. This global rise in the consumption of added sugars has been linked to obesity which causes the prevalence of most Non-Communicable Diseases (NCDs) that have resulted in strained national health budgets [1]. Regrettably, South Africa has a population that is increasingly adopting poor dietary habits with the South African Demographic and Health Survey

(2003) reporting adult men and women across all races who are obese using their measure of body index at 29.8% and 54.7% respectively.

In a study conducted in Gauteng in 2006, health awareness and lifestyle behaviour were associated with reading nutrition labels. Habitual readers of food labels who also understood their interpretation proved to be concerned and more conscious about their health.

This research sought to investigate the level of knowledge of added sugars in sugar-sweetened beverages (SSBs) by the University of Limpopo postgraduate students.

2. Problem statement

There is a lack of understanding of nutritional labels that are contributing to a lack of usage of those labels and overconsumption of sugar [2, 3]. The consumption of sugar has increased both globally and in South Africa over the last few decades [4]. It has become increasingly necessary to assist consumers to choose healthier foods [5].

Theoretically, consumers should rely on food labels to make healthy purchasing choices, as they "provide nutritional information" [2]. However, as demonstrated by Jacobs et al., [2] and Heike & Taylor [5], this has not been the case, since the nutrition labels consist of technical language that most consumers cannot comprehend. The "lower the educational level of respondents, the less commonly they read food labels" [2]. It is against this background that the University of Limpopo's postgraduate students become relevant as the unit of analysis for this research study. There is limited research available on the South African consumer's level of knowledge of sugar in SSBs.

3. Research question

The main research question was:

1. What is the University of Limpopo postgraduate students' level of knowledge of sugar in SSBs?

Sub-questions:

1. What is the University of Limpopo postgraduate students' knowledge of nutrition labels on SSBs?

2. What is the University of Limpopo postgraduate students' use of nutrition label information on SSBs?

4. Literature review

Studies based on the impact of the level of knowledge of added sugar in SSBs point toward a global need for improved awareness and consciousness of the effects of excessive consumption of added sugars. Finkelstein, Ruhm, & Kosa [6], support this notion by suggesting that consumers are aware that the overconsumption of SSBs increases the risk of NCDs such as obesity. The prevalence of these NCDs including obesity has become public health concern [7]. The concept of added sugar in food is well clarified in several studies; however, the issue of consumers' knowledge about how sugar relates to nutrition, general nutrition knowledge and the role that food and nutrition labels play in knowledge acquirement is still unclear [3–5, 8–19].

5. The concept of added sugar in SSBs

Added sugars are sugars and syrups such as sucrose and high fructose corn syrup added to different types of food and beverages during the preparation or processing stages [16]. SSBs come in the form of drinks, from sports drinks, and fruit drinks to ice tea and coffee [8]. Sugar found in fruit, milk or nuts are naturally occurring, meaning that they are not added through an artificial process, therefore they do not fall under the abovementioned group of added sugars [16].

In a study conducted by Erzse et al. [12], and Vorster et al. [20], it was found that to reduce the risk of becoming obese, consumers should ensure that the total energy intake from SSBs does not exceed 10% of added sugars. Further, Vorster et al. [20] found that there is a 'positive correlation between the consumption of added sugar and Body Mass Index (BMI)'. Interestingly, men and women differ in their intake of sugar, which results in a difference in the relationships between their dietary intake versus their BMI.

6. Nutritional knowledge of added sugar in SSBs

The notion of nutrition knowledge has been found by Worsley [19] to be very vague and hence there is evidence of a lack of clarity between what nutritionists deem as knowledge about nutrition and what consumers think is important to know about nutrition [19]. Worsley [19] argues that nutrition knowledge cannot affect consumers' food behaviours to the extent that it can change them. For instance, once an individual is aware of the amount of added sugar in their favourite SSB they will not necessarily stop consuming the SSB purely based on the fact that they possess the nutritional knowledge [19]. However, although nutrition knowledge may not have the power to create change on its own, Worsley [19] acknowledges that if nutrition knowledge is paired with other variables, for example, if a consumer has nutrition knowledge but also has goals to lead a healthier lifestyle, their food behaviours have a good chance of changing [19]. This is confirmed by Grunert et al. [21] that nutrition knowledge is associated with being able to understand the nutrient content depicted on the food label.

7. Food and nutritional labelling

Food and nutrition labels are one of the most common sources of knowledge about food products [3, 9, 13]. These labels are essential as they assist consumers in making healthy choices [22]. Therefore, consumers are encouraged to use food and nutritional labels as part of their healthy dietary habits.

Debates have emerged that added sugars tend to be hidden in the food label [23]. This contributes to consumers having difficulties in comprehending the level of added sugars by looking at the food label, as this is usually not depicted [24].

Emerging questions from food label studies range from looking at the use of food labels, whether that information is translated into knowledge and if that knowledge is of any practical value to the purchasing power of a consumer [25–28]. The use of food and nutrition labels is attributed to the nutrition knowledge of a consumer and is affected by socio-demographic factors [29].

The ineffectiveness of labels to perform the functions that they are supposed to can be attributed to two factors, the motivation to use the information and the confusing information on food and nutrition labels [3, 5, 9, 10, 15, 19, 30].

Consumers are influenced by various social factors; this is especially concerning their food behaviour and choices. An individual's background, personal beliefs, values and opinions play an important role in not only what they choose to purchase and consume but also whether food and nutrition labels can influence their food behaviour [5]. Therefore, consumers have been found to take from food labels what is most relevant and convenient for them and disregard information that they may not believe or makes them uncomfortable [5]. A study conducted by Graham and Laska [31] discovered that there was a relationship between the frequent use of nutrition labels and food behaviour. By frequently using nutrition labels, consumers value their health and dietary intake [31].

The level of knowledge of added sugar in food is linked to the use of nutritional labels. Often the frequent use of these labels influences the purchasing power of the consumers which helps them in making healthier choices about their beverage intake. Demographic factors such as gender and the body mass index (BMI) are considered when assessing the level of knowledge of added sugar in SSBs. This is due to the difference in their nutritional needs as it is recommended that men consume slightly more sugar than women.

8. Research hypothesis

The research hypotheses that were tested are as follows:

- Hypothesis (*H0*): There is no relationship between gender and the knowledge of added sugar in SSBs among the University of Limpopo postgraduate students.

- Hypothesis (*H1*): There is a relationship between gender and the knowledge of added sugar in SSBs among the University of Limpopo postgraduate students.

- Hypothesis (*H0*): There is no relationship between body mass index (BMI) and the knowledge of added sugar in SSBs among the University of Limpopo postgraduate.

- Hypothesis (*H2*): There is a relationship between body mass index (BMI) and the knowledge of added sugar in SSBs among the University of Limpopo postgraduate.

The literature is non-directional about the relationship between gender and knowledge of sugar in SSBs or food; it shows a 'correlation between BMI and added sugar consumption' [20].

9. Methodology

This section discusses the research and sample methods that were applied in this study. It further discusses the data collection methods and how the ethical considerations were addressed. Additionally, the data analysis procedure is discussed. The section concludes with the reliability and validity of measurements of the whole study.

10. Research design

A survey was used to conduct this study. A questionnaire was designed and pilot tested before it was emailed and self-administered by the University of Limpopo postgraduate students. This design was used for its convenience to the target population, as they had access to emails and the internet, and for cost-effectiveness for the research team, as they did not have to travel or call to collect data for this study.

11. Sample

A probability census sampling method was used, targeting all the University of Limpopo postgraduate students. A questionnaire was circulated to 359 students. Of these 300 respondents returned the survey questionnaire. The analysis and results of this study are based on only 278 respondents after removing the incomplete questionnaires from the data, constituting a 77% response rate of the target population (**Table 1**).

Sample	Frequency	%
Final sample	278	77%
Returned	300	83%
Discarded	22	6%
Population size	359	100%

Table 1.
Response rate.

12. Ethical issues

The respondents were informed of the study's purpose and that their responses will be analysed and compiled into a report solely to fulfil the requirements of independent publication. Furthermore, the respondents were informed about their right to voluntary participation, the confidentiality in which their responses will be treated and the survey ensured their anonymity by not collecting identifying information such as names, surnames or photos. By completing and submitting a questionnaire, it was taken that the respondents have consented to the ethical considerations. Ethical clearance was sourced from Turfloop Research Ethics Committee (TREC) and the certificate (TREC No: TREC/221/2019: IR) was issued on 04 September 2019.

13. Procedure

A survey questionnaire was designed on Google Form and comprised three sections. The questionnaire was first sent to the University Statistician at the Research Administration and Development. Email addresses of the University of Limpopo postgraduate students were obtained from the University's IT system. The questionnaire that comprised a consent was circulated to the respondents.

14. Survey instrument

The questionnaire comprised of three sections namely, the demographics, the knowledge of added sugar and the use of nutrition labels. The questionnaire had only two measurement scales namely, the 'simple category and multiple-choice' ([32]:105) for demographic and knowledge questions. Additionally, a picture depicted in **Figure 1** was used to test the respondents' understanding and interpretation of the terminology used on the nutrition label.

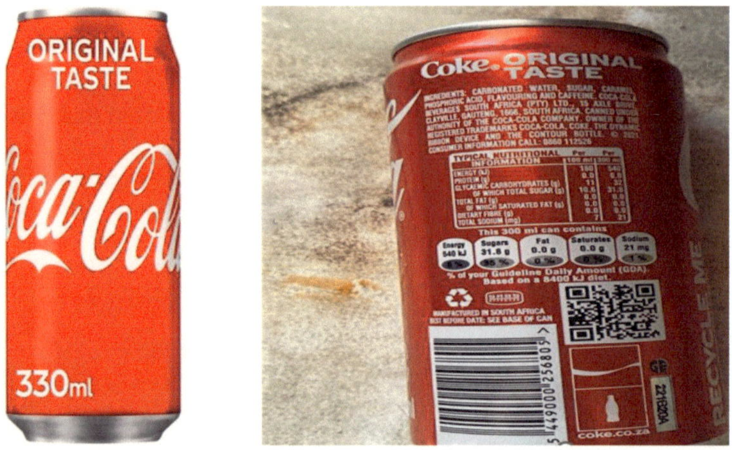

Figure 1.
Nutrition label of 330 ml Coca-Cola can.

15. Data analysis

Data obtained from the questionnaires were analysed using IBM SPSS statistics (version 26). Data analysis entailed categorising, ordering, cleaning and summarising the data. The demographic and knowledge questions were analysed through 'descriptive statistics such as mean, standard deviation, minimum and maximum values' for all scaled questions and frequency tables were used to illustrate these data [32].

The inferential statistical analysis, that is, the t-test was used to compare knowledge scores based on the independent variables of gender and BMI. Additionally, 'Cronbach's Alpha was used to test the internal consistency' of measurement used for the knowledge variable ([33]:209). Equally, data were coded for nominal scale data, replacing the text with actual values. The responses that had more than fifty per cent of data missing were removed from the data. Additionally, knowledge scores were calculated for questions measuring similar constructs.

16. Reliability and validity

16.1 Internal reliability

The internal consistency of the knowledge scale was calculated using 'Cronbach's Alpha and the average inter-item correlation' ([33]:209). These values are presented in **Table 2** below.

Although the values of 'Cronbach's Alpha and average inter-item correlation' ([33]:209) are 0.483 and 0.130 respectively, below the minimum acceptable values, they are acceptable since it was expected that the respondents would possess some knowledge on the level of added sugar in SSBs depending on their exposure and usage of nutrition labels of the SSBs.

16.2 Validity

Face and content validity were tested for this study. The face validity of the knowledge scale is the extent to which the respondents perceived that the knowledge scale is measuring the knowledge of SSBs; and content validity refers to the "extent to which the measurement was representative" of all aspects measuring the SSBs ([33]:212).

Both the 'face and content validity' ([33]:212) were tested through piloting of the questionnaire and feedback received from the respondents on the content of the questionnaire, that is, the logical flow, the ambiguity and the terminology.

Scale	Cronbach's Alpha	Average inter-Item correlation	Number of items
Knowledge	0.483	0.130	8

Table 2.
Internal consistency reliability values of scales.

17. Results

This section begins with a discussion on the data preparation procedure and then the structure of the results. The research questions for the level of knowledge of added sugar in SSBs, the knowledge of nutrition labels and its use are tested through the item level responses, as depicted in **Figure 2**. The results present the item level responses, followed by the scale level responses, the tests of the hypotheses, and lastly the effect size.

17.1 Level of knowledge of sugar in SSBs, and food and nutrition labelling

This section below discusses the knowledge scores in SSBs, and food and nutrition labelling.

17.2 Knowledge scores at item-level

To investigate the level of knowledge of added sugar in SSBs, eight questions were asked. **Figure 2** illustrates the responses to these questions.

More than a third quarter (64%) of the respondents were knowledgeable about the effect of added sugar on health, while less than half (44.5%) of the respondents

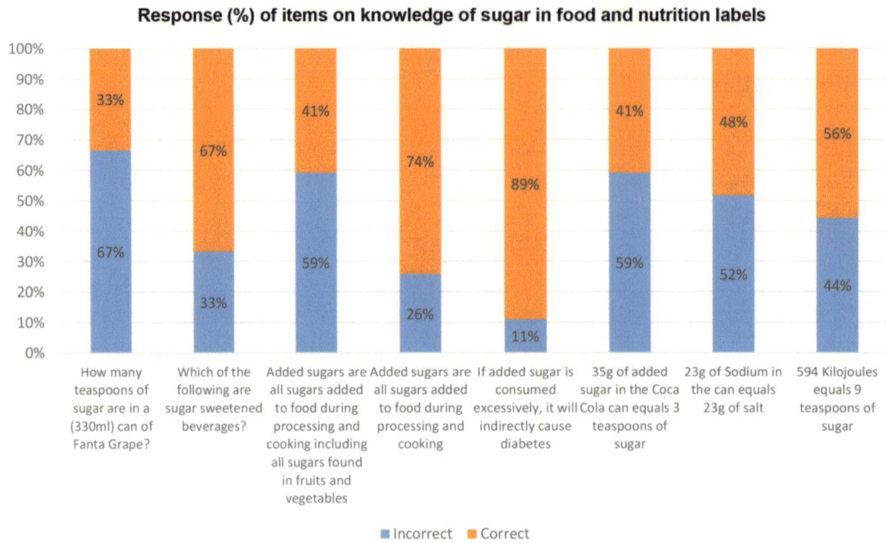

Figure 2.
Summary of responses to items measuring knowledge of sugar (n = 278).

could interpret the added sugar content of SSBs as the equivalence of teaspoons of sugar. Overall, the respondents were split between either knowing or not on questions relating to knowledge of added sugar and understanding of nutrition labels on SSBs.

17.3 Knowledge scores at scale-level

The item-level responses are summated to scale level and the summary statistics and frequency distribution are supplied in **Table 3** and **Figure 2**.

Based on the summary statistics supplied in **Table 3**, more than one-half of the respondents have knowledge of added sugar in SSBs, with M = 56.02%, SD = 22.03%. The skewness value of −58.20% is similar to its standard error (44.80%) and is thus considered significant. Furthermore, the histogram in **Figure 3** below appears to be approximately normally distributed.

	Statistic	Std. error
Mean	56.02%	4.24%
Median	62.50%	
Std. Deviation	22.03%	
Minimum	0.00%	
Maximum	100.00%	
Range	100.00%	
Interquartile Range	25.00%	
Skewness	−58.20%	44.80%

Table 3.
Summary statistics of mean knowledge scores (n-278).

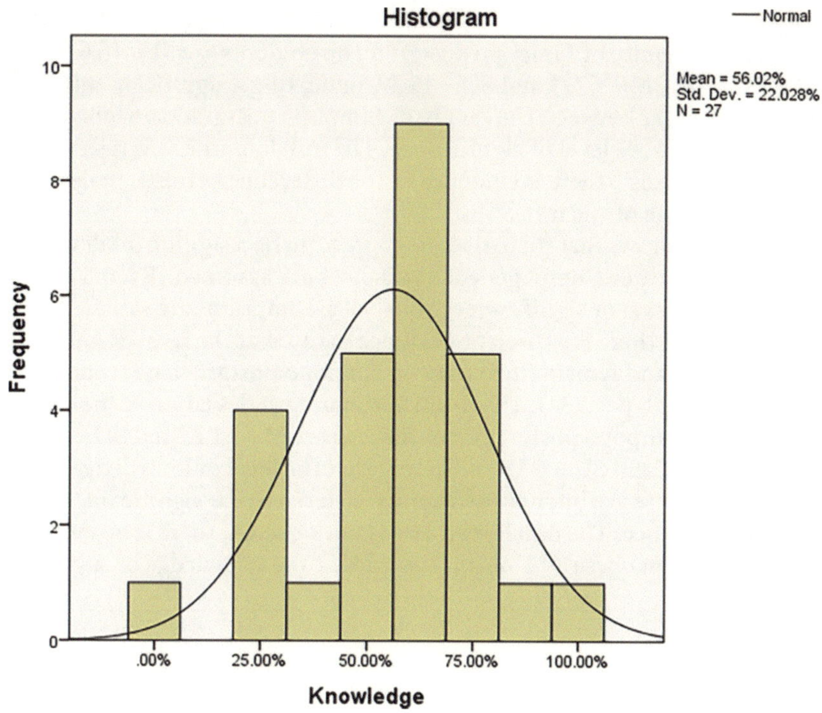

Figure 3.
Distribution of knowledge scores (n=278).

17.4 Hypothesis testing

The results of the hypotheses tests and t-test are discussed in the section below. Hypothesis:

1. H_0: There is no relationship between gender and the knowledge of added sugar in SSBs among the University of Limpopo postgraduate students

H_1: There is a relationship between gender and the knowledge of added sugar in SSBs among the University of Limpopo postgraduate students.

2. H_0: There is no relationship between BMI and the knowledge of added sugar in SSBs among the University of Limpopo postgraduate students.

H_1: There is a relationship between BMI and the knowledge of added sugar in SSBs among the University of Limpopo postgraduate students.

The assumptions of the t-test for independent samples were tested based on visual inspection of the normality of the distribution of mean level of knowledge scores (**Figure 2**) and the 'Levene's test for equality of variance' ([32]: 222). There does not appear to be a significant deviation from normality, based on the figure. Furthermore, homogeneous variances are assumed ($F = 0.598$, $p = .218$) using the 5% level of significance. Thus, all assumptions are satisfied.

Based on the results of the study, there is sufficient evidence to say that the level of knowledge of added sugar between male and female University of Limpopo postgraduate students are different ($t (25) = 2.763, p = .011$). The mean and standard deviation of male University of Limpopo postgraduate students are $M = 46.67$ and $SD = 21.89$, and for females' $M = 67.71$ and $SD = 16.39$, indicating a significant difference in the knowledge of sugar between University of Limpopo postgraduate female and male students, using the 5% level of significance. The null hypothesis is rejected, in favour of the hypothesis – there is evidence of the difference between males and females of the knowledge of sugar in SSBs.

Second hypothesis shows that there does not appear to be a significant deviation from normality. Furthermore, homogeneous variances are assumed ($F = 0.508$, $p = .483$) using the 5% level of significance. Thus, all assumptions are satisfied.

Based on the results, there is sufficient evidence to say that the level of knowledge of added sugar of male and female University of Limpopo postgraduate students are different ($t (22) = -1.228, p = .232$). The mean and standard deviation of 'normal weight' University of Limpopo postgraduate students are $M = 51.25$ and $SD = 6.58$, and for obese $M = 62.50$ and $SD = 6.15$, indicating that the level of knowledge of both 'normal weight' and obese are but not sufficiently different to be significant, using the 5% level of significance. The null hypothesis is not rejected, there is no evidence of the difference between obese and 'normal weight' of the knowledge of sugar in SSBs.

17.5 Cohen's effect size

Cohen's effect size for the knowledge of sugar of the SSBs between male and female University of Limpopo postgraduate students. The Cohen's effect size for the independent variable of gender and the dependent variable of knowledge is $d = 1.07$. The value of *d* represents a substantially big effect and difference in the knowledge of sugar of the SSBs between male and female University of Limpopo postgraduate students.

17.6 Cohen's effect size for the knowledge of sugar of the SSBS and BMI

The effect size for BMI and knowledge is $d = 0.51$. The value of *d* represents a moderate effect and difference in the knowledge of added sugar of the SSBs between BMI levels of University of Limpopo postgraduate students.

17.7 The use of nutrition labelling on SSBs

Fifty-nine percent of the respondents reported not looking at the nutrition label. The number of those reported to look at the nutrition label before they purchase SSBs is lower than the mean value, that is, $M = 56.02\%$, of the respondents knowledgeable about added sugar in SSBs.

18. Discussions

18.1 Level of knowledge of sugar in SSBs, and food and nutrition labelling

More than fifty percent of the students were knowledgeable about the sugar contents of the SSBs. Females were more knowledgeable about the sugar contents of SSBs than their male counterparts. The difference in the knowledge of added sugar was significant between the two genders and therefore, there is sufficient evidence to conclude that there is a relationship between gender and knowledge. Furthermore, the relationship between BMI and knowledge did not yield a positive result.

Just over eighty per cent of the respondents displayed knowledge of the effects of added sugar consumption on health. This supports the findings of Finkelstein et al., [6] that there is awareness among consumers that excessive consumption of sugar contributes to the risk of non-communicable diseases. However, the awareness of the risk factors of excessive consumption of sugar and knowledge of consumers of the sugar contents in food products does not necessarily translate into consumption behaviour change.

18.2 Level of knowledge and understanding of the nutrition labelling

Tierney et al., [24] reported that the technical language used on nutrition labels tends to be a barrier to serving its primary objective of ensuring that consumers know the nutrition contents of food products they purchase and then make informed consumer choices. This study tested this finding by using a picture of a Coca-Cola 330 ml can and asked questions regarding its nutrition label. The per cent of those respondents who could comprehend with this technical language used on the nutrition label ranged from forty-one to fifty-six.

Given that this study targeted Postgraduate students who do not necessarily represent the average South African, and still scored lower than 60%, as they could not interpret terminologies such as sodium, kilojoule and a number of grams of sugar, and what these mean in terms of the number of teaspoons of sugar or salt, these findings confirm that the terminology used on nutrition labels pose a challenge to consumers.

18.3 The use of nutrition labels on SSBs

The number of respondents who reported looking at the nutrition label before they purchase food products is lower (i.e., 41%) than the mean value, that is, M = 56.02% of the respondents knowledgeable about sugar in SSBs. Although this fact has not been fully established in this study, the respondents' knowledge of the sugar content in food products and consumers' understanding of nutrition labels alone seems not to be sufficient factors to influence the purchasing behaviour of consumers. Heike and Taylor [5] reported that social factors such as an individual's background, beliefs, values and opinions about what is important and not, play a very critical role in the consumers' behaviour. Therefore, nutrition literacy interventions should consider behaviour change as a key component of these interventions to influence consumer purchasing behaviour since knowledge alone is insufficient.

19. Conclusions and Recommendations

More than three-quarter of the respondents are knowledgeable about the effect of sugar on health, while only one-third of the respondents could interpret the sugar content of SSBs as the equivalence of teaspoons of sugar. More than one-half of the respondents have knowledge of sugar in SSBs, with M = 56.02%, SD = 22.03%.

There is sufficient evidence that there is a relationship between the gender of University of Limpopo postgraduate students and their level of knowledge of added sugar in SSBs, with more females having more knowledge of sugar in SSBs than their male counterparts, with the value of ($t(25) = 2.763$, $p = .011$). The mean and standard deviation of male University of Limpopo postgraduate students are M = 46.67 and SD = 21.89, and for females' M = 67.71 and SD = 16.39, indicating a significant difference in the knowledge of sugar between WSG female and male students, using the 5% level of significance. Furthermore, there is no evidence to support the hypothesis that suggests a relationship between BMI and knowledge of added sugar on SSBs.

Less than half (i.e., 41%) of the respondents reported not looking at the nutrition label before they purchase food products. Regardless of this study targeting post-graduate students, the respondents fared in a range of forty-one to fifty-six per cent to questions relating to interpreting technical language, such as sodium, kilojoules and grams of sugar, on the nutrition label confirming the findings by earlier studies that the technical language used on food products is a barrier to serve the primary purpose it was initiated, as consumers struggle to comprehend it and thus make informed purchasing decisions.

These findings similar to earlier studies recommend user-friendly language that ordinary people would understand to be used on the nutrition labels and this could be either in a form of images or a number of teaspoons of sugar, to enable ordinary citizens to understand the contents of the food they purchase.

As reported earlier, University of Limpopo postgraduate students' knowledge and awareness of added sugar in food products did not seem sufficient to influence their purchasing and consumption behaviours, thus supporting the recommendations made by Drichoutis et al. [29]; Hieke and Taylor [5], that additional focus must be on the social factors such as that knowledge and awareness consumer beliefs, values and opinions, since awareness to change consumers' behaviour.

Author details

Netshidzivhani Mmbengeni Victor*, Selepe Mosa and John Mamokhere
Department of Research Administration and Development, University of Limpopo, South Africa

*Address all correspondence to: mmbengeni.netshidzivhani@ul.ac.za

References

[1] Stacey N, Tugendhaft A, Hofman K. Sugary beverage taxation in South Africa: Household expenditure, demand system elasticities, and policy implications. Preventive Medicine. 2017;**105**:S26-S31

[2] Jacobs SA, de Beer H, Larney M. Adult consumers' understanding and use of information on food labels: A study among consumers living in the Potchefstroom and Klerksdorp regions, South Africa. Public Health Nutrition. 2011;**14**(03):510-522

[3] Temple NJ, Fraser J. Food labels: A critical assessment. Nutrition. 2014;**30**(3):257-260

[4] World Health Organization. Reducing the consumption of sugar-sweetened beverages in Cape Town. 2021. https://www.who.int/news-room/feature-stories/detail/reducing-the-consumption-of-sugar-sweetened-beverages-in-cape-town

[5] Hieke S, Taylor CR. A critical review of the literature on nutritional labeling. Journal of Consumer Affairs. 2012;**46**(1):120-156

[6] Finkelstein EA, Ruhm CJ, Kosa KM. Economic causes and consequences of obesity. Annual Review of Public Health. 2005;**26**(1):239-257

[7] Ziraba AK, Fotso JC, Ochako R. Overweight and obesity in urban Africa: A problem of the rich or the poor? BMC Public Health. 2009;**9**(1):465

[8] Bleich SN, Barry CL, Gary-Webb TL, Herring BJ. Reducing sugar-sweetened beverage consumption by providing caloric information: How black adolescents alter their purchases and whether the effects persist. American Journal of Public Health. 2014;**104**(12):2417-2424

[9] Cooke R, Papadaki A. Nutrition label use mediates the positive relationship between nutrition knowledge and attitudes towards healthy eating with dietary quality among university students in the UK. Appetite. 2014;**83**(September):297-303

[10] Cowburn G, Stockley L. Consumer understanding and use of nutrition labelling: A systematic review. Public Health Nutrition. 2005;**8**(1):21-28

[11] Emrich TE, Qi Y, Mendoza JE, Lou W, Cohen JE, L'Abbé MR. Consumer perceptions of the Nutrition Facts table and front-of-pack nutrition rating systems. Applied Physiology, Nutrition, and Metabolism. 2014;**39**(4):417-424

[12] Erzse A, Christofides N, Stacey N, Lebard K, Foley L, Hofman K. Availability and advertising of sugar-sweetened beverages in South African public primary schools following a voluntary pledge by a major beverage company: A mixed methods study. Global Health Action. 2021;**14**(1):1898130

[13] Mackison D, Wrieden WL, Anderson AS. Validity and reliability testing of a short questionnaire developed to assess consumers' use, understanding and perception of food labels. European Journal of Clinical Nutrition. 2010;**64**(2):210-217

[14] Medeiros LC, Hillers VN, Kendall PA, Mason A. Food safety education: What should we be teaching to consumers? Journal of Nutrition Education. 2001;**33**(2):108-113

[15] Spronk I, Kullen C, Burdon C, O'Connor H. Relationship between nutrition knowledge and dietary intake. British Journal of Nutrition. 2014;**111**(10):1713-1726

[16] Taubes G. Is sugar toxic? The New York Times. 2011:1-13

[17] van der Colff N, van der Merwe D, Bosman M, Erasmus A, Ellis S. Consumers' prepurchase satisfaction with the attributes and information of food labels. International Journal of Consumer Studies. 2016;**40**(2):220-228

[18] Williams P. Consumer understanding and use of health claims for foods. Nutrition. 2005;**63**(7):256-264

[19] Worsley A. Nutrition knowledge and food consumption-can nutrition knowledge change behaviour? Asia Pacific Journal of Clinical Nutrition. 2002;**11**:S579-S585

[20] Vorster HH, Kruger A, Wentzel-Viljoen E, Kruger HS, Margetts BM. Added sugar intake in South Africa: Findings from the adult prospective urban and rural epidemiology cohort study. American Journal of Clinical Nutrition. 2014;**99**(6):1479-1486

[21] Grunert KG, Wills JM, Fernández-Celemín L. Nutrition knowledge, and use and understanding of nutrition information on food labels among consumers in the UK. Appetite. 2010;**55**(2):177-189

[22] Jordan Lin C-T, Lee J-Y, Yen ST. Do dietary intakes affect search for nutrient information on food labels?. Social Science & Medicine. 2004;**59**(9):1955-1967

[23] Marí, Josep Antoni Tur. Hidden sugar in food: A risk for health . Journal of Clinical Nutrition & Dietetics. 2017;**3**:1-3

[24] Tierney M, Gallagher A, Giotis E, Pentieva K. An online survey on consumer knowledge and understanding of added sugars. Nutrients. 2017;**9**(1):37

[25] Balasubramanian SK, Cole C. Consumers' search and use of nutrition information: The challenge and promise of the nutrition labeling and education act. Journal of Marketing. 2002;**66**(3):112-127

[26] Sunley N. Nutritional information in food labelling: What does it really mean to consumers? South African Journal of Clinical Nutrition. 2012;**25**(1):7-8

[27] van der Merwe D, Bosman M, Ellis S. Consumers' opinions and use of food labels: Results from an urban-rural hybrid area in South Africa. Food Research International. 2014;**63**(March 2016):100-107

[28] van der Merwe D, Bosman M, Ellis S, de Beer H, Mielmann A. Consumers' knowledge of food label information: An exploratory investigation in Potchefstroom, South Africa. Public Health Nutrition. 2013;**16**(3):403-408

[29] Drichoutis AC, Lazaridis P, Nayga RM. Nutrition knowledge and consumer use of nutritional food labels. European Review of Agricultural Economics. 2005;**32**(1):93-118

[30] Musiker JC, Kesa H. The Impact Nutritional Information Has on Customers' Behaviours towards Their Food Choices in Restaurants. Global Review of Research in Tourism, Hospitality and Leisure Management. 2014;**1**(1):34-57

[31] Graham DJ, Laska MN. Nutrition label use partially mediates the relationship between attitude toward healthy eating and overall dietary quality

among college students. Journal of the Academy of Nutrition and Dietetics. 2012;**112**(3):414-418

[32] Wagner C, Kawulich B, Garner M. Doing Social Research: A Global Context. New York: McGraw-Hill; 2012

[33] Neuman WL. Social Research Methods: Qualitative and Quantitative Approaches. Seventh ed. Boston: Pearson; 2011

Chapter 5

Perspective Chapter: Evidence-Based Medicine – A New Approach for Medical Education and Practice

Delelegn Emwodew Yehualashet, Binyam Tariku Seboka, Tizalegn Tesfaye Mamo and Mulugeta Namaro Yawo

Abstract

The new concept is gaining worldwide recognition and acceptance in medical education and practice. Evidence-based medicine (EBM) is the term used to describe this novel approach to the teaching and practice of medicine. The purpose of this chapter is to give you a brief overview of the components of EBM, EBM principles, the steps of EBM practice, and the skills required for EBM that can shape your approach toward EBM. A review of the English-language literature was conducted in PubMed, Google Scholar, and Google to obtain EBM definitions, the components of EBM, EBM principles, the steps of EBM practice, and the skills required for EBM. EBM is the integration of the best available research evidence with clinical expertise and patient values. It consists of three basic components: the best available evidence, clinical expertise, and patient values. The integration of these three components can be effectively achieved by completing the five steps of the EBM practice. The five-step process of EBM is asking, acquiring, appraising, applying the evidence in clinical decisions, and assessing the outcome.

Keywords: evidence-based medicine, critical appraisal, levels of evidence, medical practice, medical education

1. Introduction

The new concept is gaining worldwide recognition and acceptance in medical education and practice. Evidence-based medicine (EBM) is the term used to describe this novel approach to the teaching and practice of medicine. EBM is the integration of the best available external clinical evidence with clinical expertise and individual patient values to inform clinical decision-making [1]. It is a new area of expertise that all medical learners and practicing physicians should ideally acquire to be more present in their daily practices [2, 3]. The inclusion of EBM in one's practice not only makes one a better physician but also allows one to provide the best possible medical care for their patients. Therefore, EBM can be integrated into the medical curriculum [4, 5].

The practice of EBM usually begins with patient encounters, which raise questions about diagnosis, treatment, or prognosis [6, 7]. EBM seeks to find the best answers to these questions based on a detailed review of the literature published in medical journals that apply strict criteria for research validity. Evidence does not make decisions on its own, but it helps clinicians make better decisions about the patient care process and increases the likelihood of better medical outcomes [8]. Because EBM supports the collection of evidence in an accurate, concise, and informative manner, the implementation of EBM in clinical practice provides guidance for the selection of the most appropriate patient care based on the best available evidence [9]. Therefore, all medical personnel on the cross-disciplinary medical care team must have EBM skills to appraise, interpret, and apply research findings to their clinical practice [3, 9]. The purpose of this chapter is to give you a brief overview of the components of EBM, EBM principles, the steps of EBM practice, and the skills required for EBM that can shape your approach toward EBM.

2. Methods

A literature search was conducted in PubMed, Google Scholar, and Google to retrieve definitions of EBM, components of EBM, principles of EBM, EBM practice procedures, and skills required for EBM. Numerous combinations of keywords, such as "evidence-based medicine," "evidence-based practice," "medical education," "medical practice," "clinical practice," "teaching," and "training," were employed to ensure comprehensive coverage of the EBM literature. Website pages, research articles, and commentaries were selected based on insight, accurate content, and balance to ensure non-bias. Furthermore, examples were drawn from the EBM resources for illustrative purposes.

3. Components of EBM

Contrary to its name, EBM is not just about evidence. It consists of three basic components: the best available evidence, clinical expertise, and patient values [1].

The best research evidence: The best research evidence refers to the latest scientific research in various aspects of patient care, diagnosis, treatment, or prevention.

Clinical expertise: Clinical expertise is a combination of medical skills, medical knowledge, and professional experience acquired by physicians throughout their careers.

Patient values: Patient values are the unique priorities, concerns, expectations, beliefs, hopes, and stresses that each patient brings to the clinical encounter (**Figure 1**).

4. Principles of EBM

The basic principles of EBM include: [6]

- Clinical problems should be translated into answerable clinical questions.
- Medical decisions should be based on the best available scientific evidence.
- Clinical problems should determine the type of evidence to look for.

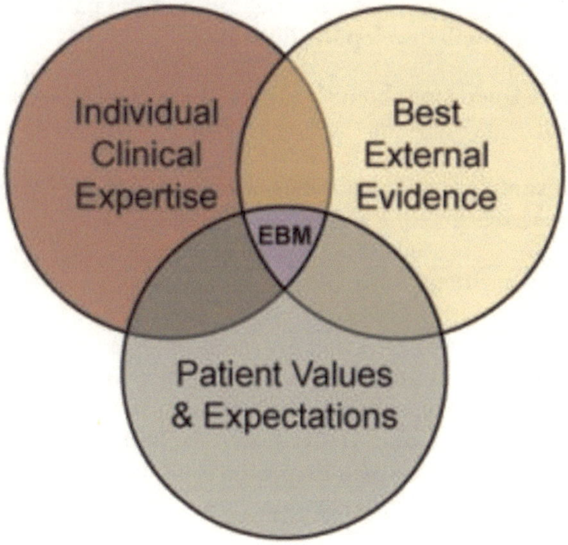

Figure 1.
The fundamental components of evidence-based medicine.

- The best evidence should be critically appraised for validity, relevance, and applicability.
- Findings from a critical appraisal of evidence should be applied in clinical practice.
- Clinical performance should be constantly evaluated.

5. Steps to practice EBM

The EBM process consists of five main steps: formulating a clinical question, acquisition of the evidence, evaluating the evidence, application of evidence to clinical decisions, and evaluation of outcomes [10].

5.1 Step 1: formulating answerable clinical questions

The first and most important step of EBM is formulating answerable clinical questions. The PICO (population (P), intervention (I), comparison (C), and outcome (O)) framework helps turn clinical problems into answerable clinical questions.

5.1.1 Types of clinical questions

1. **Therapy:** Questions about the effectiveness of treatment in improving outcomes for patients/patients with the disease.
2. **Diagnosis:** Questions about the ability of the test or procedure to distinguish between those with the disease or those without the disease.

3. **Prognosis:** Questions about the potential cause of the patient's illness or the likelihood that they will develop the disease.

4. **Etiology/harm:** Questions about the harmful effect of intervention or exposure on the patient.

Here are some examples of clinical scenarios for each type of clinical question to illustrate how you can design clinical questions using PICO.

5.1.2 PICO for therapy questions

When using PICO to formulate a therapy question, P is the patient or disease, I is medications or specific procedural interventions, C is comparison intervention (or no treatment), and O is the outcome of interest such as disease or condition management.

Scenario: Your preceptor wants you to search for literature. She is interested in whether acetaminophen is better than ibuprofen in reducing fever in young children.

PICO: P = Young children, I = Acetaminophen, C = Ibuprofen, and O = Reduced fever.

Clinical question: Is acetaminophen more effective than ibuprofen in reducing fever in young children?

5.1.3 PICO for diagnosis questions

To formulate diagnostic questions using the PICO framework, P is the population of interest or the target disease, I is a diagnostic test or procedure, C is an alternative diagnostic test or the current gold standard test for the problem, and O is a measure of the test utility such as the sensitivity and specificity of the diagnostic tool, although the outcome measures usually do not need to be included in database searches.

Scenario: You are part of a team reviewing local cervical screening guidelines. The most commonly used test is the Pap test, which detects abnormal cells but does not detect the HPV virus. In recent years, tests have been developed to detect the HPV virus. You may want to know what the latest evidence says about using HPV and Pap tests, or whether they should be used in combination.

PICO: P = cervical cancer, I = HPV test, C = Pap test, O = effect of both tests.

Clinical question: Is the HPV test or Pap test more effective in detecting cervical cancer?

5.1.4 PICO for prognosis questions

When using PICO to generate prognostic questions, P is the patient, population, or problem; I is the prognostic factor; C is usually not applicable; and O is the outcome of interest (e.g., deaths and recurrence). Many prognosis questions require only population and outcome because they are more often related to a broader population than to subgroup comparisons.

Scenario: The father of a twenty years old schizophrenic is worried about his son's future health. He asks you about possible relapses.

PICO: P = 20-year-old man with schizophrenia, I = inapplicable, C = inapplicable, O = relapse.

Clinical question: What is the likelihood of relapse in a twenty years old schizophrenic man?

5.1.5 PICO for etiology questions

When using PICO to formulate an etiology question, P is the patient or population, I is exposure to certain conditions or risk behaviors, C means not being exposed to those conditions or hazardous behaviors, and O is the outcome of interest such as the development of a particular disease or condition.

Scenario: You have a 39-year-old patient who has experienced heavy bleeding for most of her life. After considering all other options, we discuss the possibility of cervical surgery as a solution, although one may wonder if her high blood pressure in the year after surgery increases her risk of severe myocardial infarction.

PICO: P = 39-year-old woman undergoing cervical surgery, I = high blood pressure, C = normal blood pressure, and O = increased risk of acute myocardial infarction.

Clinical question: Are hypertensive women at higher risk of developing acute myocardial infarction in the first year after cervical surgery compared to non-hypertensive women?

5.2 Step 2: acquire the evidence

The second step is to search for the best available evidence in the medical literature that provides an answer to the question. This step involves identifying the search terms, selecting resources to perform your search, and developing an effective search strategy.

5.2.1 EBM pyramid: the evidence hierarchy

The EBM pyramid is a diagram that helps you understand how to weigh different levels of evidence for clinical decisions. It allows you to take a top-down approach to identify the best available evidence, by first searching for the recent systematic review, and if it is not available, search for the next level of evidence to answer your question. EBM pyramid ranks study types based on the strength and accuracy of their research methods. **Figure 2** below shows the hierarchy of evidence or the EBM pyramid.

At the top of the pyramid is filtered evidence, which represents the strongest level of evidence such as systematic reviews, meta-analyses, and critical appraisals. At the bottom of the pyramid is unfiltered evidence, including randomized controlled trials, cohort studies, and case-controlled studies. You should seek the highest level of evidence available, but be aware that filtered evidence may not be relevant to your specific clinical question. If so, you need to move the pyramid down to find strong evidence that will solve your clinical question.

5.2.2 Filtered resources

Filtered resources critically assess the quality of the study and recommend its application in practice. A critical appraisal of individual articles has already been done for you, which will save a great deal of time. As the critical appraisal is completed, the filtered literature is suitable to use for clinical decision-making during care. In addition to saving time, filtered literature often provides more accurate answers than individual research studies. Examples of filtered sources include systematic reviews from the Cochrane Database of Systematic Reviews, TRIP Database, JAMA Evidence, BMJ Best Practices, UpToDate, DynaMed Plus, ACP Journal Club, and PubMed (Medline).

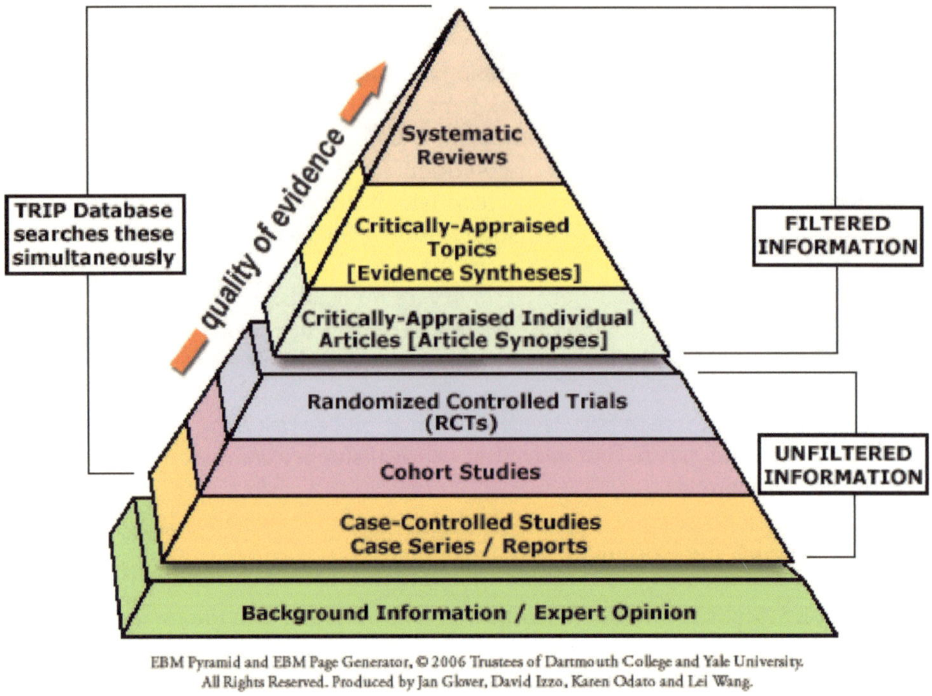

Figure 2.
Hierarchy of evidence or EBM pyramid.

5.2.3 Unfiltered resources

Unfiltered resources are primary studies that have not yet been synthesized. Therefore, they are challenging to read, interpret, and apply in practice. Examples of unfiltered resources are CINAHL, EMBASE, Web of Science, PsycINFO, and PubMed. If a current, well-designed systematic review is not available, proceed to a primary study to answer your question. The best type of primary studies varies depending on the type of clinical question. **Table 1** lists the study types suitable for the main types of clinical questions.

5.2.4 Building a search strategy

There are many ways to find information using online resources. An overview of these strategies is provided below. However, note that each database you use handles these strategies differently.

Boolean Operators (AND, OR, and NOT): Boolean operators allow you to combine search terms to identify records that contain matching words.

AND

- **AND** narrows the search.
- Retrieve documents that contain both the specified search terms or keywords.
- The more terms you connect with AND, the fewer the search results.

Type of clinical question	The ideal type of study to answer the question
Therapy	RCT > Cohort study > case–control
Diagnosis	RCT > Cohort study
Prognosis	Cohort study > case control > case series/case report
Etiology/Harm	RCT > Cohort study > case–control

Adapted from the Dartmouth Biomedical Libraries: Evidence-Based Medicine Worksheets: http://www.dartmouth.edu/~biomed/services.htmld/EBP_docs/clin_question_worksheet_EXAMPLE.pdf

Table 1.
Type of clinical questions and the ideal type of study to answer the question.

Example: Hip **AND** Fracture retrieve documents containing both hip and fracture.
OR

- Use **OR** to expand your search.
- Retrieve documents that contain either of the specified keywords or both keywords, but not necessarily both.
- The more keywords you combine with **OR**, the more search results you will get.
- Use to search for similar keywords.

Example: Renal **OR** Kidney retrieves documents that contain either renal or kidney or both renal and kidney.
NOT

- **NOT** limit your search.
- Use **NOT** to remove terms from your search and find fewer results.

Example: pig **NOT** guinea will return items containing only the term pig but eliminates items containing the 2nd term (guinea) or both terms.

Nesting or parentheses: Use parentheses to group your search terms and Boolean operators in the order in which you want to process them. Using the advanced search screen in the database is another way to group your words so that you can find more relevant documents on the topic you want. **Example:** (dental anxiety OR dental fear OR dental phobia) AND (music therapy OR music).

Truncation and Wildcards: Using truncation and wildcards is a shortcut strategy for retrieving records that contain a word variation. Truncation markers allow you to add individual word endings and spellings without listing them as search terms. For example, educat* will retrieve documents that contain words such as education, educator, educating, educated, or educational. Wildcards are often used to find alternate spellings of a word, such as wom?n for woman or woman. Be careful when using truncation and wildcard symbols as different databases use different symbols. To determine which symbol to use in the database you are looking for, find the Help screen and look for information on wildcards, truncation, or word variation.

Field search: A field is a part of an electronic record of a database. Try narrowing or broadening your search by searching specific fields such as author, subject, title, or full text.

Controlled vocabularies: Few databases contain thesauruses, but some use subject headings. If the database you are using has either, it is worth checking how the topics are grouped and the database language used. A subject title search is more accurate than a keyword search.

5.3 Step 3: appraise the evidence

Once the evidence that answers the clinical question is identified, the next step is to evaluate the evidence for its validity/closeness to truth and applicability/clinical importance. Critical appraisal of each type of study requires answers to three basic questions, which are as follows:

- Are the study results valid?
- What are the results?
- Do the results help my patient care?

There are standard questions that can be used to assess the validity and applicability of evidence. The questions that can be asked depend on the type of clinical question and the study method. To see examples of these questions, refer to the worksheet below (**Tables 2–5**).

5.4 Step 4: apply the evidence

If you find evidence that is valid, important, and generalizable to your patient, you need to decide how to apply the findings to your patient care. Applying the best evidence is undoubtedly the EBM step that requires the most skill. It is at this stage that you synthesize your medical expertise and outstanding scientific knowledge with the patient's specific values and circumstances to make a clinical decision: Before applying evidence from research to your patient, answer the questions listed in **Table 6**.

5.5 Step 5: assess the outcome

The final step is self-assessment of your performance in the EBM process. You should evaluate your application of research evidence, identify the effectiveness of the strategies you have applied, and examine whether you are able to provide a satisfactory result to the patient. Self-assessment of performance in EBM is the process of answering questions in **Table 7**.

6. Skills required for EBM practice

The five-step process of EBM requires a wide variety of knowledge and skills. To perform the first three steps, clinicians need to be able to question current clinical practice and answer clinical questions (Step 1), have knowledge of medical databases and skills in literature search (Step 2), ability to understand scientific methods and

Screening	• Does the study employ an appropriate study design? • Does the PICO match your question? • Is there a possible conflict of interest?
Validity	**Patient follow-up** • Were all patients included in the trial adequately considered and included in their conclusions (loss to follow-up should be less than 20%? • Is the follow-up of the patient complete? **Randomization** • Were the included subjects a good representative of the target population? • Was the patients' allocation to the treatment random? • Was the allocation secret? **Intention to treat analysis** • Were patients analyzed in randomized groups? • Does the data of all randomized subjects analyzed? **Baseline characteristics similar to patients** • Were the groups similar at the start of the study? **Blinding** • Were patients, health care workers, and researchers "blinded" to the treatment? • If blinding was not possible, were blinded mice and/or objective outcome measures used? **Equal treatment** • Apart from the experimental intervention, were the groups treated equally? **Summary of the validity of the article** • What are the significant research strengths, weaknesses, or concerns? • How serious are the threats to validity, and in what ways might research results be biased?
Clinical importance	• How precise were the treatment effects? (confidence interval; in its absence p-value tells statistical significance) • How large was the treatment effect? (see below) Outcome present Outcome absent Treated/exposed A = B= Control/non exposed C = D= **Experimental event rate (EER)**: The proportion of patients in the experimental treatment group who are observed to experience the outcome of interest. EER = A/(A + B) **Control event rate (CER):** The proportion of patients in the control group who are observed to experience the outcome of interest. CER = C/(C + D) **Absolute risk reduction (ARR):** The calculated absolute difference in the incidence of adverse outcomes between experimental and control participants in a trial. ARR is sometimes called risk difference. ARR = CER - EER **Relative risk reduction (RRR):** The relative reduction in the incidence of adverse outcomes between experimental and control participants in a trial. RRR = CER - EER/CER **Number needed to treat (NNT):** The number of patients who need to be treated with the specified intervention to prevent one bad outcome or produce one good outcome over the period of time specified in the study. NNT = 1/AAR

Source: Dartmouth Biomedical Libraries: Evidence-Based Medicine Critical Appraisal Worksheet for a Therapy study: http://www.dartmouth.edu/~biomed/services.htmld/EBP_docs/clin_question_worksheet.pdf

Table 2.
Critical appraisal worksheet to assess the validity and applicability of therapy studies.

statistics (biostatistics and epidemiology). In applying the evidence (Step 4), physicians rely on their medical expertise. Therefore, they need the ability to use both clinical skills and previous experience to identify a patient's personal health status and diagnosis, their patient values and assessments, and the specific risks and benefits of

Screening	• Why was the study conducted (what was the research question)? • Does the study employ an appropriate study design?
Validity	• Did the study have a clear and specific question? • Was the presence or absence of the target disease confirmed by the reference standard? • Was the comparison with an independent reference standard blinded to the results of the research study? • Was this test evaluated in a suitable range of patients? • Were reference criteria applied to all patients?
Clinical importance	Disorder present Disorder absent Positive test result A B Negative test result C D **Sensitivity:** The percentage of people with the target disease whose test is positive. Used to help evaluate and select diagnostic tests/symptoms. Sensitivity = A/(A + C) **Specificity:** The proportion of people whose tests are negative and do not have the desired disease. Used to help evaluate and select diagnostic tests/symptoms. Specificity = D/(B + D) Likelihood ratio for a positive test = sensitivity/1 − specificity Likelihood ratio for a negative test = 1 − sensitivity/specificity

Dartmouth Biomedical Libraries: Evidence-Based Medicine Critical Appraisal Worksheet for Diagnostic test study: http://www.dartmouth.edu/~biomed/services.htmld/EBP_docs/CriticalAppraisalWorksheetDiagnosis.pdf

Table 3.
Critical appraisal worksheet for a diagnosis study.

Screening	• Why was the study conducted (what was the research question) • Does the study employ an appropriate study design?
Validity	• Is the defined representative sample collected in a common (usually early) stage of the disease? • Was patient follow-up sufficient to achieve the desired clinical outcome? • Is the follow-up of the patient complete? • Do the outcomes of interest predefine? • Were outcomes measured "blind" (i.e., without knowledge of patient clinical characteristics and prognostic factors)?
Clinical importance	• What are the risks of the outcome over time? • How precise are the estimates?

Dartmouth Biomedical Libraries: Evidence-Based Medicine Critical Appraisal Worksheet for a Prognosis Study: http://www.dartmouth.edu/~biomed/services.htmld/EBP_docs/CriticalAppraisal WorksheetPrognosis.pdf

Table 4.
Critical appraisal worksheet for a prognosis study.

Screening	• Why was the study conducted (what was the research question)? • Does the study employ an appropriate study design?
Validity	• Did the study have a clear and specific question? • Were there clearly defined and similar groups of patients? • Were exposures and clinical outcomes measured in the same way in both groups? • Was the follow-up complete and long enough? • Is the proposed causal link reasonable?
Clinical importance	Adverse outcome Present (case) Absent (control)

	Exposure (yes) A B Exposure (no) C D Cohort study: Relative risk = A/(A + B)/C/(C + D) For case–control studies: Odds ratio = A*D/B*C
Dartmouth Biomedical Libraries: Evidence-Based Medicine Critical Appraisal Worksheet for an Etiology /Harm Study: http://www.dartmouth.edu/~biomed/services.htmld/EBP_docs/CriticalAppraisalWorksheetHarm-Etiology.pdf	

Table 5.
Critical appraisal worksheet for a harm/etiology study.

Similar patients	• Are my patients similar to the study patients? • Are the patients so different as the results to be inapplicable?
Realistic interventions	• Is the intervention realistic in your practice setting? • Do comparative interventions reflect your current practice? • What alternative interventions are available?
Right outcomes	• Are all relevant outcomes considered? • Are the results appropriate for the patient? • Does the intervention match patients' values and preferences?
Dartmouth Biomedical Libraries: Evidence-Based Medicine Critical Appraisal Worksheet for Applying the Evidence. h ttp://www.dartmouth.edu/~biomed/services.htmld/EBP_docs/ApplyingWorksheet.pdf	

Table 6.
Checklists to apply the evidence in clinical practice.

EBM practice steps	Self-evaluation checklists
Step 1	1. Am I asking well-formulated questions? 2. Do I have a way of identifying my knowledge gaps? 3. Do I have a working method of saving my questions for later answering?
Step 2	1. Am I searching for evidence at all? 2. Do I know the best source of current evidence for your clinical area? 3. Do I have easy access to the resources of the current evidence? 4. Are my searches more efficient? 5. Am I using truncation, Booleans, MeSH headings, delimiters, thesaurus, and intelligent free text when searching? 6. How well do my searches compare to those of librarians and research colleagues?
Step 3	1. Am I critically appraising external evidence at all? 2. Are the critical appraisal checklists/worksheets becoming easier for me to apply? 3. Am I becoming more proficient in applying critical appraisal measures? 4. Am I creating any appraisal summaries?
Step 4	1. Am I integrating my critical appraisals into my practice at all? 2. Can I adjust the critical appraisal measures to fit my individual patients? 3. Am I proactively monitoring for newly emerging evidence in my clinical discipline
Adapted from [11].	

Table 7.
Self-evaluation checklists to assess your performance.

potential interventions [12]. Finally, to evaluate performance (Step 5), clinicians must be able to self-evaluate and reflect on their own performance in the EBM stages and on the application and integration of evidence into clinical practice [10].

7. Conclusion

EBM integrates the best available evidence with clinical expertise and patient values to inform clinical decisions. Thus, EBM has three essential elements: best available evidence, clinical expertise, and patient values. The integration of these three components defines evidence-based clinical decisions. This integration can be effectively achieved by completing the five steps of EBM practice. The five-step of the EBM process requires a variety of knowledge and skills. To perform the first step (Step 1), the practitioners need the skills to question current clinical practices and frame answerable clinical questions. To acquire the evidence (Step 2), you need to have knowledge of medical databases and literature search skills. To critically appraise the evidence (Step 3), you must be able to understand scientific methods and statistics (biostatistics and epidemiology). When using evidence (Step 4), clinicians need the ability to use both clinical skills and previous experience to identify patients' health status and diagnosis, their patient values and assessments, and the specific risks and benefits of potential interventions. Finally, to evaluate the performance (Step 5), clinicians should be able to self-assess and reflect on their performance in the EBM phases and the application of evidence and its integration into clinical practice.

Conflict of interests

The authors report no conflicts of interest.

Author details

Delelegn Emwodew Yehualashet*, Binyam Tariku Seboka, Tizalegn Tesfaye Mamo and Mulugeta Namaro Yawo
School of Public Health, Dilla University, Dilla, Ethiopia

*Address all correspondence to: delelegn1244@gmail.com

References

[1] Straus SE, Glasziou P, Richardson WS, Haynes RB. Evidence-based medicine: How to practice and teach EBM. 2019. Available from: http://search.ebscohost.com/login.aspx?direct=true&scope=site&db=nlebk&db=nlabk&AN=1836719

[2] Albarqouni L, Hoffmann T, Straus S, Olsen NR, Young T, Ilic D, et al. Core competencies in evidence-based practice for health professionals consensus statement based on a systematic review and Delphi survey. Jama Network Open Internet. 2018;**1**(2):e180281

[3] Lafuente-Lafuente C, Leitao C, Kilani I, et al. Knowledge and use of evidencebased medicine in daily practice by health professionals: A crosssectional survey. BMJ Open. 2019;**9**:e025224

[4] Lehane E, Leahy-Warren P, O'Riordan C, Savage E, Drennan J, O'Tuathaigh C, et al. Evidence-based practice education for healthcare professions: An expert view. BMJ evidence-based medicine. 2019;**24**(3):103-108

[5] van Woezik TET et al. Practice-based learning: An appropriate means to acquire the attitude and skills for evidence-based medicine. International Journal of Medical Education. 2020;**11**:140-145

[6] Djulbegovic B, Guyatt GH. Progress in evidence-based medicine: A quarter century on. Lancet. 2017;**390**(10092):415-423

[7] Reddy K. Evidence based medicine: A paradigm for clinical practice. Journal of Gandaki Medical College-Nepal. 2018;**11**(02):74-81. DOI: 10.3126/jgmcn.v11i02.22989

[8] Acharya Y, Raghavendra Rao MV, Arja S. Evidence-based medicine in pre-clinical years: A study of early introduction and usefulness. Journal of Advances in Medical Education & Professionalism. 2017;**5**(3):95-100

[9] McTavish J. Negotiating concepts of evidence-based practice in the provision of good service for nursing and allied health professionals. Health Information and Libraries Journal. 2017;**34**(1):45-57

[10] Straus SE, Glasziou P, Richardson WS, Haynes RB. Evidence-based medicine E-book: How to practice and teach EBM. Edinburgh London New York Oxford Philadelphia St. Louis Sydney Elsevier Health Sciences; 2018 Feb 27

[11] Straus S, Glasziou P, Richardson W, Haynes R. Evidence-based medicine: how to practice and teach it. 4th ed. Edinburgh: Churchill Livingstone Elsevier; 2011

[12] Snibser AK. Evidence-based practice in Bachelor healthcare education. Norway: University of Bergen; 2019

Chapter 6

Awareness and Prevalence of Hepatitis B and C in Rural Areas of Lahore, Pakistan

Aqsa Sohail

Abstract

To evaluate the knowledge, attitude, and practice of participating entities toward hepatitis B and C to know about prevalence, literacy rate, and socioeconomic status of community people. A baseline survey was conducted to study the awareness, knowledge, and screening in a randomly selected population in different communities. Among common people of age above 16 years, a survey was conducted by filling out data collection forms for 560 individuals according to the plan of work designed. From the data collected, results were keenly analyzed, organized, and arranged in the form of tables for the comparison between the observed awareness about the disease and its screening. The prevalence of hepatitis B was found to be 18 (3.2%), hepatitis C 104 (18.6%), and both positive 17 (3%). It showed the high prevalence of hepatitis C. Out of 560 participants, 275 people (49.1%) knew the term hepatitis. Two hundred twenty-two (39.6%) participants did not know about the signs and symptoms of hepatitis. The descriptive statistics showed that 451 (80.5%) did not know the availability of vaccination against hepatitis B. Three hundred and thirty-six (60%) respondents strongly agreed that hepatitis can cause death. Out of 560 participants, 322 people (57.5%) strongly agreed that blood transfusion from hepatitis patients is the cause of hepatitis. Three hundred and seventy-three (66.6%) participants said that they use filtered plant water. In addition, 480 participants (85.7%) never vaccinated themselves. Chi-square test result ($p = 0.004$) showed a significant relation in the practice of male and female participants of study. A significant value of chi-square in practice domain of KAP was seen in educational qualification ($p = 0.021$) with undergraduates having better practice among all other levels of qualification. Current study concluded that people are unaware of the causes, prevention, and treatment of hepatitis B and C. People who are with positive signs and symptoms of hepatitis are reluctant to its long-term treatment. Government must arrange awareness campaigns and screening camps in communities to educate people about the importance of prevention and treatment of the disease.

Keywords: prevalence, hepatitis B and C, rural areas, awareness, KAP (knowledge, attitude, and practice)

1. Introduction

Hepatitis is a word combined of two words, “hepatic” meaning liver, and “titis” meaning inflammation. Hepatitis refers to an inflammation of the liver. It is a viral infection that affects the normal functioning of liver. Hepatitis can be caused by secondary agents like drugs, toxins, medications, and alcohol. In our body, liver performs different functions, such as bile production, filtering of toxins, metabolism of drugs, storage of glycogen, breakdown of carbohydrates, fats and proteins, activation of enzymes, and excretion of bilirubin [1]. Globally, about 1 billion people are infected by hepatitis B and among them, 400 million people are suffering from chronic HBV infection [2]. Every year, in Pakistan, 2.4% of people are affected by hepatitis B. This viral infection causes cirrhosis and hepatocellular carcinoma. Mostly pregnant women are at high risk of getting this infection confirmed by one research work done at district Bannu and 60% of babies got infection from their mothers [3]. In Europe, more than 10 million Europeans suffer from chronic viral hepatitis. The prevalence of HBV is estimated to be around 0.9% and of HCV about 1.1% [4]. In Asia, the Southeast Asia Region of WHO has an estimated 39 million people living with chronic hepatitis B and 10 million people living with chronic hepatitis C [5]. In Pakistan, hepatitis B antigen, hepatitis C infection, and antibodies weighted average were found different in both nonblood giver and blood donors [6]. In Pakistan, from epidemiological data, it was estimated that the spread of HCV will increase about 3.9% to 5.1% from 2016–30 [7]. So far, four (A, B, C, and D) out of eight reported genotypes were identified. Genotypes A, B, and C were predominant. HBV genotype C was the most predominant in this collection [8].

Why current study is a need: As Pakistan is the second largest country in the world after China, that is, with high prevalence of hepatitis B and C. People of Pakistan have a lack of knowledge and awareness regarding hepatitis. The current study is needed to evaluate the knowledge, transmission mode, vaccination available, and treatment availability of hepatitis B and C [9].

Aims and objectives: The aim of this study is to: Screen the community population for hepatitis B and C. To evaluate the knowledge and awareness of community population regarding hepatitis transmission mode, treatment, vaccination availability, and preventive measures. Educate the community population regarding hepatitis [10].

2. Literature review

A cross-sectional study was conducted in Karachi, Pakistan, to assess the knowledge and awareness of HBV infection, its prevalence, transmission, and perception of HBV vaccine and vaccination status among young females. Descriptive statistics were used and out of 550 survey questionnaires, only 434 were returned. Response rate was 78.9%. More than 90% had knowledge of HBV infection. Only 17% had received HBV vaccination during childhood. Only 24% had been tested for HBV in adulthood. Majority of respondents had some awareness of HBV and related consequences [11].

A comparative cross-sectional facility-based survey between HCV-positive and negative respondents at Taluka Hospital (OPD) Rural district of Sindh was conducted to assess the knowledge regarding risk factors of HCV transmission and options to prevent the risk factors associated with HCV transmission. Out of 520 respondents, only 66% having HCV infection were interviewed. Highest infection was present among 21–30 years of ages (39%). About 75.6% of urban population and 52.9% illiterate group were infected. Majority of HCV infected population had the misconception of water, food, heat, and mosquitoes as factors of HCV transmission [12].

A cross-sectional study was done in Nigeria, antenatal clinics in six different geopolitical zones recruited 159 pregnant women who agreed to undergo antihepatitis C virus testing, which was then validated using the polymerase chain reaction method. Out of 159, 99 pregnant women in Nigeria are not well informed about hepatitis C virus infection, and those 77, who are informed, are more likely to be young and highly educated. High hepatitis C virus infection rates serve as early support for the need for routine prenatal screening [13].

Eliminating the hepatitis C virus (HCV) requires an understanding of its obstacles and overcoming them. The current study set out to look into the prevalence of HCV disease awareness, linkage to care, and treatment uptake in a Taiwanese hyperendemic area. Residents in Tzukuan, between the years 2000 and 2018, were invited to take part in the questionnaire-based HCV interviews. Anti-HCV-seropositive participants' rates of disease knowledge, accessibility, and anti-HCV therapy were assessed. Even in the early days of direct-acting antiviral agents, found out significant gaps in disease awareness, link-to-care, and treatment uptake in the HCV care cascade in an HCV-hyperendemic area. It is critical to overcome these obstacles to achieve HCV eradication [14].

By using survey results, hepatitis B free campaign was conducted to eliminate HBV in San Francisco by increasing awareness, testing, and vaccination. The campaign conducted 306 street intercepts and telephone interviews of San Francisco patients for assessment. One-third of respondents ranked HBV as a key health issue in Asian community, second to diabetes. General HBV awareness is high. The campaign used survey results to focus efforts on more intensive provide outreach and to create messages for public media campaign [15].

A general population-based study was carried out in Nawabshah Sindh, Pakistan, to evaluate the epidemiological rate and risk factors of hepatitis B and hepatitis C. In count, 523 people were tested for hepatitis B and C, with 232 being female and 291 being male. Hepatitis C and B were found in 14.3% and 6.7% of the population, including both. Public health issues are being raised by the higher numbers of hepatitis B surface antigens and hepatitis C virus in Nawabshah. Precautionary action must be taken immediately [16].

This study aims to examine cost-effectiveness of community-born screening and early treatment with antiviral therapy for HBV in The Gambia. In Gambia, the prevalence of HBsAg is 8.8% in people older than 30 years. Adult community-born screening and treatment for HBV in The Gambia is likely to be a cost-effective intervention [17].

In the United States, a community-born study was conducted to assess attitudes about HCV screening and knowledge about HCV disease at several sites that serve high-risk populations. 140 participants were surveyed. Baseline hepatitis C knowledge was poor. However, brief educational intervention improved knowledge and raised acceptability of testing [18].

The study regarding HIV and hepatitis C viral screening practices in a geographic disease sample of American community Health Centers. It involves the complete survey of their attitudes and beliefs about HIV and HCV testing. Statistics were generated to describe the prevalence of HIV and HCV and associated demographics by CHCs. HCV prevalence ranged from 0.1–3.7%. Additional education and counseling may facilitate increased screening rates [19].

A prospective community-wide screening was conducted to assess rates of chronic HBV and HCV infections among Somali, Liberian, and Kenyan immigrants in Minnesota. Out of 853 participants, 13.5% had chronic HBV infection while 7% of them had HCV infection. Chronic HBV and HCV are major health problems among African immigrants. Community-based screening is effective to identify and provide health education for those who are at risk of viral hepatitis [20].

A street outreach study was conducted to assess the prevalence of HCV infection among many homeless PWUDs in Tel Aviv, detect risk factors for HCV infection, evaluate knowledge of the disease status, and measure the probability of connection to care. Data showed that HCV infection is very common in PWUDs who are homeless. Importantly, it was discovered there was startlingly limited access to care in this cohort despite relatively high awareness of HCV status. To stop the spread of HCV, these findings inspire new therapeutic strategies aimed at enhancing accessibility and conformity among homeless PWUDs [21].

A study conducted an evidence review to determine the burden of hepatitis C information in the immigrant population and to assess effectiveness of screening and treatment programs for chronic hepatitis C infection in Canada for the Canadian collaboration for immigrant and refugee's health. Immigrants had a high prevalence of chronic hepatitis C infection as compared to the Canadian-born population. They are also at increased risk of mortality from complications of Cirrhosis and hepatocellular carcinoma. Treatment of chronic HCV in those with Cirrhosis eliminated the risk of liver failure [22].

A cross-sectional survey-based study was conducted among healthcare workers of the Federal Medical Center Bida, Nigeria to assess knowledge, awareness, and prevalence of viral hepatitis. About 248 individuals participated in this study. Overall awareness of the various types of hepatitis was 70.6% with a marked trend over educational level. There is a need to provide education to raise awareness and knowledge among this group [23].

A cross sectional study was conducted to assess awareness and knowledge of hepatitis B infection in selected areas of Puchong, Malaysia. Out of 400 subjects, 48.5% were not aware, and 66.5% had never taken vaccine for hepatitis B. Overall, the level of awareness and knowledge was low. This low level should be improved through health education and frequent vaccination program for hepatitis B among public, especially in Puchong, Malaysia [24].

A cross-sectional study was done in Nigeria, antenatal clinics in six different geopolitical zones recruited 159 pregnant women who agreed to undergo antihepatitis C virus testing, which was then validated using the polymerase chain reaction method. Out of 159, 99 pregnant women in Nigeria are not well informed about hepatitis C virus infection, and those 77, who are informed, are more likely to be young and highly educated. High hepatitis C virus infection rates serve as early support for the need for routine prenatal screening.

3. Materials and methods

A cross sectional study was conducted including 560 people from rural areas. A nonprobability technique of sampling was used (using convenient sampling). The duration of study was from May 2018 to September 2018.

Inclusion criteria: Male and female having an age above 16 years. Who attends hepatitis screening and awareness camps?

Exclusion criteria: people below 16 years of age.

Methodology: First of all, we engaged different doctors who were gastroenterologist in their profession. They facilitated our project. Then, with the assistance of Hilton Pharmaceuticals, we arranged hepatitis screening and awareness camps in different communities of rural areas of Lahore like Taj bhag, Nawab pura, Hameed Pura, SA Rehman darogah wala, and Sadar (Naseer Hospital). In these camps, we screened approximately 600 people from which 560 people respond to our questionnaire. In every camp, we arranged three counters, at first counter, screening of hepatitis B and C was done, at second counter, questionnaire evaluating disease and knowledge was filled and at the third counter results of Screening were intimated to community population. After that, people with negative screening results were referred to our group members for awareness regarding prevention of hepatitis, and people with positive screening results were referred to doctor Jameel who is the owner of Al Maki Al Madni Trust. In this Trust, they were provided with hepatitis treatment at discount or free of charge to the needy patients.

4. Results

A total of 600 questionnaires were distributed and 560 were returned, giving a response rate of 93.3%. The very high response rate might be due to face-to-face interaction with the study participants. Non-respondents were not followed up. The demographic profile of study participants, including frequencies of gender, marital status, screening results, etc. are shown in following **Table 1**.

Descriptive statistics for each item in the questionnaire are given in **Tables 1–6**. **Table 1** is related to the demographic profile of the study participants. In our study, females participated more as compared to the males, such as 395 (70.5%) participated and from which 498 (88.9%) were married and 314 (56.1%) were housewives. Socio-economic status of 189 (33.8%) was from 10,000 to 20,000. The prevalence of hepatitis B was found to be 18(3.2%), hepatitis C 104 (18.6%), and both positive 17 (3%). It showed the high prevalence of hepatitis C.

The responses of the participants toward the hepatitis knowledge were assessed by the questions focusing on the types of hepatitis, sign and symptoms, vaccination available, and oral treatment of hepatitis, **Table 2**. Out of 560 participants, 275 people (49.1%) knew the term of hepatitis. Two hundred twenty-two (39.6%) participants did not know about the sign and symptoms of hepatitis. The descriptive statistics showed that 451 (80.5%) did not know the availability of vaccination for hepatitis B. Attitude toward hepatitis was assessed by asking ten questions as shown in **Table 3**. Three hundred and thirty-six (60%) respondents strongly agreed that hepatitis can cause death. Out of 560 participants, 322 people (57.5%) strongly agreed that blood transfusion from hepatitis patients is the cause of hepatitis. In addition, 313 (55.9%) remained neutral on asking question no 6 that is; vaccination of hepatitis is only for children.

The practice toward hepatitis was assessed and described in **Table 4**. Descriptive statistics showed that 327 (58.4%) participants respond never to question to exercise. On asking if they avoid meeting hepatitis patients 420 (75%) respond on never. Three hundred and seventy-three (66.6%) participants said that they use filter plant water. In addition, 480 participants (85.7%) never vaccinated themselves.

Out of 560 participants, majority of the people (146) obtained information regarding hepatitis from the Health Care Professionals (HCP). In addition, 206 (36.8%) found the role of government satisfactory (**Tables 7–9**).

Variables	N (%)
1. Gender	
Male	165 (29.5%)
Female	395 (70.5%)
2. Marital status	
Single	62 (11.1%)
Married	498 (88.9%)
3. Occupation	
Unemployed	73 (13%)
Government employee	24 (4.3%)
Private job	149 (26.6%)
House wife	314 (56.1%)
4. Education qualification	
Primary (upto 12 years)	379 (67.7%)
Secondary (upto 17 years)	63 (11.3%)
Undergraduate	17 (3%)
Post graduate	16 (2.9%)
Illiterate	85 (15.2%)
5. Socioeconomic status	
No income	111 (19.8%)
<5000	33 (5.9%)
5000–10,000	113 (23.8%)
10,000–20,000	189 (33.8%)
>20,000	94 (16.8%)
6. Screening Test Result	
B +ve	18 (3.2%)
C +ve	104 (18.6%)
Both –ve	421 (75.2%)
Both +ve	17 (3%)

Table 1.
Demographic profile of study participants.

Domain	Ques no.	Yes	No	Don't know
Knowledge	1	275 (49.1%)	148 (26.4%)	137 (24.5%)
	2a	66 (11.8%)	140 (25%)	354 (63.2%)
	2b	82 (14.6%)	118 (21.1%)	360 (64.3%)
	2c	6 (1.1%)	174 (31.1%)	380 (67.9%)
	3a	98 (17.5%)	106 (18.9%)	356 (63.6%)
	3b	155 (27.7%)	74 (13.2%)	331 (59.1%)

Domain	Ques no.	Yes	No	Don't know
	3c	149 (26.6%)	76 (13.6%)	335 (59.8%)
	4	65 (11.6%)	107 (19.1%)	388 (69.3%)
	5	139 (24.8%)	199 (35.5%)	222 (39.6%)
	6a	96 (17.1%)	47 (8.4%)	417 (74.5%)
	6b	69 (12.3%)	52 (9.3%)	439 (78.4%)
	6c	49 (8.8%)	58 (10.4%)	453 (80.9%)
	6d	107 (19.1%)	45 (8%)	408 (72.9%)
	6e	64 (11.4%)	55 (9.8%)	441 (78.8%)
	6f	44 (7.9%)	56 (10%)	460 (82.1%)
	7	249 (44.5%)	82 (14.6%)	229 (40.9%)
	8	39 (7%)	238 (42.5%)	483 (50.5%)
	9a	11 (2%)	74 (13.2%)	475 (84.8%)
	9b	81 (10.9%)	48 (8.6%)	451 (80.5%)
	9c	9 (1.6%)	71 (12.7%)	480 (85.7%)
	10a	4 (0.7%)	62 (11.1%)	494 (88.2%)
	10b	48 (8.6%)	46 (8.2%)	466 (83.2%)
	10c	18 (3.2%)	60 (10.7%)	482 (86.1%)
Do you think you can get hepatitis?		193 (34.5%)	367 (65.5%)	0 (0%)

Table 2.
Responses to hepatitis knowledge items.

Domain	Ques No.	Definitely agree	Moderately agree	Neutral	Moderately disagree	Definitely disagree
Attitude	1	247 (44.1%)	12 (2.1%)	247 (44.1%)	12 (2.1%)	42 (7.5%)
	2	90 (16.1%)	9 (1.6%)	307 (54.8%)	26 (4.6%)	128 (22.9%)
	3	336 (60%)	8 (1.4%)	190 (33.9%)	6 (1.1%)	20 (3.6%)
	4	316 (56.4%)	15 (2.7%)	203 (36.3%)	6 (1.1%)	20 (3.6%)
	5	322 (57.5%)	10 (1.8%)	201 (35.9%)	4 (0.7%)	23 (4.1%)
	6	79 (14.1%)	9 (1.6%)	313 (55.9%)	22 (3.9%)	137 (24.5%)
	7	171 (30.5%)	10 (1.8%)	308 (55%)	15 (2.7%)	56 (10%)
	8	245 (43.8%)	21 (3.8%)	255 (45.5%)	8 (1.4%)	31 (5.5%)
	9	277 (49.5%)	14 (2.5%)	218 (38.9%)	15 (2.7%)	36 (6.4%)
	10	341 (60.9%)	12 (2.1%)	185 (33%)	2 (0.4%)	20 (3.6%)

Table 3.
Attitude toward hepatitis.

Ranking/scoring:
0 (0%)–12 (52%) Poor
13 (56%)–18 (78%) Moderate
19 (82%)–23 (100%) Good

Domain	Ques no.	Always	Frequently	Sometimes	Rarely	Never
Practice	1	108 (19.3%)	24 (4.3%)	73 (13%)	28 (5%)	327 (58.4%)
	2	160 (28.6%)	4 (0.7%)	28 (5%)	12 (2.1%)	356 (63.6%)
	3	77 (13.8%)	17 (3%)	39 (7%)	7 (1.3%)	420 (75%)
	4	486 (86.8%)	11 (2%)	22 (3.9%)	4 (0.7%)	37 (6.6%)
	5	119 (21.3%)	18 (3.2%)	46 (8.2%)	11 (2%)	366 (65.4%)
	6	107 (19.1%)	10 (1.8%)	35 (6.3%)	12 (2.1%)	396 (70.7%)
	7	373 (66.6%)	7 (1.3%)	40 (7.1%)	8 (1.4%)	132 (23.6%)
	8	279 (49.8%)	11 (2%)	30 (5.4%)	8 (1.4%)	232 (41.4%)
	9	55 (9.8%)	7 (1.3%)	15 (2.7%)	3 (0.5%)	480 (85.7%)
	10	40 (7.1%)	16 (2.9%)	26 (4.6%)	12 (2.1%)	466 (83.2%)

Table 4.
Practice related to hepatitis.

Q No.	TV	Internet	Magazine	HCP	Relative	Friend	Poster	Brochure	No where
1	128 (22.9%)	8 (1.4%)	6 (1.1%)	146 (26.1%)	135 (24.1%)	18 (3.2%)	13 (2.3%)	2 (0.4%)	104 (18.6%)

Table 5.
Information obtained regarding hepatitis.

Ques No	Excellent	Good	Satisfactory	Unsatisfactory
1	104 (18.6%)	108 (19.3%)	206 (36.8%)	142 (25.4%)

Table 6.
Role of government in prevention and treatment of hepatitis.

Variable (N = 560)	Poor	Moderate	Good	#p-value
Gender				
Male	153 (27.3%)	12 (2.1%)	0	0.416
Female	375(67%)	19 (3.4%)	1 (0.2%)	
Marital status				
Single	57 (10.2%)	4 (0.7%)	1 (0.2%)	0.017
Married	471 (84.1%)	27 (4.8%)	0	
Occupation				
Unemployed	67 (12%)	6 (1.1%)	0	0.223
Govt. servant	24 (4.3%)	0	0	
Private job	136 (24.3%)	12 (2.1%)	1 (0.2%)	
Housewife	301 (53.8%)	13 (2.3%)	0	

Variable (N = 560)	Poor	Moderate	Good	#p-value
Educational qualification				
Primary	364 (65%)	15 (2.7%)	0	0.014
Secondary	53 (9.5%)	9 (1.6%)	1 (0.2%)	
Undergraduate	16 (2.9%)	1 (0.2%)	0	
Postgraduate	15 (2.7%)	1 (0.2%)	0	
Illiterate	80 (14.3%)	5 (0.9%)	0	
Socioecnomic status				
No income	107 (19.1%)	4 (0.7%)	0	0.465
<5000	33 (5.9%)	0	0	
5000–10,000	126 (22.5%)	7 (1.3%)	0	
10,000–20,000	177 (31.6%)	11 (2%)	1 (0.2%)	
>20,000	85 (15.2%)	9 (1.6%)	0	
Screening test result				
B+ve	18 (3.2%)	0	0	0.521
C+ve	94 (16.8%)	10 (1.8%)	0	
Both –ve	400 (71.4%)	20 (3.6%)	1 (0.2%)	
Both +ve	16 (2.9%)	1 (0.2%)	0	

Table 7.
Categorization of study population in different knowledge ranks by using chi-square test.

Variable (N = 560)	Poor	Moderate	Good	#p-value
Gender				
Male	102 (18.2%)	46 (8.2%)	17 (3%)	0.558
Female	228 (40.7%)	115 (20.5%)	52 (9.3%)	
Marital status				
Single	39 (7%)	14 (2.5%)	9 (1.6%)	0.501
Married	291 (52%)	147 (26.3%)	60 (10.7%)	
Occupation				
Unemployed	49 (8.8%)	16 (2.9%)	8 (1.4%)	0.281
Govt. servant	10 (1.8%)	8 (1.4%)	6 (1.1%)	
Private job	91 (16.3%)	41 (7.3%)	17 (3%)	
House wife	180 (32.1%)	96 (17.1%)	38 (6.8%)	
Educational qualification				
Primary	215 (38.4%)	116 (20.7%)	48 (8.6%)	0.00
Secondary	30 (5.4%)	17 (3%)	16 (2.9%)	
Undergraduate	12 (2.1%)	4 (0.7%)	1 (0.2%)	
Post graduate	7 (1.3%)	8 (1.4%)	1 (0.2%)	
Illiterate	66 (11.8%)	16 (2.9%)	3 (0.5%)	

Variable (N = 560)	Poor	Moderate	Good	#p-value
Socioecnomic status				
No income	58 (10.4%)	38 (6.8%)	15 (2.7%)	0.377
<5000	19 (3.4%)	11 (2%)	3 (0.5%)	
5000–10,000	87 (15.5%)	33 (5.9%)	13 (2.3%)	
10,000–20,000	116 (20.7%)	52 (9.3%)	21 (3.8%)	
>20,000	50 (8.9%)	27 (4.8%)	17 (3%)	
Screening test result				
B+ve	10 (1.8%)	5 (0.9%)	3 (0.5%)	0.004
C+ve	75 (13.4%)	20 (3.5%)	9 (1.6%)	
Both –ve	240 (42.9%)	125 (22.3%)	56 (10%)	
Both +ve	5 (0.9%)	11 (2%)	1 (0.2%)	

Table 8.
Categorization of study population in different attitude ranks by using chi-square test.

Variable (N = 560)	Poor	Moderate	Good	#p-value
Gender				
Male	131 (23.4%)	28 (5%)	6 (1.1%)	0.004
Female	354 (63.2%)	36 (11.4%)	5 (0.9%)	
Marital status				
Single	53 (9.5%)	9 (1.6)	0	0.375
Married	432 (77.1%)	55 (9.8%)	11 (2%)	
Occupation				
Unemployed	64 (11.4%)	8 (1.4%)	1 (0.2%)	0.001
Govt. servant	20 (3.6%)	4 (0.7%)	0	
Private job	114 (20.4%)	28 (5%)	7 (1.3%)	
House wife	287 (51.3%)	24 (4.3%)	3 (0.5%)	
Educational qualification				
Primary	331 (59.1%)	43 (7.7%)	5 (0.9%)	0.021
Secondary	53 (9.5%)	8 (1.4%)	2 (0.4%)	
Undergraduate	10 (1.8%)	5 (0.9%)	2 (0.4%)	
Post graduate	14 (2.5%)	2 (0.4%)	0	
Illiterate	77 (13.8%)	6 (1.1%)	2 (0.4%)	
Socioecnomic status				
No income	89 (15.9%)	18 (3.2%)	4 (0.7%)	0.096
<5000	31 (5.5%)	2 (0.4%)	0	
5000–10,000	121 (21.6%)	11 (2%)	1 (0.2%)	
10,000–20,000	169 (30.2%)	17 (3%)	3 (0.5%)	
>20,000	75 (13.4%)	16 (2.9%)	3 (0.4%)	

Variable (N = 560)	Poor	Moderate	Good	#p-value
Screening test result				
B+ve	17 (3%)	0	1 (0.2%)	0.126
C+ve	85 (15.2%)	15 (2.7%)	4 (0.7%)	
Both –ve	370 (66.1%)	45 (8%)	6 (1.1%)	
Both +ve	13 (2.3%)	4 (0.7%)	0	

Table 9.
Categorization of study population in different practice ranks by using chi-square test.

The results of chi-square test showed a significant difference between the knowledge of single and married participants of the study (p = 0.017). According to marital status mean score, the single people had more knowledge than the married participants of the study. Another significant finding of the study was that although there was no significant difference between KAP of undergraduates and postgraduates; however, there was a statistically significant difference between knowledge of participants (p = 0.014) belonging to different educational categories (primary, secondary, and illiterate) as compared to undergraduates. Test result shows that participants belonging to undergraduate level showed high mean score on knowledge section than participants belonging to postgraduate level. Chi-square test results revealed that there is no significant difference in knowledge of male and female (p = 0.416) but the mean score value of male participants was greater than compared to females. The other demographic factors of knowledge section, such as occupation, socioeconomic status, and screening test results also showed nonsignificant p-values of 0.223, 0465, and 0.521, respectively.

p-value calculated by using chi-square test.

0 (0%)–5 (50%) Poor

6 (60%)–7 (70%) Moderate

8 (80%)–10 (100%) Good

In the attitude section of current KAP study, two demographic factors, educational qualification, and screening test results have significant p-values. Chi-square test result of educational qualification (p-value = 0.00) showed that there was almost no significant difference between KAP of undergraduates and postgraduates; however, there was statistically significant difference between attitudes of participants belonging to different educational categories (primary, secondary, and illiterate) as compared to undergraduates and postgraduates. Chi-square results of screening test results indicate a significant difference (p = 0.004) in the attitude of people having B+, C+, and both +ve -ve. The most positive attitude was seen among the participants having positive hepatitis B and hepatitis C. The poorest attitude was seen among the participants having both hepatitis B and C negative. And the other demographic factors of attitude section, such as gender, marital status, occupation, and socioeconomic status, showed non-significant chi-square test results with p-value of 0.558, 0.501, 0.281, and 0.377, respectively.

p-value calculated by using chi-square test.

0 (0%)–5 (50%) Poor

6 (60%)–7 (70%) Moderate
8 (80%)–10 (100%) Good

The practice section also revealed significant values of three demographic factors. According to the gender section chi-square test result ($p = 0.004$), there was a significant relation in the practice of male and female participants of the study. Mean score of male shows better practice of male participants toward hepatitis B and C. Another significant value was seen among the participants associated with different levels of occupation. A significant difference ($p = 0.001$) was observed in the practice of these groups (unemployed, government servants, private jobs, and housewives). And the third significant value in practice domain of KAP was seen in educational qualification ($p = 0.021$) with undergraduates having better practice among all other levels of qualification. Other demographic factors of practice domain, such as marital status, socioeconomic status, and screening test results, showed non-significant chi-square test results with p-values 0.375, 0.096, and 0.126, respectively.

p-value calculated by using chi-square test.

5. Discussion

This study was done to evaluate the KAP toward hepatitis B and C among different community populations. Firstly, in this study, there is no age grouping for study participants, only people with age less than 16 years are not included in this study. Above 16 year of age participants are included in current study. Second prospect of this study was to evaluate knowledge, different attitudes, and practices of literate and illiterate community toward hepatitis B and C. In this study, we also look for the socioeconomic status of study participants. To evaluate how much of the community was non-affording. A scoring system was developed and scores of participants for each domain were analyzed and co-related with various demographic factors, also for each domain participants have been categorized according to their scores. Results of this study revealed that demographic factor gender showed no significant difference in knowledge and attitude of male and female candidates, but the practice of these two categories showed significant value of chi-square ($p = 0.004$). According to marital status, the single people had more knowledge than the married participants in this study. The results of chi-square test showed a significant difference between the knowledge of these two groups ($p = 0.017$), but there was no significant difference between the attitude and practice of the married and single participants in this study. Another significant finding of the study was that although there was no significant difference between KAP of undergraduates and postgraduates, there was statistically significant difference between knowledge of participants belonging to different educational categories (primary, secondary, and illiterate), as compared to undergraduates. Current study shows that participants belonging to undergraduate level showed high mean score on knowledge and practices section than participants belonging to postgraduate level. The study has attempted to shed light on KAP by engaging study participants from different levels of education (primary, secondary, undergraduates, postgraduates, and illiterate). As the p values of knowledge, attitude, and practice were 0.014, 0.00, and 0.021, respectively. These results clearly showed a significant difference between the knowledge, attitude, and practice of the participants belonging to different levels of education. One of the important findings of study was the evaluation of knowledge attitude and practice among the participants according to screening test results. Chi-square results indicate significant difference ($p = 0.004$) in the attitude of people having B+, C+, and both +ve and -ve. The most positive attitude was seen among the participants having positive hepatitis B and C. But there was no significant difference between knowledge and practice among these groups. The poorest knowledge, attitude, and practice were seen among the participants having both hepatitis B and C negative. Another significant value was seen among the participants associated with different levels of occupation. A significant difference was observed in the practice ($p = 0.021$) of these groups (unemployed, government servants, private jobs, and housewives). There was no significant difference in knowledge and attitude; however, the mean score value showed that government servants had better knowledge and attitude; whereas, according to the mean scores, the knowledge, attitude, and practice of housewives were poorest among all. According to health belief model, the perception of disease and probability of adoption of positive practices and attitude of an individual depends on four important variables, that is, perceived seriousness of a disease, susceptibility of a disease, perceived benefits of positive attitude and practice, and lastly, perceived barriers that might restrain an individual to make positive changes [25]. A common negative attitude that was observed among study participants was low perceived seriousness of hepatitis B and C, financial barriers, and lack of time and knowledge about disease treatment and vaccination. Due to these barriers and somehow due to superstitious thoughts of people about hepatitis, people did not agree to get treatment. According to a previous study of WHO in 2015, only 3–5% of infected individual receive treatment annually, worldwide. About 75% of infected individuals are not aware of their HCV positive status and remain undiagnosed. This cause a huge economic impact cost for government, society, and also for patient. As with the progression of ailment, cost also increases [26].

6. Conclusion

Current study concluded that people are unaware about the causes, prevention, and treatment of hepatitis B and C. People who are with positive signs and symptoms of hepatitis are reluctant to its long-term treatment. Government must arrange awareness campaigns and screening camps in communities to educate people about the importance of prevention and treatment of the disease.

Author details

Aqsa Sohail
Institute of Pharmacy, Lahore College for Women University, Lahore, Pakistan

*Address all correspondence to: hudafatma2626@gmail.com

References

[1] Available from: https://www.healthline.com/health/hepatitis#prevention

[2] Ali M, Idrees M, Ali L, Hussain A, Rehman IU, Saleem S, et al. Hepatitis B virus in Pakistan: A systematic review of prevalence, risk factors, awareness status and genotypes. Virology Journal. 2011;**8**: 102

[3] Awan ZUR. Sero prevalence of hepatitis B virus (hbv) infection in pregnant women of district Bannu KP, Pakistan. Fuuast Journal of Biology. 2021;**11**(2):145-149

[4] Available from: https://ecdc.europa.eu/en/publications-data/systematic-review-hepatitis-b-and-c-prevalence-eueea

[5] Available from: http://www.searo.who.int/entity/hepatitis/data/hepatitis_data_statistics/en/

[6] Mehmood S et al. National prevalence rate of Hepatitis B and C in Pakistan and it's risk factors. Journal of Public Health. 2019;**28**:751-764

[7] Lim AG et al. Curbing the hepatitis C virus epidemic in Pakistan: The impact of scaling up treatment and prevention for achieving elimination. International Journal of Epidemiology. 2018;**47**:550-560

[8] Available from: https://lms.rn.com/getpdf.php/2128.pdf

[9] Available from: http://www.who.int/features/qa/76/en/

[10] Available from: https://www.everydayhealth.com/hepatitis/diagnosing-hepatitis-tools-and-tests.aspx

[11] Shakeel S, Iffat W, Ishaq H. Assessing the level of Awareness and vaccination status of Hepatitis B among young female community of Pakistan. Bangladesh Journal of Medical Sciences. 2015;**14**(4):376

[12] Ali A, Khalid SN, Qureshi H. Assessment of Knowledge regarding risk factors of hepatitis C virus transmission and options to avoid them. International Journal of Collaborative Research on Internal Medicine and Public Health. 2015;7:9

[13] Eleje GU et al. Awareness and prevalence of hepatitis C virus infection among pregnant women in Nigeria: A National Pilot cross-sectional study. Women's Health. 2021;**17**: 17455065211031718. DOI: 10.1177/17455065211031718. PMID: 34256625; PMCID: PMC8283213

[14] Tsai P-C et al. Low disease awareness as a contributing factor to the high prevalence of hepatitis C infection in Tzukuan, a hyperendemic area of southern Taiwan. Kaohsiung Journal of Medical Sciences. 2022;**38**(7):694-702. DOI: 10.1002/kjm2.12552. Epub 2022 Apr 29. PMID: 35485737

[15] Shiau R, Bove F, Henne J, Zola J, et al. Using survey results regarding Hepatitis B Knowledge, Community Awareness and testing Behavior Among Asian to improve the San Francisco Hepatitis B free Campaign. Journal of Community Health. 2012;**37**: 350-364

[16] Samo AA et al. Prevalence and risk factors Associated with Hepatitis B and C in Nawabshah, Sindh, Pakistan. The American Journal of Tropical Medicine and Hygiene. 2020;**104**(3):1101-1105

[17] Nayagam S et al. Cost-effectiveness of community based screening and

treatment for chronic Hepatitis B in the Gambia: An economic modeling analysis. The Lancet Global Health. 2016;**4**: PE568-PE578

[18] Norton BL et al. Community-based HCV screening: Knowledge and attitudes in a high risk urban population. BMC Infectious Diseases. 2014;**14**:74

[19] Mayer KH et al. HIV and Hepatitis C viral screening practice in a geographically diverse sample of American Community Health Centers. AIDS Patient Care and STDs Clinical and Epidemiologic Research. 2016;**30**(6):237-246. DOI: 10.1089/apc.2015.0314. PMID: 27286294

[20] Mohamed EA, Giama NH, et al. Community wide outreach and screening to reduce Hepatitis B, Hepatitis C and liver cancer disparities among African immigrants in Minnesota. Cancer Epidemiology Biomarkers Prevention. 2017;**26**(2_Supplement):C76

[21] Lasmanovich R et al. Hepatitis C virus prevalence, medical status awareness and treatment engagement among homeless people who use drugs: Results of a street outreach study. Sage Journals. 26 May 2022;**16**: 11782218221095871. DOI: 10.1177/11782218221095871. PMID: 35651594; PMCID: PMC9149611

[22] Greenway C et al. Screening for Hepatitis C infection: Evidence review for newly immigrants and refugees. Canadian Medical Association or Its Licensors. 2011;**2011**. DOI :10.1503/cmaj.090313

[23] Amiwero CE, Nelson EA, et al. Knowledge, awareness and prevalence of viral Hepatitis among health care workers (HCWs) of the Federal Medical Center Bida, Nigeria. The Journal of Medical Research. 2017;**3**(3):114-120

[24] Pathmanathan H, Lakshmanan P. Assessment of awareness and knowledge of Hepatitis B among residents of Puchong, Malaysia. Tropical Journal of Pharmaceutical Research. 2014;**13**(10): 1719-1724

[25] Health Belief Model. Theory Essence Sentence, Personnel belief influence health

[26] Available from: https://epha.org/wp-content/uploads/2017/03/8.-Corina-POP_hepatita-C-.pdf

Chapter 7

Perspective Chapter: Integrating Follow-up Care Management for Assessment and Management of Rape Survivors Diagnosed with PTSD and Depression in Primary Health Care Settings

Nombulelo Veronica Sepeng, Lufuno Makhado and Leepile Alfred Sehularo

Abstract

Rape is very high in South Africa. It predisposes rape survivors to many health care problems, including the risk of contracting human immunodeficiency virus, sexually transmitted infections, falling pregnant, and long mental health effects. PTSD and depression are regarded as the most common mental health effects diagnosed among rape survivors, and they require long term mental health care management. In the current era, follow-up care management for rape survivors is mostly done at Thuthuzela Care Centres. However, rape survivors do not often go for follow-up care, because these centres are mostly far from them. Thus, this problem can be addressed by integrating the management of these long-term disorders within the primary health care settings in South Africa, because most people have access to their nearby clinics. This chapter aims to describe ways of integrating follow-up care management for continuous assessment and management of rape survivors diagnosed with PTSD and depression through task-shifting these duties to nurses working within the primary health care settings in South Africa. The chapter focuses on the mental health care status of rape survivors diagnosed with PTSD and depression. Training of nurses is essential to manage rape survivors diagnosed with PTSD and depression in primary health care.

Keywords: follow-up care, rape, PTSD, depression, primary health care settings, nursing

1. Introduction

Rape is an illegal act typically involving sexual intercourse performed forcibly or threatened by bodily harm against the survivors' will [1]. Rape is a public health concern affecting everyone worldwide, but South Africa is known as the country reporting a high prevalence of rape. South Africa reported about 10,006 cases from 2020 to 2021 [2]. Rape has many effects. It predisposes rape survivors to contract human immunodeficiency virus (HIV), sexually transmitted infections (STIs), pregnancy, physical injuries, and mental health disorders [3]. Despite this, post-traumatic stress disorders (PTSD) and depression are the commonest mental health disorders [4, 5]. PTSD is defined as a set of four clusters of symptoms that include intrusive and recurring memories of the trauma, avoidance of trauma-related stimuli, numbing and/or unfavorable changes in mood or cognitions related to the trauma, and changes in reactivity and arousal [6]. Depression is a negative affective state characterized by feelings ranging from unhappiness and discontent to extreme sadness, pessimism, and hopelessness that interfere with daily life. Various physical, cognitive, and social changes, such as altered eating or sleeping habits, lack of energy or motivation, difficulty concentrating or making decisions, and withdrawal from social activities, are also common [6].

The preferred non-pharmacological treatment given among rape survivors diagnosed with PTSD and depression includes cognitive behavioral therapy (CBT), cognitive processing therapy (CPT), family therapy, and exposure therapy (ET) [7, 8]. In South Africa, a model of post-sexual assault care has been integrated into the public health system, with dedicated sexual assault centers in major urban towns. The care model is based on intersectoral collaboration, with a collaboration between medical personnel, police, and social support services [9]. Standard of care at these facilities currently includes forensic medical examination, HIV testing with pretest and posttest counseling, pregnancy testing and emergency contraception, STD treatment, HIV post-exposure prophylaxis (PEP), and trauma debriefing [9]. However, the mental health care needs of rape survivors are not met in these services. Often they are not even referred to specialized services [10, 11]. In addition, many people who have PTSD are hesitant to seek treatment in specialized mental health care settings [12]. Therefore, there is a need to develop a strategy that can be used to cater to the mental health needs of rape survivors.

In South Africa, the decentralization and integration of the management of rape survivors diagnosed with PTSD and depression into primary health care settings must be considered to cater for their mental health care needs. One reason is that there are far too few mental health care practitioners, particularly in the public health sector (which serves 80% of the population) and particularly in rural areas [13]. Primary care is a logical setting to target early and management efforts of PTSD and depression because: (1) it facilitates the early identification of patients who require treatment; (2) most mental health services are delivered through primary care [8], so primary care provides greater access, and thus broader population coverage, than treatment delivered exclusively in specialized care populations; and (3) mental health care delivered in a primary care context may constitute a more acceptable treatment option [12].

Professional nurses are frontline workers, making up the largest number within the health care system [14] and mainly in primary health care. Professional nurses are doing mental health nursing in undergraduates. Some further their studies in advanced postgraduate mental health nursing qualifications. Those that completed their undergraduate 4-year diploma and a degree in nursing [15] and postgraduate nursing are registered with the South African Nursing Council to render care to patients [16]. Therefore, nurses need to integrate follow-up care of rape survivors for assessment and management of PTSD and depression in primary health care settings through task shifting. In this chapter, the authors described the mental health status of rape survivors diagnosed with PTSD and depression in South Africa. The skills and training of nurses in mental health nursing are described in this chapter. The importance of task-shifting mental health care for rape survivors diagnosed with PTSD and depression among nurses is described in this chapter.

2. Mental health care status of rape survivors diagnosed with PTSD and depression in South Africa

PTSD and depression are common among survivors seeking health care in Thuthuzela Care Centres post-rape experiences in South Africa [5, 9]. Several studies reported poor integration of mental health care services for rape survivors seeking treatment in Thuthuzela Care Centres in South Africa [5, 17, 18]. Many factors affect the integration of mental health services for rape survivors seeking help in Thuthuzela Care Centres. One of the factors is a significant mismatch in South Africa between the scope of the Childhood Sexual Abuse (CSA) problem and the expected psychological and the availability of services for children [9]. Despite this, the Republic of South Africa documented that all children survivors of CSA are required to get therapeutic care under the Children's Amendment Act [19]. Nevertheless, data suggest that very few children have access to or are referred to specialized services to mitigate the possible detrimental impacts of abuse [11, 20]. Furthermore, one study reported that adult rape survivors who reported rape in Thuthuzela Care Centres were not given follow-up care to screen and manage PTSD post-rape experiences [10].

Apart from that, mental health care management for rape survivors diagnosed with PTSD and depression requires about 12 sessions with the therapist when using treatment modalities such as cognitive behavioral therapy (CBT), exposure therapy (ET), and cognitive processing therapy (CPT), etc. [7, 8]. This type of care is mostly given in specialized care services such as hospitals [12]. Hence, it is impossible to manage rape survivors diagnosed with these disorders in Thuthuzela Care Centres. Most rape survivors live in poverty, are unemployed, and depend on the government to provide them with social grants [21]. Additionally, most rape survivors stay in rural areas far from Thuthuzela Care Centres because they are stationed in urban areas [21]. Hence, the need for decentralization and integration of mental health care services in the primary health care setting is to promote access to the health care system. Furthermore, while decentralized and integrated primary mental health care is at the heart of many low- and middle-income countries' (LMICs) mental health policies, implementation remains a challenge, particularly for victims of violence [22, 23]. This is also the case for rape survivors diagnosed with PTSD and depression.

Previous studies indicated that the high frequency of trauma and sexual assault in South Africa might necessitate a more extensive approach to rape management, particularly mental health consequences, to be included in existing policy [24]. The extensive approach to mental health care management among rape survivors diagnosed with PTSD and depression is the decentralization and integration of follow-up care of these services into primary health care. Primary health cares are accessible to everyone, because most villages have a nearby clinic where one can go for a consultation. In post-apartheid in South Africa, a deinstitutionalized and integrated primary health care system was crucial for enhancing access, improving service quality within a human rights framework, and reorganizing mental health services [18]. These initiatives were also outlined in the Department of Health's White Paper system

Transdoemation [25] and the new Mental Health Act (MHCA), No. 17 of 2002 [26]. Despite this, the integration and decentralization of management of rape survivors diagnosed with PTSD and depression are not implemented in South Africa.

3. The importance of task-shifting mental health care management of rape survivors diagnosed with PTSD and depression to nurses

Task shifting (also known as task sharing) is defined as "the rational redistribution of tasks among health workforce teams [27]". Task shifting as an approach has some roots in HIV and AIDS care, particularly in developing countries where human resource shortages and the burden on public health systems have been severe, limiting access to antiretroviral therapy (ART) [28].

Recent research has found that task-shifting models provide higher-quality, more cost-effective care to more HIV-infected patients than physician-centered models, and that they have increased access to ART [29]. Access to ART is good in South Africa and is led by professional nurses trained in Nurse-Initiated Management of Ante-Retroviral Treatment (NIMART) [30]. Therefore, the same model can be followed for task shifting, disseminating, and integrating mental health services for rape survivors who are diagnosed with PTSD and depression in primary health care in South Africa.

One study reported that interventions incorporating mental health into primary care or community services without utilizing specialist services were the most cost-effective in reviewing mental illness costs and the cost-effectiveness of treatments [31]. Lund and Flisher [32] created a South African context- and need-specific model for calculating the costs of implementing an integrated community mental health service, emphasizing the cost-effectiveness of addressing mental health needs in communities through task-shifting approaches. However, specialist services will always be required regardless of how innovative and effective task-shifting approaches close the mental health treatment gap [33]. Thus, most medical examinations are offered by medical doctors within the South African context. In this regard, it is worth mentioning that nurses can provide medical services such as post-exposure prophylaxis (PEP) for HIV, prophylaxis for other sexually transmitted infections, emergency contraception, treatment of injuries, and even forensic examinations for rape survivors.

Hence, it is essential to shift, if not decentralize, the management of rape survivors diagnosed with PTSD and depression to professional nurses in the primary health care clinics. Also, when the task shifting is done in the primary health care setting, the management of rape survivors diagnosed with PTSD and depression can benefit society if carried out by professional nurses. This can be aided through preservice inclusion of management of rape survivors diagnosed with PTSD and depression among nurses in undergraduate training and in-service training among all professional nurses already in practice.

4. Skills and training of nurses in mental health care management of mental health care disorders within the primary health care setting

Currently, no studies reported training of nurses in mental health care management of rape survivors diagnosed with PTSD and depression. Instead, studies have documented both lack of skills and training of nurses in mental health care management of mental health disorders. One study reported a lack of training and supervision by hospital mental health teams, resulting in a lack of knowledge in managing patients with mental disorders [34]. It was further stated that this practice has a negative impact on the integration of mental health care into primary health care [35]. Furthermore, the World Health Organization (WHO) found that most health care workers in primary health care settings do not receive adequate mental health care training [34]. Again, nurses' lack of knowledge in managing patients with mental health disorders has resulted in the underdiagnosis of most mental health conditions in primary health care [36]. The study found that primary health care nurses managing patients at the clinic were not adequately qualified to provide all of the services that are provided in clinics that use a one-stop-shop approach [37]. In addition, it was revealed that some mental health patients are treated by registered nurses who do not have Psychiatric Nursing Science qualifications. This practice may result in mental health patients being misdiagnosed, leading to mental illness relapse [18]. Although the lack of skills and training of nurses in relation to mental health care management of patients diagnosed with mental health disorders is argued from a general overview of the literature review, it may impact the decentralization and integration of rape survivors diagnosed with PTSD and depression consulting in PHC settings.

Despite this, some studies have reported that nurses are trained to provide mental health care management among patients. The nurses that register for a 4-year degree or diploma are taught psychiatric nursing, and when they complete their courses, they are placed either in the hospital or primary health care to care for the patients consulting in these settings. Furthermore, the literature review illustrated that to ensure that mental health conditions are appropriately identified and managed, primary health care clinics must have psychiatric-trained nurses on staff [15]. Furthermore, most nurses have a 4-year Diploma in Nursing, indicating that psychiatric nursing training is well represented in primary health care clinics [15]. Despite this, nurses with a 4-year diploma or degree do not have adequate skills and knowledge to manage patients presenting with mental health disorders in primary health care settings [15, 38]. These findings indicate a need for capacitating these nurses to provide mental health care among patients consulting in primary health care, considering that they were trained to provide mental health nursing. In support of this, Bowlers [39] reported that for disseminating information and guidelines and practice-based education, continuing education is required for nurses. This will aid in improving diagnostic skills and psychological therapy for psychiatric patients [39].

In addition, nurses reported that they require in-service training for empowerment, quality care, and increasing staff motivation when providing mental health care management to patients [40]. In South Africa, some nurses are trained for an advanced diploma in psychiatric nursing. However, placing nurses with advanced psychiatric nursing is uncommon in primary health care settings because they are placed in mental health care institutions when they complete their studies. Therefore, we suggest that nurses who have completed advanced psychiatry in nursing must also be placed in primary health care mainly to render mental health care services among clients reporting mental health disorders, including rape survivors diagnosed with PTSD and depression.

In addition, mental health care management of rape survivors must be done by nurses studying for a postgraduate diploma in forensic nursing. Currently, South Africa's postgraduate diploma in forensic nursing is not accredited [41]. Again, most nursing universities are re-curriculating their postgraduate courses to ensure that forensic nursing is one of the postgraduate diplomas that the South African Nursing Council accredits. Therefore, it will be imperative to include mental health care management for rape survivors in their curriculum, such as placing them in primary health care settings to offer the management of rape survivors diagnosed with PTSD and depression and working in collaboration with those that are trained for mental health care at the undergraduate and postgraduate levels, thus, improving mental health care services for rape survivors in South Africa.

5. Conclusions

The mental health care status of rape survivors diagnosed with PTSD and depression in South Africa should be prioritized and afforded the necessary attention and follow-up care to help reintegrate them back into society. There is a considerable need to improve nursing skills in providing mental health and managing depression and PTSD within the primary health care setting. The training of nurses must target the undergraduate nurses who will be doing forensic nursing diploma by including mental health care management in their curricula. The in-service training must be provided for nurses with mental health care postgraduate diplomas to improve their skills in managing PTSD and depression, particularly in primary health care settings.

Conflict of interest

The authors declare no conflict of interest.

Author details

Nombulelo Veronica Sepeng[1], Lufuno Makhado[2*] and Leepile Alfred Sehularo[3]

1 University of Pretoria, Gauteng, South Africa

2 University of Venda, Limpopo, South Africa

3 North-West University, South Africa

*Address all correspondence to: nombulelo.sepeng@up.ac.za

References

[1] World population review, rape statistics by country 2022. Available from: https://worldpopulationreview.com/country-rankings/rape-statistics-by-country, 2022

[2] South African Police Service. Police recorded crime statistics Republic of South Africa, Pretoria. 2021. Available from: https://www.saps.gov.za/services/downloads/april_june_2021_22_quarter1_presentation.pdf

[3] Abrahams N, Seedat S, Lombard C, Kengne AP, Myers B, Sewnath A, et al. Study protocol for a longitudinal study evaluating the impact of rape on women's health and their use of health services in South Africa. BMJ Open. 2017;**7**(9):e017296

[4] Mgoqi-Mbalo N, Zhang M, Ntuli S. Risk factors for PTSD and depression in female survivors of rape. Psychological Trauma: Theory, Research, Practice, and Policy. 2017;**9**(3):301

[5] Sepeng NV, Makhado L. Correlates of post-traumatic stress disorder diagnosis among rape survivors: Results and implications of a South African study. Journal of Psychology in Africa. 2018;**28**(6):468-471

[6] American Psychiatric Association. Diagnostic and Statistical Manual of Mental Disorders, DSM-5. Washington, DC: Author; 2013

[7] Foa EB, Keane TM, Friedman MJ, Cohen JA, editors. Effective Treatments for PTSD: Practice Guidelines from the International Society for Traumatic Stress Studies. Guilford Press; 2010

[8] Hopkins K, Crosland P, Elliott N, Bewley S. Diagnosis and management of depression in children and young people: Summary of updated NICE guidance. BMJ. 2015;**350**

[9] Mathews S, Abrahams N, Jewkes R. Exploring mental health adjustment of children post sexual assault in South Africa. Journal of Child Sexual Abuse. 2013;**22**(6):639-657

[10] Sepeng NV, Makhado L. Present practices of rape care management in Thuthuzela Care Centres of the North West Province. Journal of Psychology in Africa. 2019;**29**(5):516-519

[11] Christofides NJ, Jewkes RK, Webster N, Penn-Kekana L, Abrahams N, Martin LJ. Other patients are really in need of medical attention: The quality of health services for rape survivors in South Africa. Bulletin of the World Health Organization. 2005;**83**:495-502

[12] Engel CC, Litz B, Magruder KM, Harper E, Gore K, Stein N, et al. Delivery of self training and education for stressful situations (DESTRESS-PC): A randomized trial of nurse assisted online self-management for PTSD in primary care. General Hospital Psychiatry. 2015;**37**(4):323-328

[13] De Kock JH, Pillay BJ. A situation analysis of psychiatrists in South Africa's rural primary healthcare settings. African Journal of Primary Health Care & Family Medicine. 2017;**9**(1):a1335. DOI: 10.4102/phcfm.v9i1.1335

[14] Mahomed OH, Asmall S. Professional nurses' perceptions and experiences with the implementation of an integrated chronic care model at primary healthcare clinics in South Africa. Curationis. 2017;**40**(1):1-6

[15] Dube FN, Uys LR. Integrating mental health care services in primary health care clinics: A survey of primary health care nurses' knowledge, attitudes and beliefs. South African Family Practice. 2016;**58**(3):119-125

[16] Pasche S, Kleintjes S, Wilson D, Stein DJ, Myers B. Improving addiction care in South Africa: Development and challenges to implementing training in addictions care at the University of Cape Town. International Journal of Mental Health and Addiction. 2015;**13**(3):322-332

[17] Abrahams N, Gevers A. A rapid appraisal of the status of mental health support in post-rape care services in the Western Cape. South African Journal of Psychiatry. 2017;**23**

[18] Petersen I, Lund C, Bhana A, Flisher AJ. Mental health and poverty research programme consortium. A task shifting approach to primary mental health care for adults in South Africa: Human resource requirements and costs for rural settings. Health Policy and Planning. 2012;**27**(1):42-51

[19] Republic of South Africa. Children's Amendment Act, No. 30884. Government Gazette, 513. 2007

[20] Abrahams N, Mathews S. Services for child sexual abuse lacking. South African Medical Journal. 2008;**98**(7):494

[21] Abrahams N, Mhlongo S, Chirwa E, Lombard C, Dunkle K, Seedat S, et al. Rape survivors in South Africa: Analysis of the baseline socio-demographic and health characteristics of a rape cohort. Global health action. 2020;**13**(1):1834769

[22] Petersen I, Ssebunnya J, Bhana A, Baillie K. Lessons from case studies of integrating mental health into primary health care in South Africa and Uganda. International Journal of Mental Health Systems. 2011;**5**(1):1-2. Available from: http://www.ijmhs.com/content/5/1/8

[23] Andersen I, Rossi R, Yabutu MN, Hubloue I. Integrating mental health and psychosocial support into health facilities in conflict settings: A retrospective review from six african countries. Frontiers in Public Health. 2020;**8**:591369. DOI: 10.3389/fpubh.2020.591369

[24] Oshodi Y, Macharia M, Lachman A, Seedat S. Immediate and long-term mental health outcomes in adolescent female rape survivors. Journal of Interpersonal Violence. 2020;**35**(1-2):252-267

[25] Department of Health. White Paper for the Transformation of the Health System in South Africa. Pretoria National Department of Health; 1997

[26] Department of Health. Mental Health Care Act (17 of 2002). Pretoria Department of Health; 2004

[27] World Health Organization. Task-shifting: Rational redistribution of tasks among health workforce teams: Global recommendations and guidelines. 2008 [cited 2013 Jan 17] Available from: http://scholar.google.com/scholar?hl=en&btnG=Search&q=intitle:Task+shifting+:+rational+redistribution+of+tasks+among+health+workforce+teams+:+global+recommendations+and+guidelines.#2

[28] Emdin C, Millson P. A systematic review evaluating the impact of task-shifting on access to antiretroviral therapy in sub-Saharan Africa. African Health Sciences. 2012;**12**(3):318-324. *Correspondence with author

[29] Callaghan M, Ford N, Schneider H. A systematic review of task-shifting for HIV treatment and care in

Africa. Human Resources for Health. 2010:8. Available from: http://www.pubmedcentral.nih.gov/articlerender.fcgi?artid=2873343&tool=pmcentrez&rendertype=abstract

[30] Makhado L, Davhana-Maselesele M, Lebese RT, Maputle SM. Factors facilitating trained NIMART nurses' adherence to treatment guidelines: A vital matter in the management of TB/HIV treatment in South Africa. BMC Nursing. 2020;**19**(1):1-8

[31] Jack H, Wagner GRG, Petersen I, Thom R, Newton RCR, Stein A, et al. Closing the mental health treatment gap in South Africa: A review of costs and cost-effectiveness. Global Health Action. 2014;**7**:1-11

[32] Lund C, Flisher AJ. A model for community mental health services in South Africa. Tropical Medicine & International Health. 2009;**14**(9):1040-1047

[33] Kakuma R, Minas H, van Ginneken N, Dal Poz MR, Desiraju K, Morris JE et al. Human resources for mental health care: Current situation and strategies for action. Lancet. 2011;**378**(9803):1654-1663. [cited 2013 Jun 26] Available from: http://www.ncbi.nlm.nih.gov/pubmed/22008420

[34] Kigozi FN, Ssebunnya J. Integration of mental health into primary health care in Uganda: Opportunities and challenges. Mental Health in Family Medicine. 2009;**6**(1):37-42

[35] World Health Organization. Integrating Mental Health into Primary Care: A Global Perspective. WHO; 2008

[36] Siddiqi K, Siddiqi N. Treatment of common mental disorders in primary care in low-and middle-income countries. Transactions of the Royal Society of Tropical Medicine and Hygiene. 2007;**101**:957-958

[37] Hlongwa EN, Sibiya MN. Challenges affecting the implementation of the policy on integration of mental health care into primary healthcare in KwaZulu-Natal province. Curationis. 2019;**42**(1):1-9

[38] Schierenbeck I, Johansson P, Andersson L, van Rooyen D. Barriers to accessing and receiving mental health care in Eastern Cape South Africa. Health and Human Rights. 2013;**15**:110

[39] Bower P, Gilbody S. Managing common mental health disorders in primary care: Conceptual models and evidence base. BMJ. 2005;**330**(7495):839-842

[40] Letlape HR, Koen MP, Coetzee SK, Koen V. The exploration of in-service training needs of psychiatric nurses. Health SA Gesondheid. 2014;**19**(1)

[41] Duma SE, De Villiers T. Clinical forensic nursing skills and competencies for quality care to victims of crime and violence: Gender and equity. African Journal for Physical Health Education, Recreation and Dance. 2014;(20, sup-1): 360-375

Chapter 8

Perspective Chapter: Perspectives toward Overcoming Depression and Anxiety to Enhance Educational Success among Students in a Rural University Context

Angelina Maphula, Lufuno Makhado and Petunia Tsheole

Abstract

Depression and anxiety among the youth are serious mental health problems leading to suicide and causing unmeasurable negative long-term impacts, not only for the individual but also for family and friends. This chapter aims to unpack current perspectives on overcoming depression and anxiety to enhance educational success among the youth. A literature review was conducted to thoroughly address relevant content to bring forth short and long-term practical steps that might enhance educational success among youth who are continuously dealing with depression and anxiety. Given the magnitude of depression and anxiety among youth, the current trends of depression among the youth, and factors leading to anxiety and depression were unpacked. In addition, the perspectives on how family members, friends, and community members can identify signs and symptoms of anxiety and depression, guidelines about overcoming anxiety and depression, tailor-made practical guidelines to enhance educational success, and recommendations were explained. In conclusion, it is clear that in rural areas, there is a knowledge gap about mental illness in general. It is, therefore, recommended that the government focus must be on educating the community to provide knowledge and understanding. Consequently, families and friends will better identify depression and anxiety and consequently provide the necessary support.

Keywords: depression, anxiety, students, educational success, rural, context, South Africa

1. Introduction

Depression is a common mental illness marked by low mood, lack of interest or pleasure, diminished energy, feelings of guilt or low self-esteem, interrupted sleep or food, poor attention, and anxiety, leading to suicide in severe cases [1]. It is also the peak age for depression [2]. on the other hand, Anxiety is a psychological and physiological condition that includes cognitive, physical, emotional, and behavioral elements. When these elements come together, they produce an unpleasant sensation associated with anxiety, dread, or concern. Many signs of depression include persistent sadness, anxious, or "empty" sensations, thoughts of despair, guilt, worthlessness and helplessness, irritability, restlessness, and a lack of interest in activities or hobbies that were formerly joyful [3].

2. The magnitude of the problem

In order to inform health policies and programs, tailor-made strategies designed to overcome depression and anxiety among students are critical and must be explored. In emerging nations, rapid urbanization is occurring, with both negative and positive implications on health and quality of life evident. A lot of research is being done that focuses on mental health and mental illness. Still, there is a scarcity of research on the psychosocial well-being of students since this aspect of health is inextricably tied to overall health and well-being [4]. The chapter will explore perspectives on overcoming depression and anxiety to enhance educational success in a rural context.

3. Current trend of depression and anxiety among the youth

The two most prevalent mental illnesses among the youth are depression and generalized anxiety [5]. Collective estimates from a meta-analysis study revealed that during the first year of the pandemic (COVID-19), one in four youth universally experienced high levels of depression while one in five youth experienced high levels of anxiety. These estimates are evidently double compared with estimates published before the pandemic [6] and show that more than 300 million people worldwide are living with depression, and about 18 million youth worldwide above the age of 17 have been found to demonstrate symptoms of depressive disorder, and 20% of these students have made one or more suicide attempts. Globally, over 79% of suicide deaths in low and middle-income countries are among young adults aged between 15 and 29 years who suffer from major depression [7].

Research at the Medical Fayoum University, Egypt, indicated that 60.8% of students suffer from depression and found that there are few studies of mental health illnesses among South African university students; 12% of South African students experience moderate to severe symptoms of depression and 24% report suicidal ideation [3, 8]. A study of first-year students at the University of Cape Town and Stellenbosch University found that 38.5% of students reported at least one-lifetime disorder, the most common of which was a major depressive disorder of those with lifetime disorders, 81.2% met the diagnostic criteria for a disorder, which had started more than a year ago [9]. The University of Free State found 26.5% of moderate to extremely severe depression [10].

4. The literature review methodology

A systematic search approach was used for the literature review. Similarly, recruiting specialists base their information sourcing on Boolean search. The Boolean search strategy was used to do the literature search. These tools frequently include a collection of Boolean expressions that combine keywords, operators, and ontology concepts to produce a multi-line artifact known as a search strategy. Keyword searches were done using several academic search engines, such as Pubmed, Google Scholar, EbscoHost, and Science Direct.

The Boolean search approach narrows the search and enhances the accuracy and effectiveness of the information by using keywords search. Boolean search approach as a search technique that enables users to add or utilize keywords such as "students and anxiety" and "students" and "depression" in a rural university. The researcher set out to look at studies that were specifically concerned with how students at a remote university overcame anxiety and depression. Key symptoms, factors leading to depression and anxiety among the youth, perspectives on how family members, friends, and community members can identify signs and symptoms of anxiety and depression, and the tailor-made practical approaches to enhance educational success among students will bc discussed.

5. Symptoms of depression and anxiety

5.1 Depression

In recent years, depression has appeared as an issue of concern for students globally as it impacts the quality of their life and ability to complete their academic studies successfully [7]. Depression is a state of a psychiatric disorder characterized by symptoms of persistent depressed mood almost every day for a 2-week period. It is characterized by a feeling of sadness, emptiness, hopelessness, and loss of interest and pleasure. DSM-5, 2013:160 explains significant characteristics of depression where a person must present with five or more of the following symptoms and represents a change from previous functioning–including significant weight loss when not dieting or weight gain, insomnia or hypersomnia nearly every day, fatigue, psychomotor agitation or retardation, feelings of worthlessness, diminished ability to think or concentrate, and suicidal thoughts. The DSM-5 outlines the criteria for diagnosis and common features: a sad, empty, or irritable mood accompanied by somatic and cognitive changes that significantly affect the individual's capacity to function [1].

5.2 Anxiety

Anxiety also coexists with depression, and it comprises constant worry that can be extremely incapacitating. People who suffer from generalized anxiety worry excessively about the outcome of events, find it hard to concentrate on the here and now, often lose focus on what they are doing quickly and are restless, become less productive, and are characterized by indecisiveness that extends to situations with varied options and daily tasks as well, experience fatigue, irritability, and headaches. Mental tension may also aggravate muscle tension and consequently lead to recurrent body aches and pains. In addition, some come common symptoms include sweating profusely, palpitations, lightheadedness, shortness of breath, occasional loss of consciousness, struggling to breathe, recurrent insomnia where one battles to fall asleep and experiences specific fears that become too overwhelming, cramping, constipation as well as feeling bloated [1].

Given the above symptoms of depression and anxiety, a student may find it difficult to fulfill their role when experiencing depression and anxiety. Therefore, it is critical to deepen our understanding of mental illnesses to alleviate their negative outcomes on students' education success.

6. Factors leading to depression and anxiety among the youth

A known fact is that rural areas are mostly disadvantaged with limited health programs, facilities, restricted assistance from experts, and fully qualified professionals [11] experience different stressors and psychological discomfort, which is usually caused by differences in family background and their family history, including monthly household income, parental vocations and education, and their interaction with families [12]. Financial stress and family background were found to be substantial negative predictors of students' physical and psychological well-being during their academic years [13]. It is worth noting that various elements contribute to student depression: increased scholastic responsibilities, acclimation to a new environment, family structure, and social life shifts. When compared with students from urban backgrounds, university students from rural regions scored higher on depression, anxiety, and stress scales. This can be explained by the fact that students from rural areas reported having the weaker family economic conditions; in addition, students who lived in leased housing or homes of poor quality were more likely to be affected psychologically [14]. Socioeconomic variables directly influence the incidence of depression among students; for example, research shows that students from lower socioeconomic classes have a greater rate of depression due to financial hardship [15].

Other key determinants of depressed behavior include family conflicts such as divorce and parent separation, rural origins, and a lack of amenities [15]. Biological, environmental, and psychological vulnerabilities all have a role in developing depression, which, when left untreated, can have serious consequences that can affect a person's capacity to function and fulfill duties on a day-to-day basis and may even lead to suicide [16]. Similarly, studying certain courses has been linked to depression and stress. The complexity of life has risen as a result of Westernization and modernization. Students who do poorly in school cannot match their parents' or instructors' expectations, resulting in increased stress, worry, and low self-esteem, leading to depression and anxiety.

On the other hand, students with psychological illnesses, such as depression, are more likely to struggle academically. In a study by Magnúsdóttir et al. [17], rumination may be divided into brooding and pondering. Brooding refers to a passive way of comparing the present situation with more desirable and unattainable standards and is associated with more depressive symptoms. Pondering refers to more purposeful cognitive problem-solving strategies and is associated with fewer depressive symptoms over time. There was an alarmingly high degree of persistence for students who have suffered from depressive disorders and anxiety problems. This may be due to a lack of perceived need for help or a lack of services use. The further deterioration of male students' depression problems may be partly attributed to their negative attitude toward emotional openness, which means they might be reluctant to utilize mental services. Therefore, this is indicative that wellness programs in institutions of higher learning must be reviewed to pay special attention to male students' mental states and encourage them to express their emotions and seek professional help if and when needed [18].

Studies suggest varied findings regarding the association of age and gender to mental illness, especially depression. In another study, depression level was significantly related to gender and increasing age. Students over 25 years and undergraduate male students presented higher scores than others [3]. In this study, gender was associated with an increased risk of depression; female students were reported to be more prone to symptoms of depression than male students. It can be concluded that South African females are vulnerable due to risk factors such as interpersonal violence, sexual assault, trauma, social stressors such as relationship problems and insufficient social support [9, 19]. On the contrary, male students were more depressed after a stressful event than females at the University of Pretoria and Limpopo university. The reason could be that males are less likely to seek professional help when experiencing psychological problems. Culturally there is a stigma against the masculine norm of being strong and independent as opposed to being perceived as weak that males always strive to uphold [20]. This practice is to the detriment of their mental health.

7. Perspectives on how family members, friends, and community members can identify signs and symptoms of anxiety and depression

Family members, friends, and community members might encounter numerous barriers to identifying signs and symptoms of depression and anxiety if they have limited knowledge of the mental illness. In addition to people's misattributions, there are other factors to consider, such as financial issues, inadequate resources, etc.

Studies looking into the stigma associated with mental illness and its treatment in Arab culture found several ways in which various commonly held negative views might limit access to mental health care. Concerns over medicine use and unfavorable attitudes toward persons with mental illnesses and mental health practitioners were among the issues raised [21].

Individuals with mental illness are more likely to express shame or humiliation and the themes "weak," "social rejection," "difficulty talking to specialists," and "confidential/anonymous services." The former might reflect the reality that shame is present in many diseases. At the same time, the latter could imply that need is overriding worries, care is altering attitudes, or individuals who are stigmatized are better able to receive assistance. These findings are consistent with individual research on how sociodemographic factors combine with stigma to limit help-seeking behavior [22]. Students who experience stressful life events of a more severe nature and burnout are ultimately affected negatively academically [23, 24].

The lack of knowledge about depression and anxiety results in ineffective social support necessary because people lack the understanding of the magnitude of depression and anxiety. The adoption of the STAR-Caregivers program, a behavioral intervention to reduce depression and anxiety in individuals with mental illness and their family caregivers, can be beneficial if rolled out on a large scale to educate families, friends, and community members [25]. This program can be adapted to fit the need of rural communities with the sole purpose of educating people about depression, anxiety, and mental illnesses.

Recently, institutions of higher learning have parents' sessions, especially at the beginning of the year, and research found that attendance of parent education sessions was linked to a decrease in depression symptoms over time. The findings emphasize the relevance of social–emotional support and depression prevention programs, emphasizing family and community protective factors [26].

The research found that students with characteristics that set them apart from most of their peers, such as minority race or ethnicity, international status, or low socioeconomic status, are more likely to be socially isolated. Furthermore, as measured by the Multidimensional Scale of Perceived Social Support, the students with lower-quality social support were six times more likely to experience mental health problems than students with higher-quality social support, including a sixfold risk of depressive symptoms [13]. Therefore, it is imperative to have programs covering the ground regarding knowledge, which set a stage to offer effective, insightful support from family and community members. Mental illness is typically perceived as a curse or retribution, and religion has been demonstrated to substantially impact views [21].

Another mechanism recognized is social media's support and impact on mental health outcomes, which forms a massive part of students' lives [27]. In order to minimize mental health symptoms, the positive advantage can be access to services through social networks in addition to parent, friends, and community behavioral interventions.

8. Tailor-made practical approaches to enhance educational success among students

Students must effectively move from late youth to maturity during their university years. The frequency and incidence of mental illnesses are linked to long-term negative effects in later adulthood and worse academic achievement and later drop-out [23]. It is critical to investigate the disparities further in order to allow proper screening and intervention programs, particularly during orientation, to prevent mental health problems among university students; ongoing monitoring should be conducted. Not just in the first year of study, but even among senior students who may be concerned about their future transition after graduation, it is critical to identify and diagnose susceptible individuals early, give treatment, and provide intervention such as individual counseling [14]. Goals can be driven by self-control, according to [28]. Goal setting may be a useful technique for internal commitment, allowing students who lack self-control to put in more effort. Low life satisfaction was linked to poor cognitive engagement in the classroom [29]. Several researchers have discovered a substantial link between socioemotional aspects such as academic accomplishment, emotional control, behavioral regulation, academic concept, self-concept, etc.

Relaxation methods and breathing exercises can be utilized to improve academic performance by lowering study anxiety, boosting resilience, and encouraging positive coping skills. They said that good academic performance/services and educational intervention could help students establish and maintain a positive self-image, lowering the likelihood of developing emotional disorders [30]. Life crafting techniques for students in universities between the ages of 18 and 26 to help them cope with stressors are important, and it ensures successful completion of their studies. Bio-feedback is known to be superior to relaxation techniques because it focuses on psychophysiological arousal [31], which might be beneficial to enhancing a stimulated mind.

8.1 Life crafting therapy

Schippers and Ziegler [32] advocate utilizing a "life-crafting" intervention to improve students' academic achievement and overall well-being. The online life-crafting intervention is made up of numerous parts that work together. These elements are based on scientifically validated processes that help people think about their current and future lives, establish goals, create plans, and behave in ways consistent with their values [32].

8.1.1 Discovering a self-concordant passion or purpose phase

The intervention's initial stage walks participants through the process of discovering a self-concordant passion or purpose. This phase is about discovering what one values as significant and meaningful, rather than simply recognizing what one loves or enjoys (hedonic well-being). "Ikigai" is a Japanese notion that is similar to this self-awareness. When an aim is both internally and externally concordant, it is said to be self-concordant and the belief that it is worthwhile to pursue. The exercises encourage participants to set objectives that they honestly think are important to them. This increases the likelihood that one's (goal-oriented) activities are consistent with one's values leading to awareness of oneself. A goal is considered self-concordant when internally and externally concordant [32].

8.1.2 Goal ranking and mental comparison phase

Second, the planning stage involves goal ranking and mental comparison. This stage assists students in determining how their intended future differs from their existing situation. Participants compare and contrast the idealized best-case scenario for achieving the goal with an internal roadblock. Competencies, habits, social life, profession, and health are all areas where this strategy is used. Students are asked to define what competencies and habits they already have and what competencies and habits they wish and need. Simply dreaming about an ideal future can have a beneficial effect, but it reduces the likelihood that a person would make an effort to achieve the desired outcome.

On the one hand, they contrast the perfect future with the existing condition. The activities inspire people to develop goals that they truly believe are important to them. This makes it more likely that one's (goal-oriented) actions align with one's values [32].

8.1.3 Prioritizing and goal-setting process phase

Third, participants develop and prioritize their most essential goals using the goal-setting process. They are urged to balance social, career, and health-related objectives. Therefore, they are encouraged to build a harmonious passion rather than an obsessive job passion, which is linked to conflicts between different aspects of life [33]. They are advised to write ambitious yet clear and realistic goals while establishing their goals. Setting goals helps people focus their energy on goal-related activities and enhances self-control and motivation. Prior study has linked writing about one's hobbies and ambitions to improved academic achievement [32].

8.1.4 Implementation phase

Finally, participants construct the implementation intents they'll need to carry out their plans as part of the life-crafting process. Implementation intents are "if-then" strategies that help a person make goal-related decisions in a pinch. These are especially useful when individuals are confronted with difficulties or diversions, and they significantly impact goal achievement. Allowing oneself to be diverted from studying (procrastination) is a major risk factor for students and a predictor of depression, poor personal health, and poor academic performance. Self-efficacy and self-esteem are also predicted by prior performance. The self-image and esteem are therefore reinforced by a poor or strong start. When given at the study's outset, the life-crafting intervention can jumpstart self-regulated learning promptly [32].

8.2 Internet-based mental health intervention

Compared with online treatment, treating mental health issues with traditional face-to-face methods is costly. Internet-based or digital forms of mental health care can be scalable and, therefore, cost-effective [31].

Evidence shows that OEDIS (Online Educational Information Support) lowers SAD (Stress, Anxiety, and Depression), and OEMIS (Online Emotional Information Support) lowers stress and anxiety. Negative emotions can be decreased, and educational outcomes can be enhanced by offering online information. This research implies that online information support might play a new role in assisting students with emotional changes and psychiatric disorders. The research indicates that OEDIS lowers SAD and OEMIS (lowers stress and anxiety) [34]. Given that students are most on their electronic gadgets, this is beneficial for even those who will be embarrassed or opposed to face-to-face counseling as such a platform offers chat, sms, and audio calls.

8.3 Emotional freedom technique

EFT is a gentle psychological intervention that may be readily taught and given by oneself. Subjects gently touch acupressure sites on the head, body, and hands with their fingertips, relating this to speaking certain sentences. According to recent systematic evaluations, EFT is useful for several psychiatric illnesses, including lowering presentation and test-taking anxiety and improving sports performance. According to new research, EFT is a viable therapy for students' presentation and exam anxiety. For example, EFT was demonstrated to dramatically reduce presentation anxiety in university students and looked into the effects of EFT and Progressive Muscular Relaxation (PMR) on exam anxiety among Turkish university students [35]. This can be beneficial in institutions of higher learning where presentations are highly regarded as a mode of learning.

8.4 Logo therapeutic technique

The basic observation of human beings as a three-dimensional entity underpins logotherapy. The biological/physiological, psychological/mental, emotional, and social aspects are the four dimensions or areas of noetic/spiritual significance [36]. The first two dimensions are considered easily accessible as the therapy is interdisciplinary, and additional professionals' approaches will be looked at. However, there are particular human characteristics in the noetic/spiritual realm, such as self-discovery, self-detachment, and attaining our potential. A lack or low level of meaning is related to a series of negative behaviors and mental health problems, such as alcohol and drug use, boredom proneness, depression, suicide ideation, disengagement, and risky behaviors [37].

Students can find their own identities. This may be accomplished by employing the Logotherapeutic approach of Socratic Dialog [38]. The approach was named after the Greek philosopher Socrates, who utilized narrative inquiry to help his students learn about themselves via dialog. When the students' self-detachment permits them to perceive themselves objectively from the outside, they are able to find various potentials and obstacles. This helps them realize that they have the ability to make their own decisions and that they are responsible for themselves. Individuals can eventually transcend their egocentric existence and become self-transcendent. The logotherapeutic method improves four treatment goals.

1. Self-distancing from the symptoms;

2. Modification of attitudes;

3. Reduction of symptoms;

4. Orientation toward meaningful activities and experiences.

The first step assists and allows the student to disengage from the situation. Feelings of self-doubt, worthlessness, poor self-esteem, inferiority, and hopelessness are all signs of depression. The second step involves assisting the student in seeing themselves objectively, similar to looking in the mirror (where this does not occur). The Socratic Dialog can be supplemented with the use of meaning-oriented questions, such as the use of humor or metaphors be used. The lessening of symptoms is the third phase. Further Socratic Dialog can be used to help the person see themselves from a different perspective—the more an individual views themselves through the eyes of others, the better. The more patients see themselves objectively, the fewer symptoms they may experience. The fourth stage is to direct the student's attention to relevant activities and experiences that will help the person maintain a positive outlook.

8.5 Acceptance and commitment therapy

ACT is a transdiagnostic psychotherapy intervention based on the Relational Frame Theory theoretical paradigm. It is a "third wave" cognitive behavioral treatment (CBT) that encourages people to participate in values-based behaviors regardless of the presence or absence of symptoms. The basic goal of ACT is to enhance psychological flexibility, which is the ability to be attentive to current events in a nonjudgmental and accepting manner while acting according to one's ideals [39].

Even when one's thoughts and feelings resist taking the desired action, one must behave in accordance with one's values. Acceptance (i.e., willingness to open fully to unwanted experiences such as difficult thoughts, memories, or emotions), contact with the present moment (i.e., being mindful and aware of one's experiences), self as context (i.e., maintaining perspective about oneself within one's experiences), and cognitive defusion (i.e., being able to step back from unwanted experiences such as difficult thoughts, memories, or emotions) are six interrelated and overlapping processes that ACT uses to foster psychological flexibility [40] .

Many post-secondary institutions are already offering ACT-based group therapies to increase student well-being and avoid mental health disorders. Student's psychological troubles, according to ACT, are partially caused by the following mechanisms:

a) they engage in experiential avoidance behaviors aimed at changing, controlling, or avoiding certain thoughts, emotions, or painful feelings, which perpetuates their problems (e.g., anxiety); b) they are unable to separate themselves from their thoughts, believing them to be a reflection of reality, or even an extension of who they are; c) they are prisoners of the past (e.g., ruminations) or the future (e.g., preoccupations) and have difficulty being mindful [40]. ACT tries to counteract these tendencies by assisting individuals in developing more psychological flexibility, which is described as the ability to be present at the moment and take actions consistent with one's values [41].

9. Conclusion

Depression and anxiety are commonly reported among university students globally, and it is rife with suicide rates escalating daily, especially in developing countries. Students' environment is a stressful one that often bears mental health issues. Students' quality of life and psychosocial well-being upon adjusting and adapting well to the lifestyle, academic challenges, and stressors lead to depression and anxiety. Therefore, programs targeting families, friends, community members, and students are essential. Given the gap in knowledge about what depression and anxiety are among rural communities, it is recommended that programs focus on educating people and equipping them to understand, which will allow them to identify and sufficiently support those suffering from mental health illnesses. In addition, existing wellness programs in higher education institutions that target students must be continuous, and social media platforms must also be maximized for their capacity to reach students at ease. The potential for students to achieve their goals will increase when their mental health is at its optimal functioning, consequently reducing the health burden caused by depression and anxiety.

Author details

Angelina Maphula*, Lufuno Makhado and Petunia Tsheole
University of Venda, Thohoyandou, South Africa

*Address all correspondence to: angelina.maphula@univen.ac.za

References

[1] American Psychiatric Association. Diagnostic and Statistical Manual of Mental Disorders. 5th ed. Washington, DC: Author; 2013

[2] Billah SMB, Khan FI. Depression among urban adolescent students of some selected schools. Faridpur Medical College Journal. 2015;**9**(2):73-75. DOI: 10.3329/fmcj.v9i2.25678

[3] Wahed WYA, Hassan SK. Prevalence and associated factors of stress, anxiety and depression among medical Fayoum university students. Alexandria Journal of Medicine. 2017;**53**(1):77-84. ISSN 2090-5068. DOI: 10.1016/j.ajme.2016.01.005

[4] Wissing MP, Temane QM. The prevalence of levels of well-being revisited in an African context, Mental Well-Being. Dordrecht: Springer; 2013. ISBN: 978-94-007-5194-1

[5] Merikangas KR, He JP, Burstein M, et al. Lifetime prevalence of mental disorders in U.S. adolescents: Results from the National Comorbidity Survey Replication—Adolescent Supplement (NCS-A). Journal of American Academy of Child and Adolescent Psychiatry. 2010;**49**(10):980-989. DOI: 10.1016/j.jaac.2010.05.017

[6] Racine N, McArthur BA, Cooke JE, Eirich R, Zhu J, Madigan S. Global prevalence of depressive and anxiety symptoms in children and adolescents during COVID-19: A Meta-analysis. JAMA Pediatrics. 2021;**175**(11):1142-1150. DOI: 10.1001/jamapediatrics.2021.2482

[7] World Health Organisation. Adolescence Mental Health. 2019. Available from: https://www.who.int.-adolescentmentalhealth

[8] Kaminer D, Shabalala N. Developing a student mental health policy for a south African university: Consultation, contestation and compromise. South African Journal of Higher Education. 2019;**33**(5):196-212

[9] Bantjes JR, Kagee A, McGowan A, Steel H. Symptoms of posttraumatic stress, depression, and anxiety as predictors of suicidal ideation among south African university students. Journal of American College Health. 2016;**64**(6):429-437

[10] Van Zyl PM, Joubert G, Bowen E, du Plooy F, Francis C, Jadhunandan S, et al. Depression, anxiety, stress and substance use in medical students in 5 year curriculum. African Journal of Health Professions Education. 2017;**9**(2):67-72

[11] Chang JJ, Ji Y, Li YH, Pan HF, Su PY. Prevalence of anxiety symptom and depressive symptom among college students during COVID-19 pandemic: A meta-analysis. Journal of Affective Disorder. 2021;**292**:242-254. ISSN 0165-0327. DOI: 10.1016/j.jad.2021.05.109

[12] Ngin C, Pal K, Tuot S, Chhoun P, Yi R, Yi S. Social and behavioural factors associated with depressive symptoms among university students in Cambodia: A cross-sectional study. BMJ Open. 2018;**8**(9):1-13. DOI: 10.1136/bmjopen-2017-019918

[13] Hefner J, Eisenberg D. Social support and mental health among college students. American Journal of Orthopsychiatry. 2009;**79**:491-449. DOI: 10.1037/a0016918

[14] Shamsuddin K, Fadzil F, Ismail WSW, Shah SA, et al. Correlates of depression, anxiety and stress among

Malaysian university students. Asian Journal of Psychiatry. 2013;**6**(4):318-323. ISSN 1876-2018. DOI: 10.1016/j.ajp.2013.01.014

[15] Mamun MA, Akter S, Hossain I, Mohammad Thanvir M, Faisal H, Rahman A, et al. Financial threat, hardship and distress predict depression, anxiety and stress among the unemployed youths: A Bangladeshi multi-city study. Journal of Affective Disorders. 2020;**276**:1149-1158. ISSN 0165-0327. DOI: 10.1016/j.jad.2020.06.075

[16] Jadnanansing R, de Beurs E, Etwaroo K, et al. A survey of depression and anxiety disorders in urban and rural Suriname. BMC Public Health. 2022;**22**:51. DOI: 10.1186/s12889-021-12454-5

[17] Magnúsdóttir I, Lovik A, Unnarsdóttir AB, McCartney D, Helga Ask H, et al. Acute COVID-19 severity and mental health morbidity trajectories in patient populations of six nations: An observational study. The Lancet Public Health. 2022;**7**(5):e406-e416. ISSN 2468-2667. DOI: 10.1016/S2468-2667(22)00042-1

[18] Gao J, ZhengP JY, Chen H, Mao Y, Chen S, et al. Mental health problems and social media exposure during COVID-19 outbreak. PLoS One. 2020;**15**(4):e0231924. DOI: 10.1371/

[19] van Zyl PM, L. Metz ML, Joubert G, Francis C, et al. Depression, anxiety, stress and substance use in medical students in a 5-year curriculum. African Journal of Health Professions Education. 2017;**9**:2

[20] Maistry C. Cognitive vulnerability-stress model in predicting depressive symptoms amongst university students [mini dissertation] University of Pretoria and university of Limpop. 2016. Available form: https://hdl.handle.net/2263/55832

[21] Awadalla S, Davies EB, Glazebrook C. A longitudinal cohort study to explore the relationship between depression, anxiety and academic performance among Emirati university students. BMC Psychiatry. 2020;**20**(448):1-10. DOI: 10.1186/s12888-020-02854-z

[22] Clement S, Schauman O, Graham T, Maggioni F, Evans-Lacko S, Bezborodovs N, et al. What is the impact of mental health-related stigma on help-seeking? A systematic review of quantitative and qualitative studies. Psychological Medicine. 2014;**45**(1):11-27

[23] Bruffaerts R, Mortier P, Kiekens G, Auerbach RP, Cuijpers P, Demyttenaere K, et al. Mental health problems in college freshmen: Prevalence and academic functioning. Journal of Affective Disorders. 2018;**225**:97-103. DOI: 10.1016/j.jad.2017.07.044

[24] Pascoe MC, Hetrick SE, Parker AG. The impact of stress on students in secondary school and higher education. International Journal of Adolescence and Youth. 2019;**25**(1):104-112 . DOI: 10.1080/02673843.2019.1596823

[25] Logsdon R, McCurry SM, TERI L. STAR-caregivers. Alzheimer's Care Quarterly. 2005;**6**(2):146-153

[26] Singh N, Minaie MG, Skvarc DR, Skvarc DR, Toumbourou JW. Impact of a secondary school depression prevention curriculum on adolescent social-emotional skills: Evaluation of the resilient families program. Journal Youth Adolescence. 2019;**48**:1100-1115. DOI: 10.1007/s10964-019-00992-6

[27] Perry BL, Morris EW. Suspending Progress: Collateral consequences of exclusionary punishment in public

schools. American Sociological Review. 2014;**79**(6):1067-1087. DOI: 10.1177/0003122414556308

[28] Clark D, Gill D, Prowse V, Rush M. Using goals to motivate college students: Theory and evidence from field experiments. The Review of Economics and Statistics. 2020;**102**(4):648-663. DOI: 10.1162/rest_a_00864

[29] Holliman R, Blanco P, Kowalis C. Play therapy and academic achievement: A secondary analysis. International Journal of Play Therapy. 2022;**31**(2):82-96. DOI: 10.1037/pla0000160

[30] Nubli M, Awang MA, Othman A. The use of study anxiety intervention in reducing anxiety to improve academic performance among university students. International Journal of Psychological Studies. 2010;**2**(1):89-95. Available from: https://www.academia.edu/download/36362354/5064.pdf

[31] Dekker I, de Jong EM, Schippers MC, de Bruijn-Smolders M, Alexiou A, Giesbers B. Optimizing students' mental health and academic performance: AI-enhanced life crafting. Frontiers in Psychology. 2020;**11**(1063):1-15. DOI: 10.3389/fpsyg.2020.01063

[32] Schippers MC, Ziegler N. Life crafting as a way to find purpose and meaning in life. Frontiers in Psychology. 2019;**10**(2778):1-17. DOI: 10.3389/fpsyg.2019.02778

[33] Curran E, Rosato M, Ferry F, Gerard Leavey G. Prevalence and factors associated with anxiety and depression in older adults: Gender differences in psychosocial indicators. Journal of Affective Disorders. 2020;**267**:114-122. ISSN 0165-0327. DOI: 10.1016/j.jad.2020.02.018

[34] Jin X, Hahm S. Using online information support to decrease stress, anxiety and depression. KSII Transactions on Internet & Information Systems. 2021;**15**(8):2944-2958. DOI: 10.3837/tiis.2021.08.013

[35] Boath E, Stewart A, Carrier. Tapping for success: A pilot study to explore if emotional freedom techniques (EFT) can reduce anxiety and enhance academic performance in university students. Innovative Practice in Higher Education. 2013;**1**(3):1-15. Available from: http://journals.staffs.ac.uk/index.php/ipihe/article/view/33

[36] Asagba RB, Marshall M. The use of logotherapeutic techniques in the identification and intervention stages of treatment with persons with substance use disorder. African Research Review. 2016;**10**(3):39-54. DOI: 10.4314/afrrev.v10i3.3

[37] Van der Walt C. The relationship between first-year students' sense of purpose and meaning in life, mental health and academic performance. Journal of Student Affairs in Africa. 2019;7(2):109-121. DOI: 10.24085/jsaa.v7i2.3828

[38] Marshall M, Marshall E. Logotherapy Revisited. Review of the Tenets of Viktor E. Frankl's Logotherapy. Ottawa, Canada: Ottawa Institute of Logotherapy Press; 2012

[39] Nair B, Otaki F. Promoting university students' mental health: A systematic literature review introducing the 4M-model of individual-level interventions. Frontiers in Public Health. 2021;**9**(699030):1-10. DOI: 10.3389/fpubh.2021.699030

[40] Grégoire S, Lachance L, Bouffard T, Dionne F. The use of acceptance and commitment therapy to produce mental health and school engagement in university students: A multisite

randomized controlled trial. Behavior Therapy. 2018;**49**(3):360-372

[41] Nedelcu A, Grégoire S. Evaluating the implementation of an intervention based on acceptance and commitment therapy in post-secondary institutions. Journal of College Student Psychotherapy. 2022;**36**(1):95-112. DOI: 10.1080/87568225.2020.1806162

Chapter 9

Nurses' Coping Strategies When Caring for Mental Health Care Users Diagnosed with Substance Use Disorders

Leepile Sehularo, Lufuno Makhado and Nombulelo Sepeng

Abstract

Caring for Mental Health Care Users (MHCUs) diagnosed with Substance User Disorders (SUDs) is challenging and demanding as nurses reported that these users are untrustworthy. This leaves the nurses emotionally and physically drained. Some of these MHCUs are violent, aggressive, suicidal or homicidal. However, there is no literature found on the nurses' coping strategies when caring for MHCUs diagnosed with SUDS. The purpose of this chapter was to explore and describe the current literature on the nurses' coping strategies when caring for MHCUs diagnosed with SUDs. A narrative literature review was used in this chapter. JSTOR, Google Scholar, Sabinet Online, African Journals and Science Direct databases were used to search relevant and current literature using the following keywords: coping, coping strategies, nurses, care, caring, mental health care users, psychiatric patients, substance abuse, substance-related disorders and substance use disorders. Six themes emerged in this chapter namely nurses' resilience, peer support, management support, strengthening the multidisciplinary team (MDT) approach, open-door policy as well as education and training. The findings and recommendations of this chapter may assist nurses of all categories to provide quality care, treatment and rehabilitation services when caring for MHCUs who are diagnosed with SUDs.

Keywords: caring, coping strategies, mental health care users, nurses, substance use disorders

1. Introduction

The World Health Organisation (WHO) reported that there are 2 billion alcohol users and 185 million drug users worldwide in the general population [1]. Around the world, almost all people use one or more substances that affect their Central Nervous System (CNS), relieving physical and mental anguish or producing euphoria [2]. This is in spite of the fact that globally, there are approximately 250,000 deaths per year due to illicit drug use, and 2.25 million are caused by alcohol use [3]. Substances from all over the world currently flood South Africa (SA) [4]. The high prevalence of Substance Use Disorders (SUD) in SA makes it one of the top 10 substance-abusing countries globally [5]. This is a serious problem that needs to be attended to as soon as possible. The prevalence of substance use among forensic Mental Health Care Users (MHCUs) in Kenya is 74.8% [6]. Among the admitted Norwegian MHCUs, the prevalence of SUD is as high as 50% [7]. These statistics show that the high rates of SUDs among the MHCUs are well documented in literature [7]. From these statistics, it could be possible that most of the countries' SUD is above 50%. This is a problem that needs further research. These high statistics are a serious concern and there are no studies or book chapters found on the nurses' coping strategies when caring for MHCUs diagnosed with SUDs. These are the reasons that prompted us to write this chapter. This chapter might add important literature in the field of psychiatry and mental health nursing science. The chapter might also be relevant for other mental health care practitioners, researchers, educators and policymakers who are also concerned about the nurses who are caring for MHCs who are diagnosed with SUDs.

On the other hand, some of the authors refer to Nigeria as a substance culture [6]. For instance, the Nigerians use substances such as coffee or tea for waking up in the morning, they take soft drinks or smoke cigarettes for staying alert throughout the day, they take alcohol as a way of relaxation, and they take paracetamol for pain [6]. This shows that there are some Nigerians who are taking substances every day or 365 days a year. According to the authors of this chapter, there is a possibility that more countries can also be regarded as "*substance cultures*" particularly SA because literature indicates that it is one of the top 10 substance abusing countries globally [5]. Interestingly, SUD does not discriminate among its victims, it affects women, men and people of all races and ethnicities [8]. However, SUD is among the most prevalent mental disorders. This includes Alcohol Use Disorder (AUDs) [3]. The following information is the DSM-5 criteria for SUDs [2]:

Problematic pattern of use that impairs functioning. Two or more symptoms within a one-year period:

a. Failure to meet obligations.

b. Repeated use in situations where it is physically dangerous.

c. Repeated relationship problems.

d. Continued use despite problems caused by the substance.

e. Tolerance.

f. Withdrawal.

g. Substance taken for a longer time or in greater amounts than intended.

h. Efforts to reduce or control use do not work.

i. Much time spent trying to obtain the substance.

j. Social, hobbies, or work activities given up or reduced.

k. Craving to use the substance is strong.

From the above information, it is clear that SUD is a serious problem for the users, their families and nurses. As a result, we strongly recommend that something must be done as a matter of urgency. SUDs among MHCUs can be diagnosed with comprehensive interviews such as Psychiatric Research Interview for Substance and Mental Disorders (PRISM), Mini-International Neuropsychiatric Interview (MINI) as well as the Structured Clinical Interview for DSM-IV (SCID) [7]. Detecting and addressing SUDs proactively and systematically is essential for two reasons. Firstly, to protect the safety of all MHCUs and to enable healthcare professionals such as nurses to recognise problems early and intervene swiftly [9]. In many countries such as South Africa, when the MHCUs are finally diagnosed with SUDs, nurses are the ones who care for them. This includes assistants, staff and professional nurses. Caring is a hallmark of nursing and maybe the rationale why nursing has long enjoyed a high level of respect by the public [10]. However, the authors of this chapter noted that nursing is not the same anymore due to the MHCUs, particularly those who are admitted due to SUDs. It should also be noted that authors of this chapter share their experiences based on the South African context.

In spite of the above information, many studies show that caring for MHCUs who are diagnosed with SUD is challenging for the nurses and deemed demanding as nurses reported that these users are untrustworthy. This leaves the nurses emotionally and physically drained [1, 11]. Nurses caring for MHCUs who are diagnosed with SUDs experience frustration, anger, fear, burnout, occupational stress, emotional exhaustion, helplessness and demotivation [11]. Other nurses reported that MHCUs who are diagnosed with SUDs could be violent, aggressive and potentially threatening, thus providing a rationale for the negative views of some nurses toward caring for these MHCUs [1]. Health care professionals in general have negative attitudes toward MHCUs who are diagnosed with SUDs. Nurses are not excluded from this problem. This may lead to poor communication between the health care providers and MHCUs and this may taint the therapeutic alliance [1]. All these concerns show that a lot needs to be done in the area of mental health and SUDs. However, the authors of this chapter want to emphasise that nurses must respect the constitutional rights of these MHCs as enshrined in constitutions of many countries especially with regards to their rights to dignity and respect. On the other hand, it should be noted that most of the nurses are not coping when they care for MHCUs who are diagnosed with SUDs. The above discussion led to the following question:

What are the nurses' coping strategies when caring for MHCUs who are diagnosed with SUDs? This is the question that prompted the authors to write this chapter.

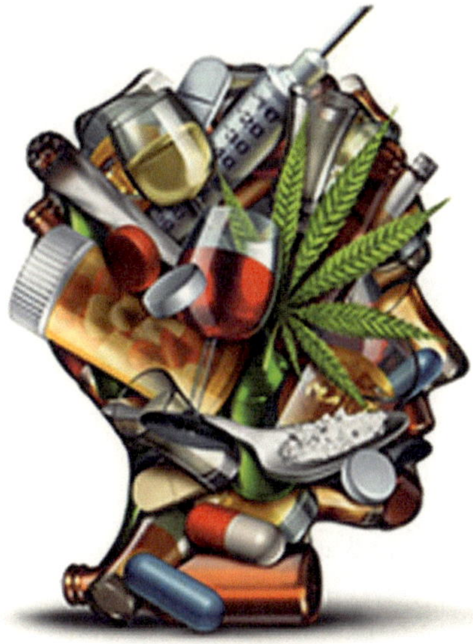

Source: William A. Haseltine.

2. Clarification of key concepts

The key concepts used in this chapter are clarified below:

2.1 Coping

Coping is defined as a combination of thoughts and actions in order to deal with a threatening situation [12]. Coping can also be defined as activities in which people use a range of cognitive and behavioural strategies to deal with, moderate or endure, situations that are demanding or surpass their routine ways of dealing with these situations [13]. Information from the introduction shows that caring for MHCUs who are diagnosed with SUDs is demanding. Coping in this chapter refers to the actions or activities that the nurses do when they care for MHCUs who are diagnosed with SUDs. It is also clear from the introduction of this chapter that nurses from different countries are dealing with stressful situations when they care for MHCUs who are diagnosed with SUDs. As a result, authors of this chapter deemed it necessary to write this chapter in order to improve coping of the nurses who are caring for MHCUs diagnosed with SUDs. It should also be noted that nurses are regarded as backbones in the health care system in most countries.

2.2 Coping strategies

Coping strategies typically involve a conscious and direct approach to problems, in contrast to defence mechanisms [12]. In this chapter, coping strategies refer to a conscious and direct approach used by nurses of all categories when they care for MHCUs who are diagnosed and admitted due to SUDs.

2.3 Mental health care user (MHCUs)

Mental health care user (MHCUs) refers to a person who is receiving care, treatment and rehabilitation services or utilising the health care services at designated health establishments that are aimed at enhancing the mental health status of users, mentally ill prisoners and state patients. When the person concerned is under the age of 18 years, or incapable of making decisions, MHCU may include the prospective user, the user's next of kin, or any person who is authorised by any law or court order to act on the behalf of that person, an executor of the diseased person's estate or an administrator appointed in terms of the Mental Health Care Act [14]. The above definition shows that MHCUs do not only include the person who is diagnosed and admitted to mental health care institutions, it also includes other people who are using the mental health care services. For the purpose of this chapter, we define MHCUs as a person who is receiving care, treatment and rehabilitation services for SUDs.

2.4 A nurse

A nurse refers to a person registered in a category under Section 31(1) of the Nursing Act in order to practice nursing and or midwifery [15]. For the purpose of this chapter, a nurse refers to a person registered with the South African Nursing Council (SANC) to care for MHCUs diagnosed with SUD.

2.5 Substance use disorders (SUDs)

Substance Use Disorders (SUDs) For the purpose of this chapter, we define SUD as the misuse of, abuse of, or dependency on substances such as alcohol, cannabis, nyaope, cocaine, tobacco and other or unknown substances. When the MHCUs are admitted to mental health care institutions for care, treatment or rehabilitation services for SUDs, they are cared for by nurses who are not coping most of the time. This is the main focus of this chapter.

3. Methodology

A narrative literature review was followed in exploring and addressing the current literature on the nurses' coping strategies when caring for MHCUs diagnosed with SUDs. Five (5) online databases were used to search for information on the nurses' coping strategies when caring for MHCUs diagnosed with SUD namely, JSTOR, Google Scholar, Sabinet Online, African Journals and Science Direct. The following keywords were used to search for the relevant literature published between 2011 and 2022: coping, coping strategies, nurses, care, caring, mental health care users, psychiatric patients, substance abuse, substance-related disorders and substance use disorders.

4. Themes

The reviewed literature revealed that there are six (6) themes that the nurses use as their coping strategies when caring for MHCUs who are diagnosed with SUDs namely nurses' resilience, peer support, management support, strengthening the multidisciplinary team (MDT) approach, open-door policy as well as education and training. The themes and sub-themes are given in the following **Table 1**:

Themes	Sub-themes
4.1 Nurses' resilience	4.1.1 Use of internal protective factors 4.1.1.2 Use of External protective factors
4.2 Peer support	4.2.1 Importance of collegial support
4.3 Management support	4.3.1 Addressing nurse-to-patient ration 4.3.2 Collaboration among employers, healthcare practitioners and researchers 4.3.3 Empowerment of nurses with relevant skills
4.4 Strengthening the multidisciplinary team (MDT) approach	4.4.1 Benefits of multidisciplinary team approach 4.4.2 Composition of multidisciplinary team
4.5 Open-door policy	4.5.1 Benefits of open-door policy
4.6 Education and training	4.6.1 Need for proper education and training 4.6.2 Continuous workshops 4.6.3 Involvement of Nursing Education Institutions in the fights against SUDs 4.6.4 Family involvement

Table 1.
Themes and sub-themes.

4.1 Nurses' resilience

It is clear from the introduction of this chapter that nurses deal with challenges in their working environment, especially those that are working at mental health establishments, or those who are caring for MHCUs who are diagnosed with SUDs. In this case, we strongly believe that nurses need to strengthen their resilience. Nurses who manage to cope and in some instances even grow in the face of omnipresent stressful experiences are described as resilient [16]. Resilience refers to a person's capacity to withstand or recover quickly from difficult conditions [16]. The same study also refers to resilience as qualities of both the individual (internal protective factors) and the environment (external protective factors) that could support positive development [16]. We also have a strong view that nurses should use both the internal and external protective factors of resilience in order to cope when caring for MHCUs who are diagnosed with SUDs. Resilience can also be defined as the ability of people to adjust to unfavourable conditions in a positive way, and bounce back from hardships and overcome negative life experiences [17]. It is clear from the information, particularly in the introduction that nurses caring for MHCUs who are diagnosed with SUDs are working in unfavourable conditions. However, they should be able to view that situation in a positive way and overcome their negative life experiences of MHCUs diagnosed with SUDs. Most of the nurses when they care for MHCUs who are diagnosed with SUDs feel angry, demotivated and dissatisfied. This resulted in some of the nurses choosing to leave South Africa in search of greener pastures [18]. Based on the above information, nurses need the opportunity to develop resilient attributes in their different specialist areas [18], particularly in the area of mental health and SUDs. Coping skills increase resilience [12].

4.2 Peer support

Peer support has been mentioned in several studies as nurses' coping strategy when caring for MHCUs diagnosed with SUD [1, 11]. Workplace support provided by peers or colleagues and the organisation is of major importance in the direct delivery of nursing care as a lack of teamwork can compromise patient care [18]. However, it should also be noted that relying on support from outside the workplace can also play an important role in the ability of nurses to cope [18], particularly when they care for MHCUs who are diagnosed with SUDs. Having collegial support from other nurses and interprofessional team members is recommended to manage uncertainty [1]. A qualitative study recently conducted in the NWP found that nurses do not collaborate with one another and as a result, they are unable to deliver quality care to MHCUs diagnosed with SUD. The above information highlights the gap that, it is imperative that nurses have role support which includes the presence of supportive, knowledgeable colleagues with whom to collaborate and gain expertise in practice [1].

4.3 Management support

Management support is one of the strategies that nurses use when caring for MHCUs diagnosed with SUDs as shown in several studies [1, 11, 19]. Participants of a qualitative study that was conducted in 2016 in the NWP of SA indicated that it would be good if the nurses were supported and motivated by their own management [11]. Nurses mentioned in a study conducted in New Jersey that they have no problem of caring for MHCUs diagnosed with SUDs for as long as the MHCU load or nurse-to-patient ratio is not too much because these MHCUs can be a handful at times [1]. This shows that the sooner the management supports the nurses by addressing the issue of nurse-to-patient ratio, the better the client outcome and the nurses' improved coping. Strengthening the prevention and treatment initiatives for addressing SUDs requires direct effort and partnership from employers (management), healthcare practitioners and researchers [19]. Managers and supervisors should create learning opportunities with the sole purpose of empowering nurses with relevant skills in providing care to mental health care users [18]. Health care practitioners should work collaboratively with the management of the mental health care institutions where they are working. The researchers should conduct more research that is aimed at assisting the nurses to cope better when they care for MHCUs who are diagnosed with SUDs.

4.4 Strengthening the multidisciplinary team (MDT) approach

Several studies mentioned strengthening the multidisciplinary team (MDT) approach as one of the strategies used by nurses who are caring for MHCUs diagnosed with SUDs [1, 8]. Nurses in collaboration with other disciplines have collective power to achieve more [10]. Two people are better off than one. Multidisciplinary team (MDT) approach is effective in caring for MHCUs who are diagnosed with SUDs. MDT approach consists of nurses, psychiatrists, pharmacists and dieticians who play a unique role in treating MHCUs who are diagnosed with SUDs [8]. For the purpose of this chapter, we suggest that the word mental health care practitioners be used to refer to MDT. According to the Mental Health Care Act 17 of 2002, mental health care practitioners also include psychologists, social workers and occupational therapists, who have been trained to provide the prescribed mental health care, treatment and rehabilitation services [14], including the care of MHCUs who are diagnosed with SUDs. Both collaboration and support with nurses and interprofessional colleagues will help manage the challenges in care and possibly mitigate the uncertainties in caring for this increasingly common patient population [1].

4.5 Open-door policy

Open-door policy is mentioned in the literature as one of the effective strategies used by the nurses who are caring for MHCUs diagnosed with SUDs. The practice of restricting the freedom of MHCUs who are diagnosed with SUDs by locking the doors of mental health care units is highly questionable [20] because everyone has the right to freedom of movement [21]. All MHCUs especially those who are diagnosed with SUDs are also protected by this right. The introduction of an open-door ward policy can reduce coercive measures like unnecessary seclusions, involuntary care, treatment and rehabilitation services, as well as incidents of aggression [20]. As a result, authors of this chapter advocate for open-door policy for all MHCUs who are diagnosed with SUDs. This will be in line with Section 21(1) of the Constitution of the Republic of South Africa (RSA) which states that "everyone has the right to freedom of movement. However, it should be noted that the MHCUs who are violent, aggressive, suicidal or homicidal, meaning those who are dangerous to themselves, or other people may be admitted involuntarily or be secluded. This is normally done after prescription by the medical doctor. The main reason for admitting these MHCUs is to protect them and other people such as families and health care practitioners. In this case, it does not mean that the MHCU's rights are violated, this is done to protect them.

4.6 Education and training

Many studies show that education and training play a major role for the nurses who are caring for MHCUs diagnosed with SUDs [1, 6, 11]. However, literature shows that some nurses do not have the necessary training and education for proper care, treatment and rehabilitation services for MHCUs who are diagnosed with SUDs. For instance, the nurses mentioned in a qualitative study that was conducted in the North West Province (NWP) of South Africa that they were taught at the university or the colleges how to care for, treat and rehabilitate MHCUs who are diagnosed with SUDs. However, the nurses maintained that caring, treating and rehabilitating an MHCU diagnosed with SUDs was not dealt with in greater detail [11]. The authors of this chapter are in agreement with this statement because substance use is presented like any other topic. There is no emphasis on it. Knowledge, skills and experience play a role in the nurses' ability to cope while providing mental health care [18]. Continuous workshops should be done for the nurses to help them deal effectively with the addicted MHCUs [12].

Another important study was conducted by two scientists from Kean University in New Jersey. The findings of the study indicated that nurses reported a lack of knowledge specific to mental disorders and SUD issues and reflected a disconnect in their ability to care for MHCUs with both physiological and psychiatric disorders [1]. The same study continues to mention that for the nurses to cope effectively with the MHCUs who are diagnosed with SUDs, nursing education programs should be created to assist nurses in developing skills in articulating and managing their uncertainty and to use evidence to guide practice [1]. This means that Nursing Education Institutions (NEIs) should also be part of the fight against SUDs.

A mixed methods study was conducted in Nigeria on the *Forex Index and Substance Abuse among Psychiatric Patients*. The findings of the study indicate that the staff in mental health care institutions including the mental health nurses should be trained on techniques of screening and detecting the use of psychoactive substances as well as on how to successfully rehabilitate MHCUs who are diagnosed with SUDs [6]. Education focusing on assessment, prevention and interventions to prevent violence and aggression, should be addressed in educational offerings, both in academia and in the clinical environment [1]. In addition, when the nurses are properly educated and trained on how to care, treat and rehabilitate MHCUs who are diagnosed with SUDs, they will be able to teach MHCUs about the dangers of substance abuse, including but not limited to the psychological and physical effects; the damage to relationships and family lives; and the impact on meeting basic needs such as holding down a job. These nurses who are well trained will also educate the MHCUs regarding treatment options, including those they can use on either an inpatient or outpatient basis and those they can use to stay substance-free long-term. The nurses might also educate MHCU's family members about what to expect from the rehabilitation process and how they can support their loved one's attempt to conquer addiction to the substances.

5. Conclusion

Caring for MHCUs who are diagnosed with SUD is challenging and demanding for the nurses as nurses reported that these users are untrustworthy. This leaves the nurses emotionally and physically drained. However, there is no documented literature on the nurses' coping strategies when caring for MHCUs diagnosed with SUDS, hence we strongly believe that this chapter is interesting and adds important literature in the field of psychiatry and mental health nursing science. Further studies should be done on the coping strategies of nurses caring for MHCUs diagnosed with SUDs. These studies should follow different methodologies such as quantitative, qualitative mixed and multi-methods, or different reviews. Different reviews can be systematic, integrated, comprehensive and scoping reviews. This chapter showed that nurses need to strengthen their resilience, they also need peer and management support, multidisciplinary team (MDT) approach, open-door policy, as well as education and training to be able to cope when caring for MHCUs diagnosed with SUDs. Nurses should specifically be trained at under and postgraduate levels on the provision of quality mental health care, treatment and rehabilitation services, management of SUDs as well as dual diagnosis. It is important for NEIs to consider development of postgraduate programs on the Management of Substance Use Disorders (SUD).

Acknowledgements

Authors acknowledge the authors of all books, articles and Acts used in this chapter.

Conflict of interest

The authors declare that they have no financial or personal relationships that may have inappropriately influenced them in writing this chapter.

Thanks

Thanks to the NWU librarians for assisting us with the literature search.

Author details

Leepile Sehularo[1*], Lufuno Makhado[2] and Nombulelo Sepeng[3]

1 Faculty of Health Sciences, NuMIQ Research Focus Area, North-West University, South Africa

2 Faculty of Health Sciences, Department of Public Health, University of Venda, South Africa

3 Faculty of Health Sciences, Department of Nursing Science, University of Pretoria, South Africa

*Address all correspondence to: leepile.sehularo@nwu.ac.za

References

[1] Neville K, Roan N. Challenges in nursing practice. The Journal of Nursing Administration. 2014;**44**(6):339-346

[2] Kring AM, Johnson SL, Davison GC, Neale JM. Abnormal Psychology. Wiley: John Wiley & Sons Inc; 2007

[3] Lucas W. The benefits of structured exercise for substance use disorders. Mental Health Matters. 2019;**6**(5):30-32

[4] Lebese RT, Ramakuela NJ, Maputle MS. Perceptions of teenagers about substance abuse at Muyexe village, Mopani district of Limpopo Province, South Africa. African Journal for Physical Health Education, Recreation and Dance. 2014;**20**(1):329-347

[5] Carelse S, Green S. Social work services by non-profit organisations for adults with substance use disorders. Southern African Journal of Social Work and Social Development. 2019;**31**(3):18

[6] Abiama EE, Ifeagwazi CM, Chukwuorji JC. Forensic index and substance abuse among psychiatric patients. IFE Psycholog IA: An International Journal. 2015;**23**(1):168-175

[7] Gundersen ØH, Mordal J, Berman AH, Bramness JG. Evaluation of the alcohol use disorders identification test and the drug use disorders identification test among patients at a Norwegian psychiatric emergency ward. European Addiction Research. 2013;**19**(5):252-260

[8] Flinter M. How health Centers engage elders with substance use disorder in treatment. Generations. 2021;**44**(4):1

[9] Monroe T, Vandoren MM, Smith ML, Cole MJ, Kenaga H. Nurses recovering from substance use disorders: A review of policies and position statements. The Journal of Nursing Administration. 2011;**41**:415

[10] Finnell DS, Tierney M, Mitchell AM. Nursing: Addressing substance use in the 21st century. Substance Abuse. 2019;**40**(4):412-420

[11] Dikobe J, Manyedi EM, Sehularo LA. Experiences of professional nurses in caring for psychiatric patients with dual diagnosis. Africa Journal of Nursing and Midwifery. 2016;**18**(1):183-197

[12] Ahmed NA, Loutfi Z, El Hamid Zaki RA. Psychosocial nursing intervention for enhancing coping skills to reduce drug craving among addicts. Ilkogretim Online. 2021;**20**:5

[13] McCann TV, Stephenson J, Lubman DI. Affected family member coping with a relative with alcohol and/or other drug misuse: A cross-sectional survey questionnaire. International Journal of Mental Health Nursing. 2019;**28**(3):687-696

[14] Republic of South Africa. Mental Health Care Act No. 17 of 2002. Government Gazette. 2002;**49**(24024):1-78

[15] Republic of South Africa. Government Gazette. Pretoria: Government Printers; 2005

[16] Mason HD. The experience of resilience among nursing students: A qualitative study. Journal for New Generation Sciences. 2018;**16**(1):62-78

[17] Du Plessis E, Nthekang SD. Resilience of auxiliary nurses providing nursing care to patients with intellectual disabilities at a public mental healthcare institution. Curationis. 2019;**42**(1):1-7

[18] Ramalisa RJ, Koen MP, Du Plessis E. Increasing coping and strengthening resilience in nurses providing mental health care: Empirical qualitative research. Health SA Gesondheid. 2018;**23**(1):1-9

[19] Harker Burnhams N, Parry CD. The state of interventions to address substance-related disorders in South African workplaces: Implications for research, policy, and practice. South Africa Journal of Psychology. 2015;**45**(4):495-507

[20] Steinauer R, Huber CG, Petitjean S, Wiesbeck GA, Dürsteler KM, Lang UE, et al. Effect of door-locking policy on inpatient treatment of substance use and dual disorders. European Addiction Research. 2017;**23**(2):87-96

[21] Republic of South Africa. Constitution of the Republic of South Africa Act No. 108 of 1996. Government Gazette; 1996. pp. 1-56

Chapter 10

Patient Feedback to Enhance Residents' Learning: A Patient and a Resident Perspective

Mana Nasori, Lindsay Bank and Fedde Scheele

Abstract

Patients are becoming more involved in healthcare, however, their involvement in postgraduate medical education (PGME) is often less prominent. We provide insight into patients' and residents' perspectives regarding possible topics for patient feedback, to increase its use and effectiveness in PGME. Semi-structured interviews with 20 purposefully sampled patients were done and 15 residents filled out a fully qualitative questionnaire. The sample size was not calculated as we aimed for data sufficiency. Content analysis was inspired by grounded theory. Topics mentioned by patients and residents were communication skills and communication of medical knowledge. While patients find organizational matters and personal aspects important topics, residents do not. Patients intend to provide feedback on task-, process-, and self-level, whereas residents do not wish to receive feedback on self-level. Topics mentioned by patients corresponded with various CanMEDS roles, that is, communicator, collaborator, professional, and leader. Feedback directed on task- and process-level would be of residents' interest, including feedback on the physician-patient relationship and communication of medical knowledge. Patient feedback should not only focus on communication skills but also on other CanMEDS roles. To provide effective feedback and ensure that it remains at the level that enhances residents' learning, patients should avoid giving feedback on self-level.

Keywords: patient feedback, residents' learning, postgraduate medical education, feedback levels, CanMEDS roles, patient feedback topics

1. Introduction

The healthcare system has put emphasis on patient-centered care [1] by empowering patients to have an active role, for example, by being involved in their personal care [2] and by contributing to improvement in the care process [3, 4]. Although patients have become increasingly involved in healthcare, their involvement in postgraduate medical education (PGME) is often less prominent. Whereas, patients' perspective and feedback on residents' performance could be valuable for enhancing residents' learning as well as the quality of healthcare in general [5]. Furthermore, expanding the involvement of patients in PGME would be in line with the current trends in healthcare. This study builds on the conception that patients are obvious members of the educational team in workplace-based learning. We aim at finding topics for patient feedback that patients and residents agree on.

Obviously, feedback and reflection are crucial aspects of residents' learning [6]. Residents receive feedback in the workplace-based learning environment, in which the relationships between patients, residents, and medical supervisors are essential [7]. Feedback is the result of observing performance and has the purpose to minimize the gap between the current performance and the desired goal [8]. Current feedback guidelines within PGME have put an emphasis on providing effective feedback for medical supervisors in order to enhance residents' learning [6, 9]. Medical supervisors give residents feedback on different competency roles based on the competency framework of the Canadian Medical Education Directives for Specialists (CanMEDS), to ensure that residents possess a range of various competencies [10]. On the other hand, Lai et al. noted additional feedback from patients as an educational tool to enhance the consultation skills of medical students as well [11]. Additionally, research has shown that patients can enlighten blind spots and suggest new opportunities for learning [12]. Furthermore, Crotty et al. reported the importance of patient feedback by means of OpenNotes in graduate medical education (GME) [13]. Whereby patients were able to look into the residents' notes and provide feedback. Although residents considered OpenNotes in GME effective, some concerns were made about the patient-doctor relationship [13].

Despite the value patients' feedback could potentially have for residents learning, there have been no studies to our knowledge that focused on the feedback topics that patients actually wish to provide feedback on in order to enhance residents learning. Studies so far have mainly focused on patient feedback regarding the communication skills of residents [3, 14–16], while medical training includes more competencies than communication skills alone [10, 17]. Even so, the current feedback systems that are in place within PGME also involve other dimensions/areas of clinical practice rather than communication skills only. Feedback from patients on other aspects of the medical profession might be valuable for learning as well. Additionally, little is known about both the patient feedback topics for resident enhancement and the effectiveness of feedback from patients.

The purpose of this study is to improve PGME by means of patient feedback. This study provides insights into both patients' and residents' perspectives regarding patient feedback topics, in order to increase its use and effectiveness in postgraduate medical education. Therefore, the research question answered in this study was: What are the feedback topics patients and residents provide for the development of patient feedback into PGME for the purpose of enhancing residents' learning?

2. Methods

2.1 Study design

In order to explore the potential content of patient feedback, a qualitative approach was chosen to investigate the perspectives of both patients and residents regarding patient feedback topics. Two different qualitative methods were used. The first perspective was gathered by means of semi-structured interviews to enable patients to explain their thoughts on patient feedback more in-depth as knowledge of patients' perspectives is limited [18, 19]. Whereas the perspective of residents was collected with the use of fully qualitative questionnaires. Qualitative questionnaires are used to collect qualitative data. The qualitative questionnaire consisted of a set of open-ended questions which allowed residents to write responses in their *own* words, instead of choosing from fixed response options. By means of this, residents' ideas on patient feedback topics were explored, while not investigating the depth [19, 20].

2.2 Setting

In order to ensure that residents possess a range of various different intertwined competencies, the CanMEDS competency framework is integrated with all PGME programs in the Netherlands [10, 21]. This framework consists of seven medical competency roles: medical expert, communicator, collaborator, health advocate, scholar, leader, and professional (**Table 1**) [10]. Residents receive feedback on these roles in order to become competent physician. This study was conducted at OLVG hospital in the Netherlands. This hospital is one of the largest teaching hospitals in the Netherlands facilitating more than 20 different PGME programs.

2.3 Sampling and recruitment

During the study period from January 2017 to May 2017, both patients and residents were sampled purposefully. Patients visiting the outpatient clinic of several departments were informed about this study and asked to participate by the main researcher (MN). After informed consent was given, the interview took place after

Competency roles	Example
Medical Expert	Disclosing patient history, performing physical examination, investigations, and setting up patient-centered management plan.
Communicator	Establish a relationship with their patients and their families in order to collect and share essential information for effective health care.
	Determine patient perspectives regarding their fears and thoughts about the disease/ treatment.
	Inform patients with the best available evidence and support patients in considering the best option.
Collaborator	Collaboration with patients, families, physicians, and other medical staff.
Leader	Contribute toward improving health care delivery by being involved in new developments.
	Demonstrate leadership in professional practice, manager planning, finances, and practice.
Health Advocate	Physicians are accountable to take responsibility for putting effort in order to improve patients' health and well-being.
Scholar	Engagement to excel in practice by continuously learning, teaching others, reflecting on evidence, and contributing to scholarship.
Professional	Demonstrate clinical competence devotion to continuous professional development.
	Commit to its own health and well-being in order to provide optimal care toward patients, including professional performance and managing influence on personal well-being.

Table 1.
CanMEDS competency roles examples.

their consultation with their medical doctor. During a resident lunch meeting, residents working at the OLVG hospital were also recruited face-to-face by the main researcher (MN). The researcher had no personal or professional ties with the participants or the medical doctors whose patients were approached. The sample size was not calculated prior to the study as we aimed for data sufficiency, which means that the data should be rich enough to answer the research question [22]. We determined data sufficiency by reaching a consensus with the research team.

2.4 Data collection

All in-depth interviews were performed with an interview guide, including example questions and probing questions (Appendix I). Frames were used in order to understand a patients' reasoning on feedback topics [18]. During the interview, the patient had the freedom to discuss their perspective on the topics they considered valuable to be discussed. Afterward, the interviews were summarized for member checking by the participants. All interviews were performed, audiotaped, and transcribed verbatim by the main researcher (MN). After transcription, the audiotapes were erased and the transcripts were anonymized.

To understand what feedback topics residents would like to receive from patients, qualitative questionnaires were handed out during a resident lunch meeting at OLVG hospital (Appendix II). The main researcher (MN) was present during completion of the questionnaires. The qualitative questionnaire consisted of six questions and took approximately 5 minutes to fill in. All questionnaires were anonymous as they did not require to fill out names.

2.5 Data analysis

A content analysis inspired by the grounded theory was used. Both the interview and questionnaire data were analyzed separately before comparison. To allow new insights, open, inductive coding was used. All transcripts were coded by the main researcher (MN). The analysis started immediately after the first interview. The transcripts were coded by attaching keywords ("codes") to all text fragments that were considered relevant to help answer the research question, subsequently, the codes were categorized. To enhance reliability, two interviews were analyzed by a second researcher (LB) using open coding and then discussed extensively. During this discussion, differences in interpretation were discussed and some codes were refined which led to the creation of the first version of the code tree. After coding 15 transcripts, no new codes were derived. The answers to the open-ended questions of the questionnaires were analyzed by the use of open coding as well. Subsequently, the derived codes were categorized, creating a separate code tree. Thereafter, the derived key themes from the interviews and questionnaire were discussed and compared in depth within the research team until a consensus was reached. All coding was performed using qualitative data analysis software (MaxQDA, version 12). We followed the consolidated criteria guidelines for reporting qualitative studies (COREQ) when writing the article [23].

After identifying the different feedback topics described by the participants, these topics were then categorized depending on which feedback level it is aimed at. Feedback can be aimed at a task level, which describes feedback about specific procedures and how well certain task is performed. Feedback on the process level is more specific to processes related to accomplishing a certain task. The self-level feedback describes feedback on the person's self, whereas self-regulation feedback includes interaction between control, confidence, and commitment [8, 9].

2.6 Ethical considerations

The study was approved by the ethical review board of OLVG hospital (WO 17–050). All participants received an information letter explaining the purpose and procedure of this study as well as the voluntary nature of participation. Informed consent was obtained from all patients.

3. Results

3.1 Participants

Between January 2017 and May 2017, 20 patients (n = 20) from OLVG hospital participated in this study. The participants were between the age of 21 and 74 years old, recruited from 12 different departments (**Table 2**) and half of them were female. The interviews lasted between 10 and 40 minutes. Four patients refused to participate due to lack of time or interest. A total of 15 residents, recruited from eight different departments, filled in the questionnaire (**Table 2**).

Below, the findings will be presented in two sections; patients' perspective and a residents' perspective, after which the two will be compared.

3.2 Patients' perspective

Generally speaking, all patients were able to put forward several topics for providing feedback to residents. However, it became apparent that patients who had mainly positive experiences with residents or other physicians had more difficulties providing topics compared to patients with rather negative experiences. Patients did not mention topics they prefer not to provide feedback on.

Involved department patients (n = 20)	Involved department residents (n = 15)
Cardiology	Cardiology
Ear, nose, and throat	Ear, nose, and throat
First aid	Internal medicine
Internal medicine	Lung disease
Lung diseases	Neurology
Neurology	Obstetrics & gynecology
Obstetrics & gynecology	Oncology
Orthopedics	Psychiatry
Pulmonary medicine	
Radiology	
Sport medicine	
Surgery	

Table 2.
Departments patients and residents were involved.

3.2.1 Involvement in medical decision making

Patients expressed that they wish to provide feedback on how a resident involves them in the process of medical decision making during which the resident gives them advice on the best options for treatments. They reported that they find it important that the final decision is up to them. This topic was explicitly mentioned because patients currently experience little room for shared medical decision-making.

"*The specialists must have all the knowledge to communicate what is best for the patient. And the patient, I think, must listen very carefully to what is being said. And weigh up the advice. [...] So yes, it is up to the patient I think to decide what he [or she] wants to do.*" (Male, cardiology department, interview 3).

3.2.2 Organizational matters

Patients mentioned waiting time as feedback residents can learn from. They have the feeling that the schedule is too tight. Ideally, patients also wish to provide feedback on making appointments and the hospital experience in general.

"*Well, I think there are a few key points which should be dealt with such as simple things like waiting time. Isn't the planning too tight? [...]there was a sign which said that the waiting time was approximately one hour, one and a half hours.*" (Male, pulmonary medicine department, interview 2).

3.2.3 Personal aspects

Additionally, patients wish to provide feedback on personal aspects such as a resident's representativeness, including a resident's personal hygiene. Furthermore, patients also mentioned their general attitude as well as their tone of voice and kindness.

"*No, not the appearance, but grooming. Yes, you could say something about that. Yes. It is very disturbing if a physician sweats a lot or smells, that's just unpleasant. You could say something about that.*" (Male, orthopedics department, interview 14).

3.2.4 Communication of medical knowledge

Patients also desire to provide feedback on a resident's ability to explain a diagnosis. The resident should be able to do this in understandable words and avoid medical jargon as much as possible. Patients also described transparency about medical uncertainties and guidance through the medical process as important topics for feedback. Patients would like to understand their medical condition and take its uncertainties into account when deciding on treatment options. However, residents do not need to explain everything in detail but should pay close attention to the information that concerns the patients and be honest about it. Furthermore, they find it important that physicians guide them and explain every action step by step in order for them to know what to expect.

"*They couldn't find anything on the MRI scan and they didn't explain further. I was overwhelmed by this. [...] I still had a lot of pain. [...] I don't think that's providing an explanation. [...] it is my body and I feel the pain.*" (Male, orthopedic department, interview 15).

3.2.5 The physician-patient relationship

Lastly, patients wish to provide feedback on the continuity of care. This involves topics such as seeing the same physician every visit and communication between physicians because it clearly influences the physician-patient relationship. Patients stated that residents should be aware of a patient's personal situation and take this into account when providing medical advice. In order to do that, residents should communicate well with each other in order to prevent patients to have to repeatedly explain their stories. Furthermore, patients find it important to provide feedback on how residents approach their patients, for example, whether a resident listens to them, takes them seriously, takes time during the consultation, and shows a real interest. In addition, patients preferred that a physician sees them as a human and not as a disease or a problem to be solved.

"It is very alienating when a physician looks at you as if you are a problem. As if you are not really there. As if the soul or the self in the body is not of interest anymore. But you are dealing with living creatures. [...] It is a human who has a problem and not a thing that's broken. I find that important." (Male, orthopedics department, interview 14).

3.3 Resident's perspective

3.3.1 Desired feedback topics

The residents mentioned physician-patient relationship and professional performance as an area they wish to receive feedback on from patients. This includes whether patients trust the resident, how the residents approach patients, and whether the patients feel the resident takes time for them. But also, whether the resident takes a patient seriously, listens to, and shows empathy toward the patient. Another area mentioned was the communication of medical knowledge, which involves giving understandable medical advice and if patients have the feeling that they can ask questions. Communication skills were also seen as a feedback topic residents would be interested in, such as information transfer, providing clear explanations, and breaking bad news.

3.3.2 Undesired feedback topics

While residents mentioned a variety of areas, they wish to receive feedback on, there are also a few areas they preferably wish not to receive feedback on from patients. These areas include feedback on their medical knowledge and personal aspects, such as the residents' kindness. Other areas mentioned were organizational matters, such as waiting time, facilities of the waiting room, the process of making appointments, and general aspects of the hospital they are working in such as the restaurant and interior design. Residents felt that these particular topics do not concern them.

3.4 Patients' feedback topics versus residents' feedback topics

When comparing both patients' and residents' perspectives regarding patient feedback topics clear similarities were seen (**Table 3**). For instance, communication of medical knowledge and the physician-patient relationship was desired feedback topics for both. However, differences between the two groups were identified as well.

	Feedback topic mentioned by...		
	Only patients	**Only residents**	**Patients and residents**
Desired feedback topics	• Involvement in medical decision making[B]	• Professional performance	• Communication of medical knowledge[A]
	• *Organizational matters*	• Physician-patient relationship[B]	
	• *Personal aspects*[C]		
Undesired feedback topics		• *Organizational matters*	
		• *Personal aspects*[C]	
		• Medical knowledge	

[A]*Task level.*
[B]*Process level.*
[C]*Self-level.*

Table 3.
Feedback topics mentioned by the participants. An overview of feedback topics mentioned by both patients and residents is presented along with the identified feedback levels. The feedback topics in italics represent topics about which patients and residents would or would not like to receive feedback, respectively.

While patients wish to provide feedback on organizational matters, such as waiting time, facilities of the waiting room, and process of making an appointment, residents wish not to receive feedback on any of these matters. Furthermore, patients also wish to provide feedback on personal aspects, such as kindness, representativeness, attitude, and tone of voice, whereas residents wish not to receive feedback on kindness either. Additionally, residents put forward their professionalism and medical knowledge as topics they would and would not like to receive feedback on, respectively. Both these topics were not pointed out by patients altogether.

3.5 Feedback level

For the purpose of residents' learning, the level of feedback provision has been identified as well (**Table 3**). Generally, patients intend to provide feedback at the task level, process level, and self-level, whereas residents do not wish to receive feedback at the self-level. Providing or receiving feedback at the self-regulation level was not mentioned by the participants altogether.

4. Discussion

4.1 Discussion

In this qualitative study, insights were gathered about both patients' and residents' perspectives regarding patient feedback topics. These insights may direct the development and involvement of patient feedback in PGME.

4.1.1 Feedback topics

Topics patients wish to provide feedback on, touch elements of the current competency framework of CanMEDS used in PGME. For instance, the communicator role (**Table 1**) which includes among others, listening to patients, taking a patient seriously, and taking enough time for patients are topics mentioned by both patients and residents as possible feedback topics [10]. Furthermore, both patients and residents put forward the value of feedback on the physician-patient relationship, including establishing trust, empathy exhibited toward a patient, and the ability to clearly explain medical knowledge and attitude toward the patient. Moreover, these topics were also identified by physicians as areas that could be changed and improved on when receiving feedback from patients making them suitable feedback topics to enhance a resident's learning [24].

In line with current trends in healthcare that put emphasis on shared decision-making and patient-centered care, the CanMEDS communicator role clearly describes that residents are ought to provide the best available evidence and support patients in their decision-making [3, 4, 10]. Indeed, patients have stated they would like to provide feedback on their involvement in the medical decision-making process. The fact that none of the residents mentioned shared decision-making or related topics in the questionnaire may be explained by cultural issues and their early phase in the development of professional identity [25].

Indeed, studies so far have either focused on residents' communication or interpersonal skills in light of patient feedback, assuming that patients can only provide feedback on these topics [3, 16, 24, 26, 27]. However, the results of this study have shown otherwise. For instance, patients also mentioned the continuity of care, which involves communication between physicians as well as seeing the same physician each visit, as an important topic to provide feedback on. Indeed, the importance of this subject is recognized in the collaborator role of CanMEDS. This role involves, among others, handing over patients' care safely to other physicians, whereby a sufficient transfer of written or verbal communication is used [10]. Although residents are trained in achieving this role, topics related to the continuity of care were not mentioned altogether. This might be explained by the fact that residents think that this could only be assessed and judged by their peers.

Although this study showed similarities between the desired feedback topics mentioned in both groups, a difference between the groups was found as well. Organizational matters, such as waiting times and the process of making an appointment, are something patients intend to provide feedback on to residents, while the latter wish not to receive feedback on this particular topic. At first glance, it may seem obvious that these topics do not concern a resident as it might not always be his or her responsibility alone. However, when looking at the leader role of CanMEDS (**Table 1**) it could be stated that residents are ought to take responsibility in organizational matters in order to improve healthcare delivery in general, which according to the CanMEDS framework involves management, financial matters and organizational matters (**Table 1**) [10].

Additionally, personal aspects were mentioned by patients to provide feedback on, that is, representativeness, tone of voice or attitude, and kindness. These aspects can be recognized in the CanMEDS role of professional as well as the role of communicator. The role of a professional particularly reflects on society's belief in physician's professionalism, which requires them to commit to their own personal health and well-being. Moreover, physicians are ought to demonstrate accountability toward society [10]. However, residents mentioned personal aspects as an undesired feedback topic. It might be argued that based on the CanMEDS roles as well as their accountability toward the public, residents should accept some feedback on personal aspects [10].

4.1.2 Feedback levels

The effectiveness of feedback depends on the level of feedback aimed at, and whether the given feedback is indeed similar to the feedback level a recipient wants to receive feedback on [8]. This study has also led to insights into what level patients intend to provide feedback and thereby helps to determine its effectiveness. First of all, patients intend to provide feedback at the task-level, which describes how well a certain task is performed, which is in line with what residents wish to receive feedback at. From the literature, we know that providing corrective feedback at this level enhances learning [8]. Therefore, patients' feedback at the task level might be effective to enhance residents' learning. Patients also intend to provide feedback at the process-level which describes the process needed in order to fulfill certain tasks [8, 9]. Residents wish to receive feedback at this level as well, suggesting patient feedback at this level may enhance residents' learning as well. Moreover, Hattie and Timperley (2007) argue that receiving feedback at this level enhances deeper learning as it is an effective way of shaping one's strategy [8]. Lastly, patients also intend to provide feedback at the self-level, which involves feedback at a personal level and includes statements about a resident, such as feedback on his or her attitude, representativeness, kindness, or tone of voice. However, providing feedback at this level generally contains little task-related information and has too little value of enhancing learning [6]. Indeed, residents in this study did not wish to receive feedback at self-level, suggesting that patients providing feedback at this level might not enhance residents' learning. As expected, feedback provision at the self-regulation level was not identified. This level describes the way residents learn, direct, and have applied previous feedback, something patients are unable to monitor over time.

4.1.3 Effectiveness of patient feedback

Residents did not wish to receive feedback on the self-level. Kluger and Denisi (2000) have shown that feedback directed on the self-level negatively affects one's performance [28]. If negative feedback is directed at the self-level, one may redirect attention to the self and become distracted from what matters, the task at hand [28]. Besides, it is important to take into account that the effectiveness of feedback might even be more influenced by the way it is delivered. Among others, effective feedback is delivered in an appropriate setting, specific, based on observation, and in nonjudgmental language [29]. Additionally, results have shown that patients who have had positive experiences with residents or physicians had difficulties providing feedback topics. Paternotte et al. (2017) also argued that patients who think positively about their physicians have difficulty reflecting on the consultation at a deeper level and provide feedback for improvement [28]. Others have also shown that these patients are not capable of providing critical feedback and are therefore less crucial to enhance change in a resident's behavior [30]. This suggests feedback from patients with rather positive experiences might be less effective in order to enhance residents' learning. Nevertheless, to ensure that residents obtain a variety of both positive and negative feedback from patients, it is recommended to involve a range of patients when seeking patient feedback. This could be achieved by assigning, for example, an assistant to collect feedback from patients instead of the residents or collect feedback regularly on a specific part of the day, for instance, a morning per month.

5. Conclusion

To our knowledge, this is the first study that explores which feedback topic patients wish to provide. In PGME, residents are medically trained based on the CanMEDS framework which includes seven different roles. Patients in this study were able to point out feedback topics that corresponded with various CanMEDS roles. It showed that patients and residents see possibilities to use patient feedback for competence development of residents on subjects other than the communicator role alone. To ensure that patients provide effective feedback, it is recommended to avoid feedback on the self-level and collect a diversity of feedback by involving a variety of patients when seeking feedback.

Currently, when patient feedback is sought, this is mainly focused on communication skills. However, in this study patients have provided potential feedback topics corresponding with four CanMEDS competency roles. This insight provides ground to extend the subjects on which feedback is sought from patients rather than a focus on communication skills alone. In order to provide effective feedback to residents and ensure that such feedback remains at the level that enhances residents' learning, it is recommended that patients avoid giving feedback at the self-level. To ensure that residents obtain a variety of both positive and negative feedback, it is recommended to involve a variety of patients when feedback is sought.

Acknowledgements

The authors wish to thank all the participating patients and residents for their input and the time they invested.

Conflict of interest

The authors declare no conflict of interest.

Appendices and nomenclature

PGME	postgraduate medical education
GME	graduate medical education

Author details

Mana Nasori[1*], Lindsay Bank[1] and Fedde Scheele[2]

1 Faculty of Sciences, Department of Healthcare Education, OLVG Hospital, Athena Institute for Transdisciplinary Research, VU University, Amsterdam, The Netherlands

2 Faculty of Sciences, Department of Healthcare Education, OLVG Hospital, Athena Institute for Transdisciplinary Research, VU University, Amsterdam UMC, Amsterdam, The Netherlands

*Address all correspondence to: mananasori@gmail.com

References

[1] Delaney LJ. Patient-centred care as an approach to improving health care in Australia. Collegian. 2018;**25**(1):119-123

[2] Candace Lind RN, Carla Ginn RN. Patient empowerment: An evolutionary concept analysis. International Journal of Caring Sciences. 2019;**12**(2):1-8

[3] Bogetz AL, Rassbach CE, Chan T, Blankenburg RL. Exploring the educational value of patient feedback: A qualitative analysis of pediatric residents' perspectives. Academic Pediatrics. 2017;**17**(1):4-8. [Internet]. DOI: 10.1016/j.acap.2016.10.020

[4] Park M, Lee M, Jeong H, Jeong M, Go Y. Patient-and family-centered care interventions for improving the quality of health care: A review of systematic reviews. International Journal of Nursing Studies. 2018;**87**:69-83

[5] Björklund K, Stenfors T, Nilsson G, Leanderson C. Learning from patients' written feedback: Medical students' experiences. International Journal of Medical Education. 2022;**13**:19

[6] Adkoli BV. The role of feedback and reflection in medical education. Journal of Basic, Clinical and Applied Health Science. 2018;**2**(1):34-40

[7] Dornan T, Conn R, Monaghan H, Kearney G, Gillespie H, Bennett D. Experience based learning (ExBL): Clinical teaching for the twenty-first century. Medical Teacher. 2019;**41**(10):1098-1105

[8] Hattie J, Timperley H. The power of feedback. Review of Educational Research. 2007;**77**(1):81-112

[9] Boor K, Teunissen PW, Brand PLP. Richtlijn feedback in de medische vervolgopleiding. Tijdschrift voor Medisch onderwijs. 2012;**30**(S2):37-42 [Internet] Available from: http://link.springer.com/10.1007/s12507-011-0033-9

[10] Frank JR, Snell L, Sherbino J, editors. CanMEDS 2015 Physician Competency Framework. Royal College of Physicians and Surgeons of Canada: Ottowa; 2015

[11] Lai MMY, Roberts N, Mohebbi M, Martin J. A randomised controlled trial of feedback to improve patient satisfaction and consultation skills in medical students. BMC Medical Education. 2020;**20**(1):1-10

[12] Haney S, Rowland P, Ginsburg S. Patients' perspectives on medical students' professionalism: Blind spots and opportunities. Medical Education. 2022;**56**(7):724-735

[13] Crotty BH, Anselmo M, Clarke DN, Famiglio LM, Flier L, Green JA, et al. Opening residents' notes to patients. Academic Medicine. 2016;**91**(3):418-426 [Internet] Available from: http://content.wkhealth.com/linkback/openurl?sid=WKPTLP:landingpage&an=00001888-201603000-00040

[14] Mitchell JD, Ku C, Wong V, Fisher LJ, Muret-Wagstaff SL, Ott Q, et al. The impact of a resident communication skills curriculum on patients' experiences of care. AA Case Rep. 2016;**6**(3):65-75

[15] Murante AM, Vainieri M, Rojas D, Nuti S. Does feedback influence patient-professional communication? Empirical evidence from Italy. Health Policy (New York). 2014;**116**(2-3):273-280

[16] Marsh M, Lauden SM, Mahan JD, Schneider L, Saldivar L, Hill N, et al. Family-centered communication:

A pilot educational intervention using deliberate practice and patient feedback. Patient Education and Counseling. 2021;**104**(5):1200-1205

[17] Mickelson J, MacNeily A. Translational education: Tools for implementing the CanMEDS competencies in Canadian urology residency training. Canadian Urological Association Journal. 2008;**2**(4):395

[18] Busetto L, Wick W, Gumbinger C. How to use and assess qualitative research methods. Neurological Research and Practice. 2020;**2**(1):1-10

[19] Braun V, Clarke V, Gray D. Innovations in qualitative methods. In: The Palgrave Handbook of Critical Social Psychology. London, UK: Springer; 2017. pp. 243-266

[20] Braun V, Clarke V, Gray D. Collecting textual, media and virtual data in qualitative research. In: Collecting Qualitative Data: A Practical Guide to Textual, Media and Virtual Techniques. Cambridge, UK: Cambridge University Press; 2017:1-12

[21] Federatie Medische Specialisten. Competentiegericht opleiden [Internet]. [cited 2019 Nov 24]. Available from: https://www.medischevervolgopleidingen.nl/

[22] Varpio L, Ajjawi R, Monrouxe LV, O'Brien BC, Rees CE. Shedding the cobra effect: Problematising thematic emergence, triangulation, saturation and member checking. Medical Education. 2017;**51**(1):40-50

[23] Tong A, Sainsbury P, Craig J. Consolidated criteria for reporting qualitative research (COREQ): A 32-item checklist for interviews and focus groups. International Journal for Quality in Health Care. 2007;**19**(6):349-357

[24] Reinders ME, Blankenstein AH, Van Der Horst HE, Knol DL, Schoonheim PL, Van Marwijk HWJ. Does patient feedback improve the consultation skills of general practice trainees? A controlled trial. Medical Education. 2010;**44**(2):156-164

[25] Spinnewijn L, Aarts J, Verschuur S, Braat D, Gerrits T, Scheele F. Knowing what the patient wants: A hospital ethnography studying physician culture in shared decision making in the Netherlands. BMJ Open. 2020;**10**(3):e032921

[26] Dubosh NM, Hall MM, Novack V, Shafat T, Shapiro NI, Ullman EA. A multimodal curriculum with patient feedback to improve medical student communication: Pilot study. The Western Journal of Emergency Medicine. 2020;**21**(1):115

[27] Mahoney D, Bogetz A, Hirsch A, Killmond K, Phillips E, Bhavaraju V, et al. The challenges of multisource feedback: Feasibility and acceptability of gathering patient feedback for pediatric residents. Academic Pediatrics. 2019;**19**(5):555-560

[28] DeNisi A, Kluger AN. Feedback effectiveness: Can 360-degree appraisals be improved? Academy of Management Executives. 2000;**14**(1):129-139

[29] Schartel SA. Giving feedback- an integral part of education. Best Practice & Research. Clinical Anaesthesiology. 2012;**26**(1):77-87

[30] Black N, Jenkinson C. Measuring patients' experiences and outcomes. BMJ. 2009;**339**(jul02 1):b2495-b2495 [Internet] Available from: http://www.bmj.com/cgi/doi/10.1136/bmj.b2495

Chapter 11

Perspective Chapter: Strengthening and Empowering Professional Health Educators' Capacity and Practice

Carol A. Cummings and Rosemary Reilly-Chammat

Abstract

Professional health education practice includes supporting and building **health literacy skills** needed to promote individual and community health and address barriers that inhibit the attainment of health. Mitigating poor health outcomes is where health and education converge. The Social Determinants of Health underscore the role of community contexts and community-driven approaches to address health disparities and the role of empowering and activating communities to that end. A comprehensive and social justice approach to health education in school and community settings helps all people develop health-promoting skills and values and is critical to educational success. This chapter aims to examine professional practice and development for health educators from a social justice lens that includes addressing inequities in health, and a growth mindset where professionals learn, apply skills, evaluate beliefs that hinder equitable learning, reflect, and improve competency and self-efficacy. Methodologies that drive more forward-thinking approaches for supporting effective practice across the lifespan are explored. The Whole School Whole Community Whole Child model, the World Health Organization Health Promoting Schools, and Health Literacy Skills will be used to frame opportunities to consider health education and the bidirectional influences to reinforce and reimagine the connections between education and health.

Keywords: health education, health literacy, health equity, health, health educator

1. Introduction

This chapter will focus on how supporting the learning and health of children and youth everywhere is essential for improving health outcomes and quality of life across the lifespan. Healthy children and youth learn better, and healthy children and youth grow into healthy adults [1–3]. Approaches that address not only the student but families, the whole school, and the community positively impacts academic achievement and health status. Using multiple approaches to address health disparities linked with inequities in education increases the ability to make healthy decisions and use health information and services [4].

The authors of this chapter will use the following questions to share our perspective on the field of health education and how empowering educators' capacity and practice improves health outcomes and educational success.

- What kind of health education do children and youth want?
- What do we owe children and youth, and what commitment should they expect from the educational system including teachers, administrators, school boards, policymakers, parents, and community organizations?
- Regardless of the setting, what should a visitor see or look for if they were to stand in the doorway of a health education classroom or workshop?

These questions may cause some trepidation because health education should not look the same for all audiences. However, we believe there are some main ideas that should always be considered when planning and teaching health education to children and youth, and when providing professional development for health educators.

2. The intersection between health and education

Let us start with, what we owe children and youth and the commitment they should expect from the educational system. The intersection of health and education, profoundly impacts well-being and quality of life. Research has shown this powerful connection, that education leads to improved health [5–7]. A gain in personal control and an increase in agency are two outcomes of education that positively impact personal health [8]. Education, both a process and a product occur in formal and informal (outside the school) settings provides children and youth with the knowledge, skills, and capacity to be healthy and productive as young people and in adulthood [9].

Children and youth, throughout the world should expect a commitment to their overall health and well-being and learning success through a comprehensive and coordinated approach. Two frameworks, that provide this approach are the United States (US) Centers for Disease Control and Prevention's Whole School, Whole Community, Whole Child Framework (WSCC) [10]. The other is the World Health Organization's (WHO) Health Promoting Schools (HPS) [11]. Frameworks create a context for the work that allows for site specific application based on the needs of the school community.

The WSCC framework puts the student at the center and the school and community surround and support the students. This model is built on the role the community has in supporting the school, the link between health and academic success, and the need for evidence-based school policies and practices [10]. The framework centers around the five tenets of the Whole Child: healthy, safe, engaged, supported, and challenged. Schools play a critical role in supporting healthy behaviors in school children. It is easier to establish good health practices in children than to try to change unhealthy behaviors in adulthood [5]. The 10 components of the WSCC model are found in **Table 1** and they mirror the HPS efforts outlined by the WHO [10, 11]. The WHO introduced the concept of a health-promoting school, a whole school approach, over 25 years ago, and the principles are based on eight global standards, which are also found in **Table 1**. These principles posit that for educational systems to be truly

U.S. CDC Whole School, Whole Community, Whole Child Framework (WSCC)	**WHO Health Promoting Schools Eight Global Standards (HPS Model)**
Five Tenants – Each student:	Six Pillars:
1. Healthy. enters school healthy and learns about and practices a healthy lifestyle.	1. healthy school policies,
2. Safe. learns in an environment that is physically and emotionally safe for students and adults.	2. healthy physical school environments,
3. Engaged. is actively engaged in learning and is connected to the school and broader community.	3. healthy school social environments,
4. Supported. Has access to personalized learning and is supported by qualified, caring adults.	4. health skills, and education,
5. Challenged. Each student is challenged academically and prepared for success in college or further study and for employment.	5. links with parents and the school community 6. access to school health services
Health education. "When provided by qualified, trained teachers, health education helps students acquire the knowledge, attitudes, and skills they need for making healthy decisions."	**School curriculum.** "The school curriculum supports physical, social–emotional and psychological aspects of student health and well-being." (Standard 5)
Nutrition environment and services. "School nutrition services provide students with opportunities to learn about and practice healthy eating."	
Physical education and physical activity. "Physical education helps students develop motor skills, knowledge, and behaviors."	
Health services. "School health services provide first aid, emergency care, and assessment of and planning for chronic conditions. In addition, services provide wellness promotion, referral to prevention services (such as HIV testing), and student and parent education. The services also ensure access or referrals to outside health care providers."	**School health services.** "All students have access to comprehensive school-based or school-linked health services that meet their physical, emotional, psychosocial, and educational health-care needs." (Standard 8)

Table 1.
A comparison of the US CDC whole school, whole community, whole child framework, and the WHO health promoting schools.

successful, they must commit to supporting and promoting the health and well-being of everyone linked to our schools including students, teachers, administrators, staff, and the community. In addition, there are bidirectional influences that impact health and well-being. For example, schools that have safe, supportive, and predictable environments are likely places where students report strong connections to staff and report that there are adults in the building who care about them.

In both the US and globally, the relationship between health and learning outcomes is being recognized more and more [11–13]. This became even more evident during the COVID-19 pandemic [14, 15]. Millions of children and youth shifted to online learning if they had the technology, and many were isolated from social, education, and supportive services and systems located in the schools. School closures, reliance on remote learning, learning loss, inequalities in educational systems, and mental health issues are examples of the impact the pandemic had on students' health and learning [16]. Healthy students are better learners and building capacity in schools for healthy living, learning, and working benefits everyone. The COVID-19 pandemic revitalized the importance and commitment to the linkages between education and health including unmet mental health needs and limited or no access to services.

Let us explore the similarities between the US CDC WSCC model, and the WHO HP model. Both approaches include collaboration across many sectors and levels. Key school, public health, government, and community stakeholders and leaders at the local, state, and national levels work together to coordinate policies, operations, and practices that champion health and learning outcomes for all students [10, 11]. The aim of both models is cohesive and collaborative efforts that are strategically planned and implemented between health, government, and educational sectors, and engage community stakeholders in the process. What does this mean? There is better coordination and access to services for students and their families, opportunity to address social determinants of health, more efforts to build students' health knowledge and skills and an inclusive learning environment, and a commitment to working together to improve and support student health and well-being. Both models provide guidance for implementing and sustaining this approach. In **Table 1**, you will notice, some of the similarities and differences. The HPS approach separates out three standards on government and school policies and school governance and leadership, which are woven through the WSCC model and are found in each of the 10 components [10, 11]. Each component of the whole child is distinct yet interconnected. If a school is challenging and does not feel safe and supportive, every child will not be able to reach their full potential. Schools that provide safe and supportive environments without challenging curricula will risk perpetuating a bias of low expectations.

Research on the impact of HPS and the WSCC models reveal improvements in health and learning outcomes [12, 17–20]. Findings reported included improved measures of depression, bullying, violence, sexual health knowledge and beliefs around gender equity for secondary students, and school and social connectedness decreased risky healthy behaviors including drug use and had a positive impact on mental health [17, 18]. Incorporating the WSCC model had led to changes in several US states' health education practices and policies where student health is more at the center of the education system, there is more support from policymakers and administrators, and community health organizations collaborate with the educational system better [20]. Finally, both modules are built on increasing health literacy skills in students and the larger community. Advancing health literacy skills increase the capacity for making health-related decisions and actions for oneself and others [21].

2.1 Takeaways: what is the significance for health educators? How do we continue to build our skills and improve our practice?

Both the WSCC and HPS frameworks provide a comprehensive public health approach for school health that supports the development of health literacy. Both link policies, programs, and practices to ensure school environments are healthy, safe, and supportive for all students and staff. While the WSCC model is child centered with a macro focus, the HPS is systems oriented. The WSCC models inner circle demonstrates how policies, programs and practices are connected. Individually, both provide a useful framework to consider robust and comprehensive school health efforts. Collectively, they are powerful tools to ensure that systems, policies, practices, and programs meet the health and academic needs of all students. We (health educators) can drive change and improve the quality and impact of health education on individuals, families, and communities by ensuring that there is a commitment and comprehensive approach to all health education efforts. This practice allows us to continue to learn about and reflect on, the value of incorporating components of national and global comprehensive models and determine if current policies, programs, and practices support health outcomes for all.

3. Health and health literacy

Health, a complex and multi-dimensional concept is built on behaviors that usually do not occur in a vacuum; and an array of variables influences one's health. There is no single consensus on the definition [22–24]. Establishing good health requires knowledge, skills, capacity, and resources at both the individual and community levels to support all the dimensions of health (physical, mental, social, political, economic, and spiritual) and remove the barriers to good health [23, 25]. Social determinants of health, the context in which people live, impacts health status and health outcomes. These determinants include a) health literacy skills and access to health care, b) educational attainment, c) where people live and work, d) job status, food security, and housing security, and e) a well-resourced healthy living environment (e.g., access to transportation, air, and water quality, safe neighborhoods) [26, 27]. Educational status has proven to be a predictor of health outcomes in the US and internationally [3, 25, 28].

Health literacy is an often-ignored social determinant of health [21]. This complex phenomenon focuses on providing individuals with the knowledge and skills to access and understand health information and services needed to make health-enhancing decisions for themselves, their family, and their community. Similar definitions of health literacy have been developed that provide further visualization of this concept and keywords used to define this term include confidence, empowerment, skills, a resource, and understanding of health messages [29–32]. Common to all these definitions is the expectation that health literacy means more than having knowledge or understanding of health content, but also enacting a healthy lifestyle by acting on knowledge and skills.

These skills are developed over a lifetime and enable individuals to use information gained for making well-informed decisions that lower health risks and promote quality of life [33]. Health education focused on health literacy not only helps children and youth adopt and maintain healthy behaviors, but they also learn to become self-regulated learners, critical thinkers, problem solvers, productive citizens, and effective communicators [34]. Further, leading with health literacy, within the WSCC framework highlights the importance of environments that support health enhancing behaviors. Health education programs need to be developed within the context of the whole school environment. Across the world, the development of health literacy skills in students improves health outcomes, reduces health risks, and increases academic success [35] Health literacy skills enable learners to "know and do."

The US federal government Healthy People 2030, health objectives for the nation recently updated the definition of health literacy for individuals and organizations [36]. Health literacy is the degree to which individuals can find, understand, and use information and services to inform health-related decisions and actions for themselves and others. Organizational health literacy is the degree to which organizations equitably enable individuals to find, understand, and use information and services to inform health-related decisions and actions for themselves and others [37]. Acquisition of health literacy skills represents a shift away from health content exclusively, to the development of skills to support healthy lifestyles inclusive of accessing scientifically accurate and developmentally appropriate health information.

Reading proficiency at the fourth-grade level is another Healthy People 2030 indicator. This measure underscores the importance of a literate population overall. Fourth grade reading proficiency includes the ability to comprehend and apply information. It is an important development point in the acquisition of literacy skills. Further children who struggle with fourth grade reading skills are more likely to struggle academically throughout their schooling. Youth who struggle academically are more likely to engage in risky behaviors. While, this relationship is not correlational, there is concordance across those domains [1].

The new definition of health literacy, emphasizing the use of health information from a public health perspective, is intended to prompt new ways of studying and promoting personal health literacy. It offers a focus on skills to help people move from an understanding of concepts and content to individual action and a focus on health within communities. Further quality school health education that emphasizes skills that teaches students how to learn about their health, how to use skills that have utility across various facets of life, and why these skills are important is foundational to health literacy [38]. Academic missions, structures, and systems need to align to support effective school health education versus as an add-on [39]. Health education is a distinct subject from physical education. Dual certification in both subjects requires sound preservice preparation in both disciplines. This needs to inform preservice programs in health education as well as state certification requirements [40]. Health education has also been identified by the US Department of Health and Human Services as a mechanism for building health literacy [21].

3.1 Takeaways: what is the significance for health educators? How do we continue to build our skills and improve our practice?

When health literacy skills are considered outcomes of the health education and school health programs, student health literate citizenry is advanced. Health literacy is supported by a skills-based health education approach. As health educators, we should be committed to this goal, student health literacy citizenry and our collective practice should reflect this commitment at the national, state, and community level.

4. Health education

In both school and community settings, health education, takes many different forms yet is built on similar principles and understanding. Educating for health means planning authentic learning experiences to support learners' and communities' development of the health skills essential for adopting and maintaining health-enhancing behaviors [23, 41, 42]. These planned efforts should be equitable and allow learners to a) adjust new learning and skills to their lived experiences without compromising healthy outcomes, b) acquire functional knowledge (essential health facts and concepts), and c) apply evidence-based and evidence-informed practices. Learners can learn and practice health skills to build the self-efficacy and agency necessary for maintaining a healthy life. Health education is also described as efforts to improve health literacy skills, health information and other health skills, and voluntary behaviors that promote health outcomes in individuals, groups, and communities [43]. One of the Core Beliefs of the American School Health Association is, "Core Belief 1:

Health and learning are directly linked and essential to the development of healthy, resilient citizens. Academic success is an excellent indicator of the overall well-being of youth and a primary predictor of adult health outcomes. This belief addresses the issue of disparities and the achievement gap and offers solutions" [44].

Schools, where children and youth learn, and grow are one of the best settings for health education. Frameworks like the WSCC model, the WHO HPS model, and United Nations Educational Scientific and Cultural Organization's (UNESCO) education for health and wellbeing approach demonstrate the importance of student-centered learning focused on well-being and dignity, engaging all stakeholders (learners, teachers, and administrators, parents, the community, etc.), and providing health education to promote student health, well-being and academic achievement [1, 10, 11] UNESCO's approach specifically focuses on the intersectionality of health, education, and gender equality. However, they all emphasize school health education as a fundamental part of a much broader school program that supports learners' health, well-being, and academic achievement.

In the US, the National Health Education Standards guide and drive comprehensive school health education throughout the nation [45, 46]. These standards assist schools and health educators with planning curriculums and lessons around functional knowledge to support acquisition of health skills. Building these health skills advances health literacy where students are more adept at accessing and navigating health information, supports, and services in ways that are health enhancing. Health education strives to create learning experiences that promotes individual, family and community health. This is the goal of health education or the end in mind when building curriculums and planning lessons. The eight standards which serve as a guide for health educators can be found in **Table 2**.

Health education in US schools, pre-kindergarten through 12th grade, and in community settings is taught across many health topics, and comprehensive and

National Health Education Standards	
What students will **KNOW an BE ABLE TO Do** following a health education lesson or unit.	
Planning with the END in MIND – Health Literacy	
Standard 1 - Know Functional Knowledge	Students will **comprehend concepts** related to health promotion and disease prevention to enhance health. (Functional Knowledge)
Standard 2 - Do Health Skill	Students will **analyze the influence** of family, peers, culture, media, technology, and other factors on health behaviors.
Standard 3 - Do Health Skill	Students will demonstrate the ability to **access valid information, products, and services** to enhance health.
Standard 4 - Do Health Skill	Students will demonstrate the ability to **use interpersonal communications skills** to enhance health and avoid or reduce health risks.
Standard 5 - Do Health Skill	Students will demonstrate the ability to **use decision-making skills** to enhance health.
Standard 6 - Do Health Skill	Students will demonstrate the ability to **use goal setting** to enhance health.
Standard 7 - Do Health Skill	Students will demonstrate the **ability to practice health-enhancing behaviors** to avoid or reduce health risks.
Standard 8 – Do Health Skill	Students will demonstrate the **ability to advocate for personal, family, and community health.**

Table 2.
National Health Education Standards.

US CDC's Healthy Schools Characteristics of an Effective Curriculum
1.Focuses on clear health goals and related behavioral outcomes.
2.Research-based and health behavior and learning theory-driven.
3.Addressed values, attitudes, and beliefs.
4.Addresses individuals and group norms that support health-enhancing behaviors.
5.Reinforces protective factors and increasing one's perception of personal risk and harmfulness linked with unhealthy practices and behaviors.
6.Addresses social pressures and influences.
7.Builds personal competence, social competence, and self-efficacy through development of health skills.
8.Provides functional knowledge that is basic, accurate, and directly contributes to health-promoting decisions and behaviors.
9.Uses strategies to personalize information, engage students and provide opportunities to practice health skills.
10.Provides age-appropriate and developmentally appropriate information, learning strategies, teaching methods, and materials.
11.Incorporates culturally inclusive learning strategies, teaching methods, and materials.
12.Provides adequate time for instruction and learning include time to practice.
13.Provides opportunities to reinforce skills and positive health behaviors
14.Provides opportunities to make positive connections with influential others.
15.Includes professional development to enhance teaching and learning.

Table 3.
The US CDC's healthy schools characteristics of an effective curriculum [46].

effective curriculums are encouraged. The US Healthy People Objectives, which guide efforts to improve health outcomes, include objectives for increasing health education courses for students in grades six through twelve and increasing health literacy among populations of all ages [47]. School leadership should view health education as a vital link between student health and academic success. The US CDC's characteristics of an effective curriculum (**Table 3**) and UNESCO's strategy on education for health and well- being further unpack vital components of health education programs [3, 46]. UNESCO developed an educational strategy to support health and well-being. "To achieve a vision where all learners can fulfill their potential, UNESCO will:

- Create and support school systems that promote physical and mental health
- Empower learners with good quality comprehensive sexuality education that includes HIV, life skills, family, and rights; and
- Nurture safe and inclusive learning environments that are free from all forms of violence, bullying, stigma, and discrimination."

Examples of UNESCO program elements including the importance of a) children and youth learning to building healthy, respectful and gender-equitable relationships, b) teacher training and development, c) gender equality and comprehensive sexual health education; d) the value of online learning; and e) inclusive education and safe inclusive learning environments.

4.1 Takeaways: what is the significance for health educators? How do we continue to build our skills and improve our practice?

Development of learners' functional knowledge and health skills, along with the characteristics of effective health education curriculums should guide our work as health educators. These characteristics enable conditions to drive implementation with an emphasis on skills infused with developmentally appropriate and scientifically accurate health content. We need to keep this in mind when developing, implementing, and evaluating health education lessons, unit, and programs.

5. Educating for health and health education pedagogy

Education for health empowers people and communities and occurs on a global level. A constructivist and social justice approach using the socio-ecological model as a lens is a foundational core for framing education for health [48–50]. Learners build and co-construct knowledge in a social setting through engaging learning activities. Social constructivism considers that learners obtain knowledge through socialization, however; various cultures would result in different learning and produce very different narratives. The socio-ecological model (SEM) posits that factors shape an individual's health status, related behaviors, and choices at the intrapersonal, interpersonal, organizational, community, and policy levels [50]. Health education practice is best when learning is dynamic and interactive. Students learn in groups or with a partner, share prior knowledge, curiosities, and assets, and knowledge. Health education practice has historically examined health equity issues through needs assessment and learning experiences that foster voluntary health-related behavioral and social change.

A culturally responsive teaching approach where students make meaningful connections between learning, their cultures, and life experiences, increases students' ownership of learning [51, 52]. Educators use cultural responsiveness to guide and elevate their practice and help students build their own person agency, so they have a more direct influence over health promoting actions. Understanding the identities and challenges students experience, and that cultivating learners' cultural assets improves learning because students feel seen and heard [52]. Too often the power in the educator-learner bond is with the educator, and the experience, knowledge, and ideas of the learner are assumed or disregarded.

Health education supports engaged citizenry, which takes many forms including individual and group actions aimed at addressing problems that are of public interest and concern. Health literate people are focused not only on improving and maintaining their own health but also on the health of others. What does this mean? Incorporating social justice into health education provides opportunities for higher-order critical thinking skills as well as engaging pedagogical practices. Addressing social determinants of health in education allows for inclusion of underlying social justice issues that influence health such as racism, xenophobia, sexism, heterosexism, transphobia, ableism, ageism, and income and wealth disparities [53]. The National Academies of Medicine's call to action stresses the upstream, systems-level changes that strengthen the integration of both health literacy and school health education to improve the health of future generations [54]. For example, using school level data to advocate for policies, programs, and practices to create equitable environments. We know that students identifying as Lesbian, Gay, Bisexual, Transgender, Queer or Questioning (LGBTQQ) experience bullying more than their heterosexual identifying peers. Students may recommend the development or strengthening of Gay, Straight Alliances or other groups that support understanding and acceptance of all students [55].

Health educators must also be adept working with adult learners. This group wants to know the "why," behind learning about a particular issue or topic, are more self-directed than younger groups, and learning should involve them in the planning and be relevant to their lives [56]. Pedagogical approaches or health education planning should ensure learning goals are linked to learners needs and interests and incorporate the learners' life experience and knowledge into the learning environment.

5.1 Health education in schools

What should school health education look like? When should children first start developing health literacy skills? An ecological approach to health literacy acknowledges that the development of these skills is influenced by factors that interact and affect health behavior and ultimately health status. For example, parents and guardians initiate this learning through indirect (modeling, establishing value systems and standards) and direct learning (intentional conversations) during their time together. These individual and social environmental factors, which include social networks, organizations, communities, and populations, should be targets for interventions aimed at improving health status [50]. Schools are one of the primary places for the delivery of current, engaging, well-planned health education lessons and curricula. Developing health literacy skills through school-based efforts should commence during the pre-school years and continue until high school graduation [37, 57]. Hu et al. [58] found that health education, focusing on nutrition, for both kindergarten children and their parents, significantly improved healthy eating behaviors. This evidence supports the role school-based health education efforts can have on student learning. Healthy students will engage in learning better and learning about how to stay healthy keeps students healthy. As individuals become more adept with these health literacy skills, confidence in accessing and navigating literate environments will increase along with self-efficacy [59].

As stated in a previous section, effective planning for school health education begins with this end in mind: Health Literacy. This approach emphasizes that students should learn about and practice healthy behaviors while at school [34]. As active participants in learning, students build critical thinking, communication, problem-solving, and other skills that support health.

There are many learning strategies or activities to consider when planning health education. In the US elementary schools, classroom teachers may serve as the health educator. Some health topics are easily integrated into other subject areas such as English Language Arts, Math, and Science. In others, health education is a stand-alone content area. We would suggest that the approach is secondary to the intentionality of implementation of one approach or a combination of approaches. First and foremost, is to ask yourself, what is the purpose of the health education lesson? What learning outcomes do I want my learners to achieve by the end of the lesson, unit, or program? What health education standards or skills are my learners working toward achieving? Once these questions are answered, the health educator can then explore the various learning strategies. Health education professional preparation and ongoing professional development need to be based on a meaningful approach to skills-based health education [40].

When the selection of learning strategies is based on learner engagement centered on the emergence of agency that builds on lived experiences, there is room for building trust between the educator and students, critical thinking, and student and community voice. In practice, the health educator should purposefully intent for students, along with themselves, to grow during the learning process. Learning should be interactive where students learn in groups or with a partner, share prior knowledge, curiosities, and assets, and knowledge is perceived as dynamic and changes with our experiences [51, 60, 61]. We recommend the following when selecting learning strategies:

a. Be purposeful and intentional when selecting engaging learning strategies that allow for developing functional knowledge, and learning, practicing and mastering health literacy skills outlined in the national health education standards [62]. There are a multitude of strategies to select from that allow learners to accomplish learning outcomes. These strategies should address the cultural composition of the group, resonate with students of all sexual orientations and gender identities, bear in mind learners' literacy levels, and represent diverse groups. Participatory methods allow learners to observe, model, and practice health skills in authentic contexts. Student centered learning strategies put the student at the center of constructing their learning and the health educator facilitates from the outside. In small or large groups, students are actively participants in their learning. This could be through student choice projects, brainstorming (in-person or online), role plays, gallery walks, online or in-person discussion groups, games, or collaborative work, interviewing others, case studies, creating personal, family or community health plans, using social media to address a health issue, share family or cultural health stories through a media composition, research common solutions and create new way to solve a health problem, etc.

b. Plan for and present intention questions that require critical thinking. This allows learners to take charge of their learning, ask questions, and become problem solvers [60]. How do you know this, how would you think differently if you had another perspective, do you agree or disagree and why, does everyone act that way, why or why not, what questions would you ask if you could meet this person, is there a better solution to this problem? Giving learners opportunity to think about their thinking help construct new knowledge and skills.

c. Provide opportunity to determine students' prior knowledge or what the students know about a health topic, or what they want to learn. This helps pique and restore interest. What questions or hypotheses do students have about this topic?

d. Identify ways to personalize learning to maximize student engagement and ownership of learning [63]. Examples include support or scaffolding students based on learning competency through conferencing and small group work, self-paced assignments, and giving students choice in what they will learn and how they will learn. These efforts allow students to develop more agency during in-person and online learning. The educator meets them where they are, which helps maximize learning.

e. Allow students to express what they are experiencing when learning. What are they thinking, noticing, feeling?

f. Provide students with time to make sense of thoughts, revelations, or discoveries as they relate to their lives. How are they different because of what they have learned?

g. Make time to give feedback, which allows the health educator to address misunderstandings and improve practice while learning from the student.

h. Wierman [64] identified 5 brain-based learning strategies to boost learning, retention and focus including the creation of a safe and supportive learning environment, establishing turn and talk time to enable students to process information and skill development; incorporate visual elements that support topical areas, break learning into chinks and incorporate movement into lessons.

5.2 Takeaways: what is the significance for health educators? How do we continue to build our skills and improve our practice?

We need to remain learner centered in our planning and educating. Our practice should incorporate personalizing learning for our students as much as possible and acknowledge what our students brings to the learning relationship. When we can help our students build or construct their health knowledge and health literacy skills, they deliberately add new knowledge to their previous knowledge. This elevates them to a more powerful degree of knowing and doing. We need to design lessons and experiences that actively engage them as learners. As health educators, we should learn with our students, earn their trust as they share knowledge, ideas, aspirations, fears, and success.

6. The health education profession and ongoing professional development

The formation of a health educator's professional identity is not static and should evolve with continued efforts to grow and change as a learner, educator, and leader. In today's world, the health education landscape needs educators to create opportunities for learners to freely exchange ideas to share stories, discipline knowledge, and new learnings [40, 51] Health education across the globe centered on the emergence of learner agency that builds on lived experiences as mechanisms for improving health outcomes can transform learning by creating space for individual and community voice.

Developing functional knowledge needed for the profession and examining the complexities of health behavior and promoting health on an intrapersonal, interpersonal, institutional, and community level are fundamental concepts that health educators must employ. In the US, The National Commission for Health Education Credentialing (NCHEC) designated eight responsibilities for health educators and each responsibility has competencies and sub-competencies [65]. The eight areas are a) Area I: Assessment of Needs and Capacity, b) Area II: Planning, c) Area III: Implementation, d) Area IV: Evaluation and Research, e) Area V: Advocacy, f) Area VI: Communication, g) Area VII: Leadership and Management, and h) Area VIII: Ethics and Professionalism. Professionals responsible for implementing health education and health promotion should understand health literacy and its impact on health outcomes. Health literacy is embedded in several of the health education specialists' professional areas of responsibility. The health education and health promotion profession, in the US and globally, strive to provide an impetus for change to promote health-literate individuals and organizations [66].

What constitutes quality professional development? We in believe professional development that allows for a growth mindset approach, where professionals learn, apply skills, evaluate beliefs that hinder equitable learning, reflect, and improve competency. Safe learning formats should allow for health educators to explore personal perspectives and vulnerabilities. Professional development models where educators learn, analyze, dialog, assess competence with standards, and evaluate beliefs improve self-efficacy. Ollis [67] and Bogler [68] demonstrated that professional development had favorable results on teacher self-efficacy and that training increased perceived self-efficacy in pedagogical methods and subjects taught. Learning opportunities focused on capacity-building support educator self-efficacy.

Professional development can take the form of in-person learning, online learning, online communities, and access to online resources and tools. Addressing learner and professional teaching standards is critical for successful professional development. Resources and effective strategies for addressing barriers, including comfort with health education topics, personal perspectives, should also be covered. These efforts and support for self-reflection and growth will increase self-efficacy and educator agency. The following professional development recommendations can serve to build health educators' capacity and continue to improve practice [69].

1. Gauge health educators' professional development interests, needs, and ideas including formats for learning.

2. Select professional development formats to maximize engagement and buy-in, develop deep content knowledge, apply, and practice pedagogical skills, and include a variety of learning methodologies.

    a. Examples include independent self-study, video analysis, case study, professional learning communities (where we all contribute to learning while gaining knowledge and skills), observing a lesson, coaching, peer observation and feedback.

3. Create your professional development with clear outcomes that identify the expected results of professional learning.

4. Assess health educators' strengths, comfort and confidence with health topics, populations, and pedagogies, using a growth mindset approach. How can we reflect on how we view our own growth and failures as opportunities to learn and do better? What makes us uncomfortable with teaching health education? Why is it important to disclose what we know to each other?

5. Incorporate learning and using technology in health education. More research is being conducted to determine the values of how technology can support health education learning [70, 71].

6. Plan for and cultivate a professional development setting where health educators learn through sharing, talking, building, collaborating, practicing new skills, and leading.

7. Provide a forum where health educators' voices are heard.

8. Include learning and discussion on best practices and research backed health education and learning strategies for learning success.

a. Include opportunities to continue master planning for authentic health education lessons based on standards and skills development that foster health literacy and well-being.

b. Identify pedagogical skills and learning strategies that engage learners in higher-order thinking. Example include having educators participate in a variety of educational activities and report on what they learned and if participation raised any questions. Have them evaluate self-efficacy with implementing

c. Pose the following questions: What does learning really look like? What does it mean for a student to meet the learning outcomes (objective)?

9. Plan for opportunity for health educators to personalize learning, practice new skills including reflective practice, and create a support plan.

10. Pose the following questions: How has your identity as a professional health educator evolved? What do you need to continue to cultivate your identity formation and reflective practitioner practice?

11. Create space where health educators critically think about and formulate ways to best acknowledge their learners. How can they continue to recognize the strengths and contributions their learners can make and not focus solely on deficits.

12. Conduct assessments of professional development to learn if outcomes were met, garner support for future opportunities and make changes based on feedback.

    a. Explore and identify contacts for support, ideas, and collaborations. These include colleagues, professional associations, non-profit, community and government organizations.

Provide opportunities to learn from and collaborate with international health educators and professionals. Some examples are provided in the **Table 4** below.

6.1 Takeaways: what is the significance for health educators? How do we continue to build our skills and improve our practice?

Professional development for health educators should focus on capacity building and not fixing deficits. Opportunities should build comfort, develop deep content knowledge, apply, and practice pedagogical skills and engage learners. We should expect and demand for opportunities to build the skills necessary for planning and implementing effective and engaging health education lessons or interventions. Identify your partners that can support your efforts. Health education professionals should consider joining professional associations to support your practice. This will connect you to like-minded professionals nationally and across the globe.

American School Health Association	International Union for Health Promotion and Education	Society for Public Health Education	Global Health Education
American Public Health Association (APA)	National Commission for Health Education Credentialing	Society of Health and Physical Educators	World Health Organization
AAHE	Society of State Leaders of Health and Physical Education	APA Public Health Education and Health Promotion	

Table 4.
US and international professional health education associations.

7. Conclusion: next steps and looking forward

How do we continue to inform key stakeholders and the larger community that health education creates opportunities for improved health and well-being? Healthier students learn better and poor health impacts educational attainment [72, 73]. We much continue to engage in this ongoing work to link the health and education sectors. We must create cohesion and alignment at the national, state, community, and school levels and use a more comprehensive model for health education. There are great benefits in using the WSCC and UNESCO model to continuously develop and refine coordinated school health efforts that support rigorous health and education outcomes for all youth. This can reverse the causality. As we move to create more health-literate societies in our countries and beyond, we must stay vigilant to the conditions of individuals and communities lives that impact both health and education. Health literacy is one of the social determinants of health. This work along with the implementation of skills-based health education can inform pedagogical practices that address the social determinants of health and create environments that support healthy literacy and healthy behaviors for all.

Now more than ever, there is a need for highly qualified health educators. Building confidence and competence in our health educators' practice improves health outcomes for all. We must invest in high quality preservice education and ongoing professional development to support the growth of all health educators. The WSCC model and the HPS model should be used to frame opportunities to consider health education and the bidirectional influences on each component of the model to reinforce and reimagine the connections between education and health. We anticipate that ongoing opportunities to connect health education and social justice will continue to evolve. We look forward to new learning that enables conversion of these relevant domains to improve delivery of health education. Continuing to create systems, policies and practices that put students and their health at the center of the educational system builds health literate individuals and thus, a health literate society.

Conflict of interest

The authors declare no conflict of interest.

Author details

Carol A. Cummings[1*] and Rosemary Reilly-Chammat[2]

1 Rhode Island College, Providence, RI, United States

2 Rhode Island Department of Elementary and Secondary Education, Providence, RI, United States

*Address all correspondence to: ccummings@ric.edu

References

[1] Hawkins GT, Lee SH, Michael SL, et al. Individual and Collective Positive Health Behaviors and Academic Achievement Among U.S. High School Students, Youth Risk Behavior Survey 2017. American Journal of Health Promotion. 2022;**36**(4):651-661. DOI: 10.1177/08901171211064496

[2] Murray NG, Low BJ, Hollis C, Cross AW, Davis SM. Coordinated school health programs and academic achievement: A systematic review of the literature. The Journal of School Health. 2007;**77**:589-600

[3] United Nations Educational, Scientific and Cultural Organization [UNESCO]. UNESCO Strategy on Education for Health and Well-Being. Paris: France: United Nations Educational, Scientific and Cultural Organization; 2022

[4] Centers for Disease Control and Prevention [CDC], National Center for Chronic Disease Prevention and Health Promotion. Social Determinants of Health: Achieving Health Equity by Addressing the Social Determinants of Health. Updated 19 May 2022. Available from: https://www.cdc.gov/chronicdisease/programs-impact/sdoh.htm

[5] Centers for Disease Control and Prevention. CDC Healthy Schools. Updated. 21 Jun 2022. Available from: https://www.cdc.gov/healthyschools/index.htm

[6] National Academies of Sciences, Engineering, and Medicine. Promoting Positive Adolescent Health Behaviors and Outcomes: Thriving in the 21st Century. Washington, DC: The National Academies Press; 2020. DOI: 10.17226/25552

[7] Hawkins JD, Kosterman R, Catalano RF, Hill KG, Abbott RD. Effects of social development intervention in childhood fifteen years later. Archives of Pediatrics & Adolescent Medicine. 2008;**162**(12):1133-1141. DOI: 10.1001/archpedi.162.12.1133

[8] Mirowsky J, Ross CE. Education learned effectiveness and health. London Review of Education. 2005;**3**:205-220

[9] Hahn RA, Truman BI. Education improves public health and promotes health equity. International Journal of Health Services: planning, administration, evaluation. 2015;**45**(4):657-678. DOI: 10.1177/0020731415585986

[10] Birch D, Videto D. Promoting Health and Academic Success: The Whole School, Whole Community, Whole Child Approach. Champaign, IL: Human Kinetics; 2015

[11] World Health Organization and UNESCO. Making every School a Health-Promoting School: Global Standards and Indicators. Geneva: World Health Organization and UNESCO; 2021

[12] Basch CE. Healthier students are better learners: A missing link in school reforms to close the achievement gap. Journal of School Health. 2011;**81**(10):593-598

[13] Owen KB, Parker PD, Astell-Burt T, Lonsdale C. Regular physical activity an educational outcome in youth: A longitudinal study. The Journal of Adolescent Health. 2018;**62**(3):334-340

[14] United Nations. Policy Brief: Education during COVID-19 and beyond. NY: United Nations; 2020

[15] Nearchou F, Flinn C, Niland R, Subramaniam SS, Hennessy E. Exploring the impact of COVID-19 on mental health outcomes in children and adolescents: A systematic review. International Journal of Environmental Research and Public Health. 2020;**17**(22):8479

[16] Engzell P, Frey A, Verhagen MD. Learning loss due to school closures during the COVID-19 pandemic. Proceedings of the National Academy of Sciences of the United States of America. 2021;**118**(17):e2022376118. DOI: 10.1073/pnas.2022376118

[17] Shinde S, Weiss H, Varghese B, Khandeparkar P, Pereira B, Sharma A, et al. Promoting school climate and health-related outcomes: A cluster randomized controlled trial of the SEHER multi-component secondary school intervention in Bihar, India. Lancet. 2018;**392**(10163):2465-2477

[18] Bond L, Butler H, Thomas L, Carlin J, Glover S, Bowes G, et al. Social and school connectedness in early secondary school as predictors of late teenage substance use, mental health, and academic outcomes. The Journal of Adolescent Health. 2007;**40**(4):357.e9-357.18

[19] Johnson Chiang R, Meagher W, Slade S. How the whole school, whole community, whole child model works: Creating greater alignment, integration, and collaboration between health and education. Journal of School Health. 2015;**85**(11):775-784

[20] Rasberry C, Slade S. Lohrmann D, & Valois R lessons learned from the whole child and coordinated school health approaches. Journal of School Health. 2015;**85**(11):759-765

[21] U.S. Department of Health and Human Services, Office of Disease Prevention and Health Promotion. National Action Plan to Improve Health Literacy. Washington, DC: National Academies Press; 2010

[22] Sartorius N. The meanings of health and its promotion. Croatian Medical Journal. 2006;**47**(4):662-664

[23] Sharma M. Theoretical Foundations of Health Education and Health Promotion. Burlington, MA: Jones & Bartlett Learning; 2022

[24] Simons-Morton BG, KR ML, Wendel ML. Behavior Theory in Health Promotion Practice and Research. Sudbury, Mass: Jones & Bartlett Learning; 2012

[25] Zimmerman EB, Woolf SH, Blackburn SM, Kimmel AD, Barnes AJ, Bono RS. The case for considering education and health. Urban Education. 2018;**53**(6):744-773. DOI: 10.1177/0042085916682572

[26] Centers for Disease Control and Prevention. Social Determinants of Health: About Social Determinants of Health (SDOH). Updated 10 Mar 2021. Available from: https://www.cdc.gov/socialdeterminants/about.html

[27] U.S. Department of Health and Human Services, Office of Disease Prevention and Health Promotion. Social Determinants of Health: What Are Social Determinants of Health? (n.d.). Available from: https://health.gov/healthypeople/priority-areas/social-determinants-health

[28] Montez JK, Berkman LF. Trends in the educational gradient of mortality among U.S. adults aged 45 to 84 years: Bringing regional context into the explanation. American Journal of Public Health. 2014;**104**(1):e82-e90

[29] Australian Bureau of Statistics. Health Literacy. Australia: ABS

Publication No. 4233.0: Australian Bureau of Statistics; 2006

[30] Canadian Public Health Association. A Vision for a Health Literate Canada: Report of the Expert Panel on Health Literacy. Ontario, Canada: Canadian Public Health Association; 2008

[31] Nutbeam D. The evolving concepts of health literacy. Social Science & Medicine. 2008;**67**(12):2072-2078

[32] Kickbusch I, Pelikan J, Apfel F, Tsouros, A. Health literacy: the solid facts. World Health Organization Regional Office for Europe Copenhagen: Denmark; 2013. Available from: https://apps.who.int/iris/handle/10665/326432

[33] Zarcadoolas C, Pleasant AF, Greer DS. Advancing Health Literacy: A Framework for Understanding and Action. New Jersey: Jossey Bass; 2006

[34] Joint Committee on National Health Education Standards. National Health Education Standards. Achieving Excellence 2nd edition. The American Cancer Society; 2007

[35] Okan O, Bauer U, Levin-Zamir D, Pinheiro P, Sorensen K, editors. International Handbook of Health Literacy: Research, Practice, and Policy across the Lifespan. Bristol, UK: Policy Press; 2019

[36] U.S. Department of Health and Human Services, Office of Disease Prevention and Health Promotion. Healthy People. Building a healthier future for all. (n.d.); 2030. Available from: https://health.gov/healthypeople

[37] Center for Disease Control and Prevention. What Is Health Literacy? Updated 2 Feb 2022. Available from: https://www.cdc.gov/healthliteracy/learn/index.html#:~:text=Personal%20health%20literacy%20is%20the,actions%20for%20themselves%20and%20others

[38] Videto DM, Dake JA. Promoting health literacy through defining and measuring quality school health education. Health Promotion Practice. 2019;**20**(6):824-833. DOI: 10.1177/1524839919870194

[39] Mann MJ, Lohrmann DK. Addressing challenges to the reliable, large-scale implementation of effective school health education. Health promotion practice. 2019;**20**(6):834-844. DOI: 10.1177/1524839919870196

[40] Birch DA, Goekler S, Auld ME, Lohrmann DK, Lyde A. Quality Assurance in Teaching K-12 health education: Paving a new path forward. Health Promotion Practice. 2019;**20**(6):845-857. DOI: 10.1177/1524839919868167

[41] Benes S, Alperin H. The Essentials of Teaching Health Education: Curriculum, Instruction, and Assessment. 2nd ed. Champaign, IL: Human Kinetics; 2022

[42] Videto D, Dennis D. Report of the 2020 joint committee on health education and promotion terminology. Health Educator. 2021;**53**(1):4-21

[43] Green L, Kreuter M. Health Program Planning: An Educational and Ecological Approach. 4th ed. New York: McGraw Hill; 2005

[44] American School Health Association. Core Beliefs in Action (n.d); Available from: https://www.ashaweb.org/wp-content/uploads/2022/10/ASHACoreBeliefs_Rev.pdf

[45] Joint Committee on National Health Education Standards. National

Health Education Standards: Achieving Excellence, 2nd ed. American Cancer Society; 2007

[46] Centers for Disease Control and Prevention. Characteristics of an Effective Curriculum. Centers for Disease Control and Prevention. Updated 29 May 2019. Available from: https://www.cdc.gov/healthyschools/sher/characteristics/index.htm

[47] U.S. Department of Health and Human Services, Office of Disease Prevention and Health Promotion. Healthy People Objectives (n.d.); 2030. Available from: https://health.gov/healthypeople/objectives-and-data/browse-objectives

[48] Vygotsky LS. Mind in Society: The Development of Higher Psychological Processes. Cambridge, MA: Harvard University Press; 1980

[49] Sensoy O, DiAngelo R. Is Everyone Really Equal? An Introduction to Key Concepts in Social Justice Education. 2nd ed. NY: Teacher's College Press; 2017

[50] McLeroy KR, Bibeau D, Steckler A, Glanz K. An ecological perspective on health promotion programs. Health Education Quarterly. 1988 Winter;**15**(4):351-377. DOI: 10.1177/109019818801500401 PMID: 3068205

[51] Ubbes VA. Educating for Health. Champaign, IL: Human Kinetics; 2008

[52] Hammond Z. Culturally Responsive Teaching and the Brain. Thousand Oaks, CA: Sage Publications; 2015

[53] Birch D. Addressing social justice through school health education: Thoughts on an expanded focus. Journal of School Health. 2021;**19**(6):439-442. DOI: 10.1111/josh.13017

[54] Auld ME, Allen MP, Hampton C, Montes JH, Sherry C, Mickalide AD, et al. Health literacy and health education in schools: Collaboration for action. NAM Perspectives. 2020;**20**(2020):1-13. DOI: 10.31478/202007b

[55] Day JK, Ioverno S, Russell ST. Safe and supportive schools for LGBTQ youth: Addressing educational inequities through inclusive policies and practices. Journal of School Psychology. 2019;**74**:29-43

[56] Knowles MS. Self-directed learning: A guide for learners and teachers. In: Englewood Cliffs. NJ, Cambridge: Prentice Hall; 1975

[57] Drummond M, Drummond C. Interview with boys on physical activity, nutrition and health: Implications for health literacy. Health Sociology Review. 2010;**19**(4):491-504

[58] Hu C, Ye D, Li Y, Huang Y, Li L, Gao Y, et al. Evaluation of a kindergarten-based nutrition education intervention for pre-school children in China. Public Health Nutrition. 2010 Feb;**13**(2):253-260. DOI: 10.1017/S1368980009990814

[59] Bandura A, Martinez-Pons M, Zimmerman B. Self-motivation for academic attainment: The role of self-efficacy beliefs and personal goal setting. American Education Research Journal. 1992;**29**(3):633-673

[60] Arends R. Learning to Teach. 10th ed. NY: McGraw-Hill; 2015

[61] Connolly M. Skills-Based Health Education. 2nd ed. Burlington, MA: Jones & Bartlett Learning; 2020

[62] Benes S, Alperin H. Health education in the 21st century: A skills-based approach. Journal of Physical Education,

Recreation & Dance. 2019;**90**(7):29-37. DOI: 1080/07303084.20191637306

[63] Rubin CS, Sanford C. Pathways to Personalization: A Framework for School Change. Cambridge, MA: Harvard Education Press (NCHES; 2018. p. 2020

[64] Weiman M. 5 Brain Based Learning Strategies to Boost Learning, Retention and Focus. TX, Richardson: Edmentum blog; 2021

[65] National Commission for Health Education Credentialing. The Health Education Profession. N.d. Available from: https://www.nchec.org/profession

[66] World Health Organization. Health Education: Theoretical Concepts, Effective Strategies, and Core Competencies. Cairo: Regional Office for the Eastern Mediterranean; 2012

[67] Ollis F. 'I haven't changed bigots but...': Reflections on the impact of teacher professional learning in sexuality education. Sex Education. 2020;**10**(2):217-230

[68] Bogler R, Somech A. Influence on teacher empowerment on teachers' organization commitment, professional commitment, and organization citizenship behavior in schools. Teaching and Teacher Education. 2004;**20**(3):277-289

[69] Centers for Disease Control and Prevention. CDC Professional Development Practices. Updated 13 Mar 2019. Available from: https://www.cdc.gov/healthyschools/tths/pd_practices.htm

[70] Kratzke C, Cox C. Smartphone technology and apps: Rapidly changing health promotion. Global Journal of Health Education and Promotion. 2012;**15**(1):72-82

[71] Satterfield H. Technology use in health education: A review and future implications. The Online Journal of Distance Education an de-Learning. 2015;**3**(2):87-96

[72] Basch CE. Healthier students are better learners: High-quality, strategically planned, and effectively coordinated school health programs must be a fundamental mission of schools to help close the achievement gap. The Journal of School Health. 2011;**81**(10):650-662. DOI: 10.1111/j.1746-1561.2011.00640.x

[73] Jiang Y, Mermin J, Perry DK, Hesser JE. The relationship of multiple, simultaneously occurring health risk behaviors to academic performance of high school students. Journal of Behavioral Health and Psychology. 2013;**2**(1):53-319

Chapter 12

Obstacles in the Nursing Training Programs

Masenyani Oupa Mbombi, Moila Dimakatso Ophilia, Mamare Adelaide Bopape and Livhuwani Muthelo

Abstract

The chapter aims to discuss obstacles that affect the successful implementation of nursing training programs from learner nurses' perspectives. The scope of the obstacles is limited to the clinical and classroom settings, where the nursing curriculum is implemented, and therefore the chapter will discuss obstacles to the nursing training program in hospitals/clinics and educational institutions. The chapter is a summary of a quantitative cross-sectional research study that collected data from all 190 learner nurses. Learner nurses were sampled with a stratified random sampling, which resulted in 129 samples of learner nurses. An electronic self-designed questionnaire written in English was sent to learner nurses *via* their university students' email to complete it. Descriptive statistics were utilized to describe the frequency of learner nurses regarding the R425 program curriculum review. The source of information, in this chapter, is the research finding obtained from learner nurses, using a quantitative research approach and literature, which highlight that the success of health education could be observed when barriers to nursing program implementation have been eliminated. The chapter provides learning opportunities to program designers and leaders of the educational and healthcare facilities where the nursing training programs are implemented.

Keywords: learner nurses, obstacles, nursing training program, implementation, healthcare management

1. Introduction

Nursing training programs play a significant role in the healthcare and educational sectors across the globe, especially since nurses continuously contribute significantly to the healthcare system [1]. At the moment, there are more than 20 nursing training programs (undergraduate and postgraduate) in existence with different significant roles in the healthcare and educational sectors. For instance, the bachelor of nursing and midwifery training program in South Africa train fundamental and general nursing care of individuals with different needs at hospitals, clinics, and occupational industries, while aiming to produce competent professional nurse and midwifery practitioner competent to function in a global context [2–4]. In contrast to this, a basic nursing program could be an intensive care nursing training program (post-basic course), which provides specialized nursing care based on the knowledge and skills of severely ill patients [5]. In South Africa, most matriculates aspire to study the bachelor of nursing and midwifery for employment purposes, while those who completed an undergraduate nursing program demonstrate intense ambitions to study post-basic courses (e.g., intensive nursing care, operating theater, trauma nursing care, and post-graduate qualifications—honors, masters, and PhD), which satisfies the career development desires [6]. However, these ambitions remain a dream for many candidates and professional nurses because of obstacles in the nursing training programs. This chapter focuses on perceived obstacles of learner nurses in the bachelor of nursing and midwifery (honors level).

To guide the process of identifying the obstacles in nursing training, we applied only 10 criteria by the council on higher education's programme accreditation of South Africa [7], which Flott and Linden [8] mentioned two environmental settings that affect the learning outcomes of the training program (classroom and clinical learning). So far, we observed unclear goal settings by candidates for studying and selection criteria for access to nursing programs in higher educational institutions as dominant obstacles in the nursing training program [9]. The chapter discusses obstacles existing in the nursing training program following the perceptions of learner nurses regarding the curriculum of bachelor of nursing and midwifery at a selected higher education institution. Notably, there are diverse benefits inherited from the nursing training programs. For instance, having more competent nursing professionals that impact positively the healthcare services provision, increases nursing staff establishment and relief of staff workload [10], and reduces high mortality [11]. Carbajo et al. [12] noted that competent nursing professionals have a significant role in improving quality healthcare service delivery and also preventing and treating disease occurrence.

According to De Rosis et al. [13], user experiences in the training program are a key element for improving quality service delivery. The findings of the study assist in improving the designing curriculum of the nursing training programs, and its implementation within higher educational institutions and clinical healthcare facilities. We believe that failure to understand the obstacles in the nursing programs could have detrimental effects on higher education and healthcare facilities. For example, one notable effect could be defeating the plan of action for scaling up quality nursing and midwifery education and practice for the African region 2012–2022 [6]. Also, we believe that learner nurses' perspective as recipients of the training programs provides an opportunity for nursing educators and institutions to monitor the quality and outcomes of the nursing training programs. Therefore, the chapter discusses the obstacles in the nursing training program—bachelor of nursing and midwifery from learner nurses' perspective about the curriculum using a quantitative research approach at selected higher educational institutions in South Africa.

2. Research methods

2.1 Research approach

The study employed a quantitative research approach to collect numerical data from learner nurses on the selected criterion for program review [14]. The quantitative research approach assisted the authors in quantifying the perceptions of learner nurses regarding the criterion for the B. Nurs R425 curriculum program.

2.2 Research design

We adopted a cross-sectional descriptive design, which is observational and collects data from a group of learner nurses at one point in time [15]. A cross-sectional descriptive research design was used to examine the perceptions of learner nurses regarding the R425 curriculum program in the Department of nursing science.

2.3 Population and sampling

A total of 190 learner nurses from the second level to the fourth level studying for the bachelor of nursing science program (R425) in the academic year 2020 constituted the population of the study. The three levels of study were the last group for training the curriculum of the R425 program in the Department of Nursing Science. Since learner nurses were from different study levels, the stratified random sampling method was the best relevant method to sample 129 learner nurses according to the Slovin formula for calculating the sample size.

2.4 Data collection and analysis

An electronic self-designed questionnaire was used to collect data from the learner nurses. The literature and criterion of CHE guided the development of the questionnaire, which was pilot tested on five learner nurses who did not form part of the study in the same study setting. An english-written electronic questionnaire was chosen because of its ability to increase the rate of responses and the quality of responses. Learners took 10 to 20 minutes to complete the electronic questionnaire. Descriptive statistics on SPSS version 27 were used to analyze the perceptions of learner nurses about the nursing training program, and which statistician took a month to return the analysis results. Summary statistics of descriptive statistics was the perfect analysis method to compare the mean regarding perceptions of learner nurses on the selected criterion for program evaluation as listed by CHE.

3. Results

3.1 Demographic profile for learner nurses

3.1.1 Gender

The study had more female learner nurses (76%), who responded to the study than male learner nurses (24%)—see **Figure 1**. The gender profile of nursing professionals is consistently dominated by female professionals.

3.1.2 Level of study

The year 2020 had only three study levels for the R425 training program, hence we present the respondents according to their study levels. Based on **Figure 2**, most learner nurses who responded were in the 3rd level of study in 2020 making 59.7% of the study, learner nurses who were in their 4th level of study made 27.1%, and 13.2% learner nurses were in their second level of study.

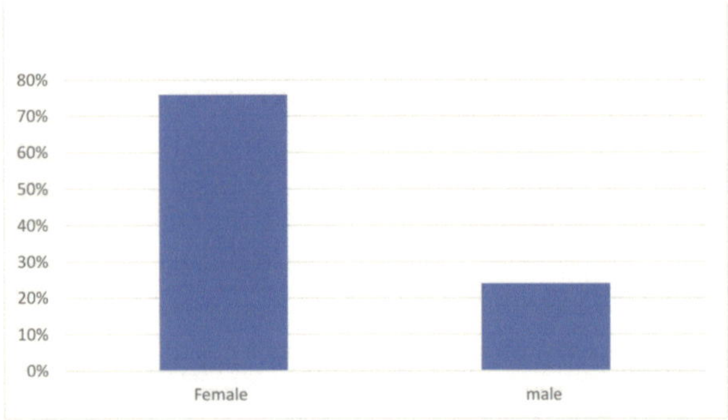

Figure 1.
Gender profile of learner nurses.

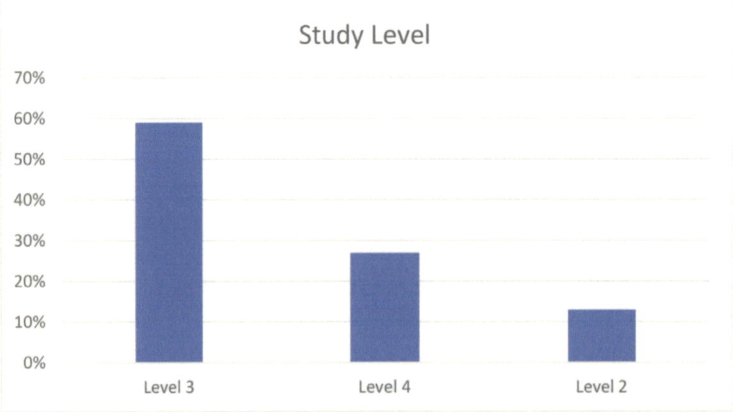

Figure 2.
Study level of learner nurses.

3.2 Perceptions of learner nurses according to the selected criteria of the council on higher education's programme accreditation

The following sections illustrate obstacles identified from selected criteria of the council on higher education's programme accreditation, which was applied to describe learner nurses' perspectives regarding the bachelor of nursing and midwifery curriculum. The obstacles were identified and quantified by 129 learner nurses of a selected higher educational institution with the use of a questionnaire. The quantitative data were analyzed using descriptive statistics as facilitated by SPSS version 27 software.

3.2.1 Lack of a clear study goal for the bachelor of nursing and midwifery

We investigated learner nurses' perspectives, regarding a reason for studying bachelor of nursing and midwifery, which is not part of the accreditation criteria. Surprisingly, only 8.5% of learner nurses said they were studying a bachelor of nursing science because it is their calling, with the remaining 91.5% of learner nurses, indicating that they chose the training program for career purposes and lack a better choice for studying at a higher educational institution.

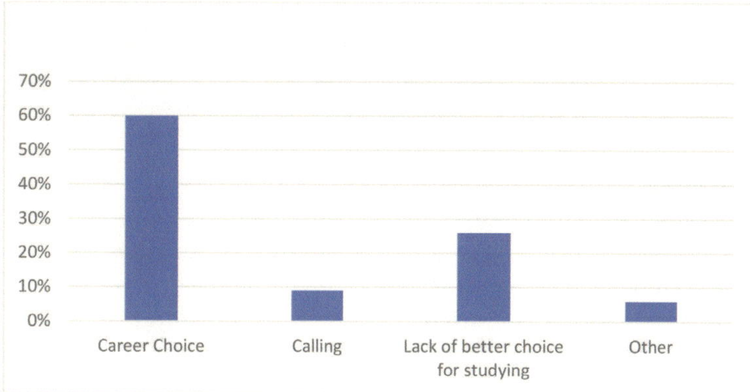

Figure 3.
Reasons for studying the R425 nursing program.

Figure 3 illustrates that most learner nurses chose to study bachelor of nursing science for a career purpose, which was expected considering the low employment rate among youth in South Africa. Based on these findings, we construe that the lack of a study goal that aligns with the nursing profession is an obstacle within the nursing training program. Raatikainen [16], in describing the nursing profession as a calling, noted that nurses who studied nursing, because it was a calling, were more devoted to their work, which translates to the provision of high-quality nursing care. Although many young people chose a study program because of employment opportunities [17], this study motive is perceived as an obstacle for the nursing profession that is described as a calling profession.

The results presented below are based on the selected Criterion for program review according to CHE. **Table 1** below illustrates these selected criteria for program review.

	D	N	A
2. Criterion 2: student recruitment, admission, and selection			
2.1. The minimum requirements required by UL for students to qualify to study for the bachelor of nursing science program are fair.	46%	10%	54%
3. Criterion 3: staffing			
3.1. There is enough staff to facilitate learning in both theory and practice within the nursing department at UL.	40%	14%	56%
4. Criterion 4: program coordination			
4.1. Hours required by the nursing council (SANC) are prioritized over anything else.	10%	25.6%	63.4%)
4.2. Time allocation for clinical learning is adequate for us to learn the outcomes of the level of study.	80%)	6.3%	13.7%

	D	N	A
5. Criterion 5: teaching and learning			
5.1. Modules offered at UL from levels 1 to 4 of the bachelor of nursing science program all contribute to the production of competent registered nurses(RNs).	70%	13%	17%
6. Criterion 6: learner assessment			
6.1 I get feedback on our work and then do corrections with our facilitators.	52%	10%	38%
7. Criterion 7: infrastructure and resources			
7.1. There are enough resources for me to practice the procedures demonstrated.	56%	10%	44%
7.2. Our skills lab is structured in a way that is convenient for me to practice the procedures demonstrated by our facilitators.	66%	0%	44%
7.3. The capacity of our skills lab is sufficient enough to accommodate all learners and makes learning easier.	56%	10%	44%
8. Criterion 8: coordination of experiential learning			
8.1. My lecturers and registered nurses are always there for us at our practice area to help and support us to abide by our scope of practice.	51%	6%	43%
9. Criterion 9: learner retention, student throughput, and program impact			
9.1. The program has high expertise within the department.	76%	2%	22%
9.2. The second level of nursing science is a the level where most students fail a subject and carry it to the next level.	2%	0%	98%
10. Criterion 10: program reviews			
10.1. Nursing has not been able to prepare adequately prepared nurses to provide safe high-quality services.	58%	8%	34%
10.2. It can be beneficial to the nursing department, the university of Limpopo, SANC, and the health care system at large to review the bachelor of nursing science program.	45%	47%	8%

Table 1.
Perceptions of learner nurses based on criteria.

3.2.2 Criterion 2: student recruitment, admission, and selection

According to council on higher education accreditation criteria, criterion 2 focuses on "recruitment, access, and selection procedures are effected in line with the University's policies and procedures. They are appropriate for the program's academic requirements, within a framework of widened access and equity. The number of students selected takes into account the program's intended learning outcomes and its capacity to offer good quality education." Learner nurses (56%) perceived one of the minimum standards of criterion 2 (requirements for admission) as an obstacle to the nursing training program. For instance, A total of 89% of learner nurses confirmed that minimum requirements constituted by high levels in mathematics and physical science are an obstacle for many matriculates' to pursue a bachelor of nursing and midwifery. The concern about minimum requirements for nursing qualifications has been discussed by several authors [9, 18–20]. The findings indicate continuous trends of concern regarding minimum entry requirements that require urgent attention.

3.2.3 Criterion 3: staffing

We acknowledged the role of staffing in ensuring good outcomes of the nursing curriculum by asking how learner nurses perceived staffing for support of their classroom and clinical learning for the bachelor of nursing and midwifery training program. A total of 54% perceived staffing as inadequate to support their clinical learning for the bachelor of nursing and midwifery training program. Furthermore, learner nurses perceived modules facilitated by one nurse educator as a barrier to their learning. Similarly, Mlaba and Emmamally [21], with other scholars [22–24], also reported inadequate clinical staff support and a lack of clinical educators for mentoring learner nurses' clinical learning as an obstacle within the nursing training program.

3.2.4 Criterion 4: program coordination

Criterion 4 ensures that the program is effectively coordinated to facilitate the achievement of its intended purpose and outcomes. The majority of learner nurses (63.4%) reported a concern regarding one of the minimum standards—stating that the regulatory body (South African nursing council) requires lots of clinical hours, which is a challenge to accumulate due to various factors. Learner nurses (86.3%) also reported concern about the duration of clinical allocation, which is perceived as short to meet the required clinical hours. In contrast, the South African nursing Council (SANC) requires 4000 clinical hours in clinical learning experiences under supervision over four years for a bachelor of nursing and midwifery [2]. There are fewer or limited scholarly studies that aimed to challenge the requirement of SANC.

3.2.5 Criterion 5: teaching and learning

The majority of learner nurses (83%) reported that some of the modules offered from levels 1 to 4 for the bachelor of nursing and midwifery program seem to be not related to the nursing profession. For example, learner nurses struggle to understand why their training program requires them to study chemistry and sociology. Learner nurses expressed concerns as they fail these modules offered outside the nursing disciple than those under the nursing. Similarly, Lewis [25] deliberated on the implications of failing modules, which included emotional, social, and financial consequences as well as the impact on the student, institution, and nursing profession at large.

3.2.6 Criterion 6: learner assessment

Suganya [26] explained that feedback is one of the essential components of the nursing curriculum. For the feedback to be effective, it should be given in a regular manner and in a supportive environment. However, our findings demonstrate that 62% of learner nurses fail to receive assessment feedback, thus being an obstacle to the successful implementation of the nursing training program. Nursing educators and supervisors should ensure they provide feedback promptly and specific to the learner's performance. Specific and high-quality feedback comments make feedback effective and valued by the learner nurses when compared to nonspecific evaluative feedback [27]. It provides an opportunity to self-assess their skills and capabilities and also it provides direction that increases motivation, confidence, self-esteem, cognitive skills, and behaviors. Effective feedback gives confidence and reassurance to the learner nurses. So, nursing professionals should give importance to feedback in their learning process and implement a mechanism by which the quantity and quality of the feedback are monitored [26].

3.2.7 Criterion 7: infrastructure and resources

The criterion requires that suitable and sufficient venues, IT infrastructure, and library resources be available for students and staff in the program. Efficient provision of infrastructure and resources is needed for the proper implementation of the nursing training program by creating well-established academic support centers [28] and keeping up with the demands of the healthcare system [6]. Leary et al. [29] also note that the provision of adequate infrastructure and resource allocation is a strategic way for enhancing the innovation of the nursing training program. Pesut and Greig [30] emphasized that the existence of proper resource allocation has fruitful results in the implementation of the nursing training program. However, most learner nurses (66%) perceived infrastructure design and allocations of resources (staff and materials) as not adequate to assist them with their learning needs. In contrast, Mothiba et al. [31] regarding the role of infrastructure in the nursing program noted a diverse positive impact of the newly established clinical skills laboratory on the clinical learning of learner nurses in the study setting. Therefore, inefficient provision of proper infrastructure and resource allocation hinders the successful implementation of the nursing training program. Subsequently, this deters the plan of action for scaling up quality nursing and midwifery education and practice for the African region 2012–2022, which requires adequate resource allocation. There is a continuous need for nursing regulators, institutions/schools, and educators to invest in proper infrastructure and adequate resource allocation to ensure effective implementation of the nursing training program.

3.2.8 Criterion 8: coordination of experimental learning

According to the council on higher education of South Africa, criterion 8 ensures that the coordination of work-based learning should be done effectively in all components of applicable programs. This includes an adequate infrastructure, effective communication, recording of progress made, monitoring, and mentoring. Learner nurses (51%) reflected a shortage of clinical nurse educators that impact negatively on clinical learning. During the clinical exposure, most learner nurses reported monitoring and mentoring for clinical learning. Clinical learning is a significant component of the nursing training program, as such, failure to achieve the component defeats the purpose of the whole nursing training program. Flott and Linden [8] reported similar concerns, regarding factors that influence clinical learning, including the physical space, psychosocial and interaction factors, the organizational culture, and teaching and learning components. Najafi Kalyani et al. [32] reported inadequacy of the educational environment faced by learner nurses that resulted in "confusion of professional identity." The aforementioned authors emphasized improving the clinical environment by identifying professional models and increasing their influence on management, education, and clinical education.

3.2.9 Criterion 9: learner retention, student throughput, and program impact

The criterion indicates that the program should take steps to alleviate shortages of expertise in relevant nursing, in cases where these are the desired outcomes of the program. However, learner nurses (76%) reflected that this is not the case within the nursing training program, where expertise is sourced outside the department. For example, expertise in sociology, chemistry, physiology, anatomy, and psychology is offered by non-nursing professionals. Sourcing of expertise outside the department contributed to the slow throughput rate of the nursing program, with more learner nurses failing at the second level. Therefore, failure to alleviate shortages of expertise is an obstacle for the nursing training program. Similarly, Fawaz et al. [33] noted the desire for growing nursing experts that occurred from a shift in the age of the nursing workforce to ensure the successful implementation of the nursing training program.

3.2.10 Criterion 10: program review

Nursing programs aim to prepare nurses who can deliver safe and high-quality care and would be able to adapt to the evolving environments of practice. However, according to learner nurses (58%), nursing has not been able to prepare adequately prepared nurses to provide safe high-quality services due to various factors that impacted the implementation of the nursing program. A few of these various factors include an increased disease burden, an overloaded healthcare system, and a shortage of nurses in schools and clinical healthcare settings. Few of the learner nurses (8%) expressed the desire of having program evaluations annually to improve the implementation. To adapt to the rapidly varying and advancing healthcare settings; nurse educators must regularly assess and review education curricula, teaching-learning strategies, and programs [33].

4. Conclusions

To our best knowledge, this chapter presented a unique perspective of learner nurses based in a rural university regarding the implementation of the nursing training program using selected criteria by CHE in South Africa. Based on the selected criterion of the council on higher education, there are obstacles to the implementation of the nursing training program, which indicate the required support from different stakeholders involved in nursing education. We recommend that program designers and educational and healthcare managers consider these obstacles in the nursing training program as a baseline reference for a successful implementation of the program.

Acknowledgements

We would like to acknowledge the learner nurses who participated in the study. Also, to the faculty of health sciences at a selected university for granting permission to conduct the study.

Conflict of interest

The authors declare no conflict of interest.

Author details

Masenyani Oupa Mbombi*, Moila Dimakatso Ophilia, Mamare Adelaide Bopape and Livhuwani Muthelo
Department of Nursing Science, University of Limpopo, Polokwane, South Africa

*Address all correspondence to: masenyani.mbombi@ul.ac.za

References

[1] Meyer SM, Naude M, Shangase NC, van Niekerk SE. The Nursing Unit Manager: A Comprehensive Guide. 3rd edn. South Africa: Pearson; 2018

[2] South African Nursing Council. South African Nursing Council (SANC), 2007, Regulations Relating to Performance of Community Service, Regulation No. R. 765. Pretoria: SANC; 2007

[3] University of Limpopo. Bachelor of Nursing: Department of Nursing Science. 2020. Available from: https://www.ul.ac.za/index.php?Entity=Nursing%20 Sciences

[4] University of Pretoria. Bachelor of Nursing Science (BNurs): Nursing Science Bachelor of Nursing Science (BNurs). 2020. Available from: https://www.up.ac.za/nursing_science/article/50612/bachelor-of-nursing-science-bnurs

[5] Ervin JN, Kahn JM, Cohen TR, Weingart LR. Teamwork in the intensive care unit. The American Psychologist. 2018;**73**(4):468-477. DOI: 10.1037/amp0000247

[6] Bvumbwe T, Mtshali N. Nursing education challenges and solutions in sub Saharan Africa: An integrative review. BMC Nursing. 2018;**2018**(17):3. DOI: 10.1186/s12912-018-0272-4

[7] Council on Higher Education of South Africa. Criteria for Programme Accreditation. 2012. Available from: http://nronline.che.ac.za/html_documents/CHE_Programme_Accreditation_Criteria_Revised_2012.pdf

[8] Flott EA, Linden L. The clinical learning environment in nursing education: A concept analysis. Journal of Advanced Nursing. 2016;**72**(3):501-513. DOI: 10.1111/jan.12861. Epub 2015 Dec 9

[9] Mbombi MO, Mothiba TM. Exploring barriers that nurses experience to enrolment for a postgraduate nursing qualification at a higher education institution in South Africa. African Journal of Health Professions Education. 2020;**12**(1):41-45. DOI: 10.7196/AJHPE.2020.v12i1.1126

[10] Ortega M, Cecagno D, Llor AM, de Siqueira HC, Montesinos MJ, Soler LM. Academic training of nursing professionals and its relevance to the workplace. Revista Latino-Americana de Enfermagem. 2015;**23**(3):404-410. DOI: 10.1590/0104-1169.0432.2569

[11] Haegdorens F, Van Bogaert P, De Meester K, et al. The impact of nurse staffing levels and nurse's education on patient mortality in medical and surgical wards: An observational multicentre study. BMC Health Services Research. 2019;**19**:864. DOI: 10.1186/s12913-019-4688-7

[12] Carbajo P, Castrodeza J, Gual A, López-Blanco JA, Martín-Zurro A, Sánchez-Biezma E. Desarrollo, seguimiento y evaluación de la formación especializada en el modelo troncal: conclusiones del seminario realizado el 24 de septiembre de. 2014. Escuela de Salud Pública, Llatzaret, Menorca. FEM.[Internet]. 2014;**17**(4):193-197. DOI: 10.4321/S2014-98322014000400004 [Google Scholar] [Ref list]

[13] De Rosis S, Barchielli C, Vainieri M, Belle N. The relationship between healthcare service provision models and patient experience. Journal of Health Organization and Management.

2022;**36**(9):1-24. Emerald Publishing Limited 1477-7266. DOI: 10.1108/JHOM-06-2021-0242

[14] Bhatia S. Predicting risk perception: New insights from data science. Management Science. Articles in Advance. 2018;**1**(1):1-24. Available from: http://pubsonline.informs.org/journal/mnsc/. ISSN 0025-1909 (print), ISSN 1526-5501 (online)

[15] Cherry K. Cross-Sectional Research Method: How Does It Work? Advantages and Challenges. 2018. Available from: https://www.verywellmind.com/what-is-a-cross-sectional-study-2794978

[16] Raatikainen R. Nursing care as a calling. Journal of Advanced Nursing. 1997;**25**(6):1111-1115. DOI: 10.1046/j.1365-2648.1997.19970251111.x

[17] Marcinowicz L, Owlasiuk A, Slusarska B, Zarzycka D, Pawlikowska T. Choice and perception of the nursing profession from the perspective of polish nursing students: A focus group study. BMC Medical Education. 2016;**2016**(1):243. DOI: 10.1186/s12909-016-0765-3

[18] Dam SA. What Matters Most? Factors Influencing Choice of a Student Affairs Master's Program. Master's thesis. Lincoln: University of Nebraska; 2014. Available from: http://digitalcommons.unl.edu/cehsedaddiss/176. [Accessed: 6 March 2020]

[19] Matsolo MP, Ningpuanyeh WC, Susuman AS. Factors affecting enrolment rate of students in higher education. Journal of Asian and African Studies. 2018;**53**(1):63-80. DOI: 10.1177/0021909616657369

[20] Smith AN, Boyd LD, Rogers CM, le Jeune RC. 2016. Self-perceptions of value, barriers, and motivations for graduate education among dental hygienists. Journal of Dental Education. 2016;**80**(9):1033-1040

[21] Mlaba ZP, Emmamally W. Describing the perceptions of student nurses regarding barriers and benefits of a peer-mentorship programme in a clinical setting in KwaZulu-Natal. Health SA Gesondheid. 2019;**24**(0):a1118. DOI: 10.4102/hsag.v24i0.1118

[22] Al-Hamdan Z, Fowler J, Bawadi H, Norrie P, Summer L, Debbie D. 'Student nurses' perceptions of a good mentor: A questionnaire survey of student'. International Journal of Humanities and Social Science. 2014;**4**(3):248-256. viewed 14 June 2015. Available from: https://www.researchgate.net/publication/260793487

[23] Dennison S. Peer mentoring: Untapped potential, educational innovations. Journal of Nursing Education. 2010;**49**(6):340-342. DOI: 10.3928/01484834-20100217-04

[24] Joubert A, De Villiers J. The learning experiences of mentees and mentors in a nursing mentoring programme. Curations. 2015;**38**(1):1-7. DOI: 10.4102/curationis.v38i1.1145

[25] Lewis SL, Bucher LB, Heitkemper MM, Harding MM. Medical-Surgical Nursing: Assessment and Management of Clinical Problems. 10th edn. St. Luis: Elsevier; 2020

[26] Panneerselvam S. Feedback Among Nursing Professionals: A Narrative Review. 2018

[27] Zhao X, Cox A, Ally L, Alsuhaibani A. A comparison of student and staff perceptions and feelings about assessment and feedback using cartoon annotation. Journal of Further and Higher Education. 2022;**46**(5):586-604

[28] Hawnkins S, Fogg N, Wilson C, Browne J. Establishing a tutoring and academic support center: Collaborating with nurse educator students. 2022;**39**(11):19-25. DOI: 10.1016/j.profnurs.2021.12.014

[29] Leary A, Villarruel AM, Richmond TS. Creating an innovation infrastructure in academic nursing. Journal of Professional Nursing. 2022;**38**:83-88. DOI: 10.1016/j.profnurs.2021.12.005

[30] Pesut B, Greig M. 2018. Resources for educating, training, and mentoring nurses and unregulated nursing care providers in palliative care: A review and expert consultation. Journal of Palliative Medicine. 2018;**21**(S1):S50-S56. DOI: 10.1089/jpm.2017.0395

[31] Mothiba TM, Bopape MA, Mbombi MO. The emergence of a clinical skills laboratory and its impact on clinical learning: Undergraduate nursing students' perspective in Limpopo Province, South Africa. AJHPE. 2020;**12**(4):197-200. DOI: 10.7196/AJHPE.2020.v12i4.1375

[32] Najafi Kalyani M, Jamshidi N, Molazem Z, et al. How do nursing students experience the clinical learning environment and respond to their experiences? A qualitative study. BMJ Open. 2018;**2019**(9):e028052. DOI: 10.1136/bmjopen-2018-028052

[33] Fawaz MA, Hamdan-Mansourb AM, Tassia A. Challenges facing nursing education in the advanced healthcare environment. International Journal of Africa Nursing Sciences. 2018;**9**:105-110. DOI: 10.1016/j.ijans.2018.10.005

Chapter 13

Baseline Analysis for Effective Diabetes Intervention

Mabitsela Mphasha, Linda Skaal and Tebogo Maria Mothiba

Abstract

Diabetes is a fast-growing disease that is costly to manage, leading to both financial and non-financial burdens. These burdens are worsened in the presence of diabetes complications, so improved interventions are critical. Prior to developing new interventions, a baseline analysis should be conducted to gain insight into the strengths and weaknesses of current interventions. Furthermore, a baseline analysis helps in identifying discrepancies to be addressed and outlining how the environment impacts diabetes management. A comprehensive literature review was adopted to collect data regarding the importance of a baseline analysis in diabetes interventions. The findings of the literature review indicated that a baseline analysis is a critical step for the development of effective diabetes interventions. Knowledge, attitudes, practices, and anthropometric factors such as quality of life and social determinants of health, should be assessed when conducting a baseline analysis. A baseline analysis is affirmed as a fundamental prerequisite for the development of diabetes interventions for better outcomes. There is also a need to assess the capacity of healthcare providers to conduct a baseline analysis to determine the need for support and in-service training. An inappropriately-conducted baseline analysis may lead to inappropriate solutions and misdiagnosis. The implementation of wrongful solutions would defeat the objective of improving diabetes outcomes.

Keywords: diabetes, baseline analysis, interventions, development, effectiveness

1. Introduction

It is essential to diagnose and gain insight into the current state of health prior to the development of disease-managing interventions. Therefore, a baseline analysis should be conducted. A baseline analysis is a critical step that informs the development of healthcare interventions, including improving diabetes management [1]. The purpose of a baseline analysis is to compile details about discrepancies in existing healthcare practices and assess the strengths and weaknesses in current interventions in order to improve practices [2]. The data obtained from a baseline analysis may motivate healthcare providers to create better management strategies with innovation and a sense of urgency. Moreover, a baseline analysis may provide information regarding how the environment surrounding patients impacts their health outcomes.

In the healthcare sector, a baseline analysis is conducted through a health needs assessment. The health needs assessment involves the evaluation and identification of health issues confronting the people, developing strategies, and allocating resources to improve health and reduce inequalities. A health needs assessment becomes a fundamental prerequisite for effective diabetes interventions. It assists in defining what ought to be done and the accomplishment of the intention [3]. A needs assessment further informs the plan, and identifications of strategies and resources needed in developing the intervention [3]. It is essential to conduct a health need assessment prior to the intervention to envision interventions that are tailored to the target group.

Diabetes is the fastest-growing disease in the world. It is often poorly managed, resulting in complications. Patients diagnosed with diabetes require ongoing evaluation of complications and should regularly monitor glucose levels [4]. The National Institute of Diabetes [5] recommends that patients should be examined 2–3 times a year to acquire information on nutrition, exercise, and overall management of diabetes, including diabetes-related complications. The costs of providing care to patients with diabetes are escalating and place a burden on personal and state budgets. There is a need for interventions to curb diabetes prevalence and its complications. Less developed countries have limited resources to address the economic burden of diabetes management. Conducting a health need assessment at the onset will therefore assist in the effective use of limited resources.

2. Diabetes as global public health problem

According to the International Diabetes Federation (IDF) [6], Diabetes Mellitus remains a public health problem. About 537 million people are living with diabetes, constituting a global prevalence rate of 10.5%. Recent reports indicate that more than 1 in 10 adults is diagnosed with diabetes globally. In some countries, one in five person adults is diagnosed with diabetes [6]. It is projected that 643 million and 783 million persons may have diabetes in 2030 and 2045, respectively. Over this period, diabetes estimation is said to increase by 46%, surpassing the estimated world population growth. In Africa, there are 24 million persons living with diabetes [4]. About 360 million residing in urban areas have diabetes, with a prevalence rate of 12.1%, compared with 176.6 million people in rural areas with a prevalence of 8.3%. Diabetes has been reported to be more prevalent among men compared to women. The Middle East and North Africa regions have the highest prevalence of diabetes at 18.1%. However, Africa has the lowest global diabetes prevalence rate, at 5.3%. China, India, and Pakistan have the highest prevalence of diabetes globally [6].

Undiagnosed diabetes poses serious a threat, with global estimates of 87.5% of cases in low- and middle-income countries. However, low-income countries have the highest estimation of undiagnosed diabetes at 50.5% compared to 28.8% in high-income countries [6]. Africa has the highest estimates of undiagnosed diabetes at 53.6%, followed by Western Pacific at 52.8% and South-East Asia at 51.3%. North America and the Caribbean region have the lowest estimate of undiagnosed diabetes at 24.2% [6].

Diabetes has recently been found to be a high-risk Non-Communicable Disease (NCD) linked to Coronavirus Disease-2019 (COVID-19) deaths worldwide. Higher susceptibility to COVID-19 among patients with diabetes is attributed to an impaired immune response due to chronic metabolic dysfunction [7].

Patients with diabetes may develop complications or other health problems such as cardiovascular disease, hypertension, erectile dysfunction, retinopathy, and kidney disease [8]. It has been reported by several studies that the identification of risk factors can serve as benchmarks to design appropriate prevention measures and minimize the risk and severity of complications [9–10]. The next section discusses the cost of managing diabetes as a sub-topic to illustrate the severity of diabetes as a global public health problem.

2.1 Costs of managing diabetes

The World Health Organization (WHO) [11] reports that diabetes is costly to manage, more so in the presence of complications. In 2017, the total cost of managing diabetes was $327 billion in direct medical costs, as well as $90 billion in reduced productivity [12]. It has been reported that patients with diabetes incur medical costs 2.3 times higher than those of non-diabetics [12]. When diabetes patients develop complications resulting in hospitalization, the cost of care increases. Hospitalization costs of diabetes are the principal driver of the total costs of managing diabetes. As a result, funds that could have been used for other developmental reasons may be channeled to fighting diabetes. The financial costs of diabetes rise with the rising prevalence of the disease, which is projected to increase in 2045. This increase would strain the healthcare budget, including the overall budgets of governments. Therefore, there is a need for governments to introduce new interventions to manage and prevent diabetes.

3. Developing diabetes interventions

Various studies have reported poor diabetes outcomes among patients [13, 14], including rising prevalence rates. This calls for new interventions and strategies to manage and curb the prevalence of diabetes. For effective intervention, developing diabetes intervention includes identifying and prioritizing health issues and needs, choosing ways to cope with them, and committing support and resources for quality health promotion activities [15]. The process of developing intervention should be an inclusive and participatory process involving the targeted group [16]. The target population should include patients living with all types of diabetes, age groups, and gender. Health needs assessment is hereby discussed as a subheading of developing diabetes intervention.

3.1 Health needs assessment

A health needs assessment is a critical and systematic approach to identifying the unmet healthcare needs of the population and making changes to meet those unmet needs [3]. In this context of diabetes management, it could be used to identify what needs to be done for better outcomes. Health needs assessments are done for the effective use of health services and resources to improve health and the quality of life of patients. A health needs assessment encourages cooperation or partnership and innovation. Needs assessments are the backbone of public health and must be conducted properly. The process of conducting a health needs assessment involves the identification of health problems and inequalities, and a determination of appropriate interventions to address the problems. The requirements for conducting successful health needs assessments are an understanding of what is involved, and the time, and resources to undertake assessments. The cost of managing diabetes and its related complications is increasing [17]. It is essential to conduct a health needs assessment properly for effective intervention. Without a clear and well-conducted health needs assessment, intervention could result in the misuse of funds. A mixed-method needs assessment study conducted in Tanzania involving diabetes patients with retinopathy demonstrated low levels of stigma and self-efficacy along with high levels of anxiety and depression [18]. Moreover, the study showed inadequate knowledge regarding a healthy diet. On those grounds, a comprehensive diabetes education program was developed to improve diabetes control and prevent complications including retinopathy [18].

According to the WHO [19], diabetes interventions are dietary therapy, increased physical activity, and pharmacological therapy consisting of oral hypoglycaemic drugs or insulin. There is a need to empower diabetes patients and their family members with skills and knowledge related to diabetes. This would help in attaining better diabetes outcomes and an improvement of quality of life, including reducing the chances of family members developing diabetes [20]. Family members of patients diagnosed with diabetes are already at risk due to family history. In South Africa, the Department of Health adopted WHO guidelines for diabetes management [21]. However, implementation has been a challenge. A baseline analysis of factors contributing to poor implementation may be necessary. Behavioral changes among patients with diabetes are difficult to implement due to the inaccessibility of the following: healthy food, an enabling environment for physical exercise, and essential self-management resources [22]. Patients diagnosed with diabetes are from various cultural backgrounds, which influences their behavior. It is therefore essential to conduct a baseline analysis to design and develop diabetes interventions that are sensitive to cultural beliefs. Behavioral changes are influenced by factors including knowledge and attitudes [23]. Education programs incorporating behavior change approaches are extra effective. Behavioral change is a complex process and should be based on a theoretical framework. The use of theory enables a greater understanding of the relationships among factors that influence behavioral change [24].

3.1.1 How to conduct a health needs assessment

According to the Centers for Disease Control and Prevention [25], there are five critical steps on how to conduct a health need assessment, which are as follows:

Plan and design: The first step involves defining the scope and objectives of the assessment. This includes defining who, what, and where.

Logistics and resources: The availability of resources impacts health needs assessment activities, so it is important to have sufficient funds to carry out the assessment. The most important resource is capacitated healthcare providers who understand the importance of the need assessment and how to conduct it.

Review and rate data: Before capturing and analyzing data, a review of the data must take place for team members to reach a consensus. At this point, the team discusses data, shares individual results, and identifies evidence to support collective rating. This step helps in identifying strengths and weaknesses.

Record and summarize data: Following an agreement on rating, data is analyzed to produce findings that will guide the action to be taken.

Action plan: Based on the findings of the data analysis, an action plan should be developed to close identified gaps. At this stage, summarized data is transformed into measurable action items.

3.1.2 Components to assess during need assessment

3.1.2.1 Knowledge regarding diabetes care

Diabetes knowledge is one of the key elements motivating individuals to follow a healthy lifestyle [26]. Nutrition and exercise are essential in diabetes outcomes. Poor knowledge in this regard contributes fundamentally to increasing the prevalence of poor control of diabetes [26], leading to complications and a high mortality rate. Not empowering patients and their family members with knowledge may increase diabetes prevalence among family members who are already at risk due to family history. Poor nutrition and exercise knowledge also normalize poor lifestyle choices, which contribute to obesity. A lack of knowledge about diabetes management often leads to non-compliance to treatment [27].

According to Ajzen et al. [28], having adequate knowledge does not guarantee the adoption of healthy behavior. The combination of knowledge and motivation to change behavior is what yields positive behavioral change [29]. Knowledge enables patients to assess diabetes risk, seek proper treatment and care, and inspires them to lead a healthy lifestyle to manage their disease. Patients with adequate diabetes knowledge tend to take appropriate measures to control the disease [30], by honoring their medical appointments. Adequate diabetes knowledge among patients minimizes comorbidities, which improves their quality of life. Having adequate knowledge about self-care practices leads to better diabetes control for a prolonged period and adherence to self-management practices [31]. Nonetheless, international knowledge and awareness of diabetes stay low [32]. A cross-sectional South African study conducted in the Vhembe district of Limpopo Province has reported poor diabetes knowledge among patients [33]. A mixed method study on diabetes knowledge conducted in Senwabarwana in Limpopo province also reported poor knowledge [34]. It is therefore important to conduct a baseline analysis regarding diabetes knowledge involving a target population.

3.1.2.2 Attitudes regarding diabetes

Attitudes are considered the most important determinants of behavior and behavior change among patients with diabetes. Attitudes towards diabetes and its treatment are associated with self-care, including adherence to a diabetes dietary plan, exercise, and medication [35]. Positive attitudes toward diabetes and its treatment may lead patients to adopting an active lifestyle and changing their behavior to control their diabetes, in contrast to patients with negative attitudes [23]. A cross-sectional study conducted in the Free State province of South Africa among Type-2 Diabetes Mellitus (T2DM) patients reported negative attitudes towards diabetes among patients, which may contribute to morbidity and mortality [36]. Another South African study reported positive attitudes among patient towards diabetes treatment and lifestyle modifications, which may contribute to better diabetes outcomes [37].

3.1.2.3 Practice related to diabetes

Practice related to diabetes management is critical and involves adherence to new treatment regimens [38]. Practice includes remembering and administering medication, honoring medical appointments, adhering to diabetes self-care practices, monitoring glucose levels, and adhering to dietary treatment and physical activity [39]. Behavioral changes and intensive lifestyle interventions are key components in the management of T2DM [36]. Poor practices, such as non-adherence to treatment, are a great concern to public health. A cross-sectional South African study reported poor practices among patients with diabetes-related to healthy lifestyle modifications [36]. Poor practices related to unhealthy eating among patients were reported in Lebanon [40]. Similar findings of poor practices related to diabetes management were also reported by a cross-sectional study conducted in Mpumalanga [41]. There is therefore a need to employ new measures to improve practices for improved diabetes outcomes.

3.1.2.4 Quality of life

Living with diabetes negatively impacts the quality of life (QoL) of patients, which is worsened in the presence of complications [42]. The negative way that diabetes impacts the patient's QoL includes the psychological impact of being chronically ill, dietary restrictions, changes in social life, symptoms of inadequate metabolic control, chronic complications, and ultimately lifelong disabilities [43, 44]. Diabetes patients from low-income countries can maintain a high QoL when treated with insulin [45]. An Argentinian study reported that the scores of QoL did not differ from those of patients in high-income countries where there is access to a high level of diabetes care [42]. An Indian observational study reported that nearly half of the diabetes patients (48.6%) had a good QoL [44]. An Iranian study reported that men living with diabetes compared to females, non-insulin-treated patients compared with insulin-treated patients had better QoL [46]. Further findings show that patients with Hemoglobin A1c (HbA1c) less than 7% had a better quality of life compared with those with a higher HbA1c [46].

Variables such as age, gender, socio-economic status, obesity, type of diabetes, treatment, chronic complications, health insurance, quality of care, and patient education have been associated with diabetes patients' Health-Related Quality of Life (HRQoL) [42]. Studies have shown that HRQoL is associated with the duration of diabetes, age, gender, diabetic complications, comorbid diseases, and the severity of the disease itself [42, 43]. A South African study that assessed the HRQoL using a Diabetes 39 (D-39) questionnaire reported an association between HbA1c and HRQoL, and no association was found between HRQoL and other clinical parameters such as the number of insulin units used per day, exercise, body mass index (BMI), lipogram and the use of oral hypoglycemic agents (OHAs) [43]. An Indian observational study reported that diabetes had significantly affected HRQoL, especially in the social relationship domain [44].

3.1.2.5 Anthropometric assessment

Anthropometric measurements estimate risk factors of different diseases [47], including diabetes and obesity. Body Mass Index is used to assess obesity, which reflects total body fat but does not reflect patterns of fat distribution [48]. Being overweight is only linked with T2DM morbidity, while obesity is linked with increased morbidity and mortality from diabetes and its complications [48]. The BMI characterization is similar across genders and ethnic groups [47]. The cut-offs for anthropometric indexes of abdominal adiposity, called waist circumference, vary by gender [45]. A high waist circumference is associated with cardiovascular risk, prevalence of diabetes, and incidences of hypertension [49]. High waist circumference and high body mass index (BMI) are considered risk factors for T2DM, though the relationship may differ with populations [47]. Several studies have reported that central obesity, which is measured through waist circumference, is an important and superior risk factor for developing diabetes, compared to the general obesity which is measured through BMI [47, 48].

Other anthropometric measurements for central obesity are Waist-to-Hip Ratio (WHR) and Waist-to Height Ratio (WtHR). According to Awasthi et al. [48], a Chinese population-based study reported that WtHR was the best anthropometric index for predicting diabetes mellitus. The WHR considers that waist circumference might over- or under-assess the dangers of different heights of individuals with the same waist circumference, while WtHR corrects waist circumference for height and can be used in different ethnic, age, and gender for central obesity [48].

3.1.2.6 Social determinants of health

Social determinants of health are non-medical factors that have an impact on health outcomes, well-being, and quality of life. These include conditions in which people are born, grow, live, work, and age [50]. Social determinants of health contribute significantly to health disparities and inequalities. For instance, a South African family of 5 adults and 4 children, depending only on an R1 890 old-age pension grant provided by the government may not have access to healthy food or good nutrition. Good nutrition is central to the development and progression of diabetes, including its management [12]. In addition, persons with less income and education were found to be 2–4 times more likely to develop diabetes compared to those with higher income and education [51, 52]. Within and outside the health sector, there are initiatives to mitigate the impact of social determinants of health through the adoption of health promotion and equity policies. For example, the introduction of social grants in South Africa is aimed at addressing social determinants of health. It is important for governments to prioritize the introduction of policies to address the social determinants of health in diabetes care, considering the increasing prevalence, complications, and management costs [53].

3.1.2.7 Examples of social determinants of health impacting diabetes

Housing: Access to proper housing is crucial in diabetes management. Improper housing creates a lack of the control and consistency needed for the daily management of diabetes, including diet, which is essential in glycemic control [54]. A lack of proper housing has been linked with increased blood glucose levels and the use of healthcare resources due to hospitalization. In addition, it impacts cholesterol and blood pressure levels, as well as the quality of life of patients with diabetes [55]. It was reported that persons in unstable housing are at a greater risk of developing diabetes, compared to those in stable housing [54]. Improved or stable housing may reduce disparities in diabetes outcomes while also helping with the initiation and maintenance of preventative care, minimizing the risk of diabetes, and improving outcomes overall [54].

Social and economic factors: Social and economic factors include income, education, employment, community safety, and social support; all of which affect the health and quality of life of persons and their life expectancy. These social and economic factors impact patients' ability to make healthy choices such as appropriate eating and active lifestyle, which are important in diabetes care. Employment or income could help in acquiring better houses, education, food, and medical treatment required in diabetes care. Unemployment or lack of income limits these options, leading to unhealthy eating and poor medical diabetes treatment [56]. Social support which includes family members is fundamental in diabetes care because most of the care happens at home [30]. Family members help with daily living activities including meal preparation and consumption, physical activity, collection of medication, bathing and clothing, distribution of household chores, and honoring of medical appointments. Family members may help patients with diabetes to cope with the disease and help with the finances needed for patients to perform their daily diabetes care activities [33]. Living alone is linked with increased depression, poor diabetes outcomes, and increased mortality [57].

4. Conclusion

A baseline analysis is affirmed as a fundamental prerequisite for the development of diabetes interventions for better outcomes. It also helps in identifying and addressing medical and non-medical factors which could impact diabetes care activities. Therefore, a baseline analysis is a foundational and critical step toward comprehensive healthcare intervention for better diabetes outcomes. There is a need to assess the capacity of healthcare providers to conduct a baseline analysis to determine the need for support and in-service training. An inappropriately-conducted baseline analysis may lead to inappropriate solutions and misdiagnosis. The implementation of inappropriate solutions would defeat the objective of improving diabetes outcomes.

Acknowledgements

The authors acknowledge existing literature regarding the baseline analysis in development of diabetes interventions, particularly the authors. Citation and full reference list have been provided. The language editor is hereby also acknowledged.

Conflict of interest

The authors declare no conflict of interest financial or otherwise.

Notes/thanks/other declarations

The authors declare that this manuscript is based on the existing literature regarding baseline analysis in development of diabetes interventions.

Author details

Mabitsela Mphasha[1*], Linda Skaal[2] and Tebogo Maria Mothiba[3]

1 Department of Public Health, University of Limpopo, South Africa

2 School of Health Sciences, University of Limpopo, South Africa

3 Faculty of Healthcare Sciences Executive Dean's Office, University of Limpopo, South Africa

*Address all correspondence to: pitso85@gmail.com

References

[1] Helmink JH, Gubbels JS, van Brussel-Visser FN, de Vries NK, Kremers SPJ. Baseline predictors of maintenance of intervention-induced changes in physical activity and sitting time among diabetic and pre-diabetic patients: A descriptive case series. BMC Research Notes. 2013;**6**(190):1-10. DOI: 10.1186/1756-0500-6-190

[2] Moullin JC, Dickson KS, Stadnick NA, Alberts B, Nilsens P, Broder-Fingert S, et al. Ten recommendations for using implementation frameworks in research and practice. Implementation Science Communications. 2020;**1**(42):1-12. DOI: 10.1186/s43058-020-00023-7

[3] Bani IA. Health needs assessment. Journal of Family & Community Medicine. 2008;**15**(1):13-20

[4] International Diabetes Federation (IDF). IDF Diabetes Atlas. 7th ed. Brussels: IDF; 2015

[5] National Institute of Diabetes. Prevent Diabetes Problems: Keep Your Diabetes under Control. NID; 2015. Available from: http://www.niddk.nih.gov/health-information/health-topics/Diabetes/prevent-diabetes-problems/Pages/index.aspx

[6] International Diabetes Federation. IDF Diabetes Atlas. 10th ed. Brussels: IDF; 2021

[7] Krause M, Gerchman F, Friedman R. Coronavirus infection (SARS-CoV-2) in obesity and diabetes comorbidities: Is heat shock response determinant for the disease complications? Diabetology and Metabolic Syndrome. 2020;**12**(63):1-9. DOI: 10.1186/s13098-020-00572-w

[8] van Wyk H. Complications of diabetes mellitus. South African Pharmacological Journal. 2015;**82**(10):16-20

[9] Shiferaw WS, Akalu TY, Aynalem YA. Prevalence of erectile dysfunction in patients with diabetes mellitus and its association with body mass index and glycated hemoglobin in Africa: A systematic review and meta-analysis. International Journal of Endocrinology. 2020:1-10

[10] Esposito K, Giugliano D. Lifestyle/dietary recommendations for erectile dysfunction and female sexual dysfunction. The Urologic Clinics of North America. 2011;**38**(3):293-301

[11] World Health Organization (WHO). Diabetes Mellitus. 2014. Available from: http://www.who.int/mediacentre/factsheets/fs138/en/

[12] American Diabetes Association. The Cost of Diabetes. Available from: www.diabetes.org

[13] Adeniyi OV, Yogeswaran P, Longo-Mbenza B, Ter Goon D, Ajayi AI. Cross-sectional study of patients with type 2 diabetes in OR Tambo district, South Africa. BMJ Open. 2016;**6**:e010875. DOI: 10.1136/bmjopen-2015-010875

[14] Patel MR. Social determinants of poor management of type 2 diabetes among the insured. Current Diabetes Reports. 2020;**20**(67):1-6. DOI: 10.1007/s11892-020-01354-4

[15] Muchiri JW, Rheeder P, Gericke G. Development and evaluation of nutrition programme for adults with type 2 diabetes in resource limited setting of Moretele sub-district, North West Province (South Africa) [thesis of Ph.D]. Health Sciences, University of Pretoria; 2013

[16] Afemikhe JA, Chipps J, Jooste K. Development of Health Education

Programme for self-management of type-2 diabetes in Edo State, Nigeria [Doctor of Philosophy in Nursing, thesis]. University of the Western Cape; 2016

[17] Wright J, Williams R, Wilkinson JR. Development and importance of health needs assessment. British Medical Journal (Clinical research ed.). 1998;**316**(7140):1310-1313. DOI: 10.1136/bmj.316.7140.1310

[18] Hall CE, Hall AB, Kok G, Mallya J, Courtright P. A needs assessment of people living with diabetes and diabetic retinopathy. BMC Research Notes. 2016;**9**:56-69

[19] World Health Organization (WHO). Global report on diabetes. Geneva: World Health Organization; 2016. Available from: https://apps.who.int/iris/handle/10665/204874

[20] Gómez-Velasco DV, Almeda-Valdes P, Martagón AJ, Galán-Ramírez GA, Aguilar-Salinas CA. Empowerment of patients with type 2 diabetes: Current perspectives. Diabetes, Metabolic Syndrome and Obesity. 2019;**6**(12):1311-1321

[21] Society for Endocrinology, Metabolism, and Diabetes of South Africa (SEMDSA). SEMDSA type 2 diabetes guidelines expert committee. Journal of Endocrinology, Metabolism and Diabetes of South Africa. 2017;**22**(Supplement 1):S1-S196

[22] Peek ME, Ferguson MJ, Roberson TP, Chin MH. Putting theory into practice: A case study of diabetes-related behavioral change interventions on Chicago's south side. Health Promotion Practice. 2014;**15**(20):40S-50S

[23] Muchiri J, Gericke GJ, Rheeder P. Impact of nutrition education on diabetes knowledge and attitudes of adults with type 2 diabetes living in a resource-limited setting in South Africa: A randomised controlled trial. Journal of Endocrinology, Metabolism and Diabetes of South Africa. 2016;**21**(2):26-34. DOI: 10.1080/16089677.2016.1200324

[24] Dombrowski SU. Form of delivery as a key 'active ingredient' in behaviour change interventions. British Journal of Health Psychology. 2016;**21**(4):733-740

[25] Centers for Disease Control (CDC). National Center for Chronic Disease Prevention and Health Promotion. National Diabetes Statistics Report: Estimates of Diabetes and Its Burden in the United States. Atlanta, GA: U.S. Department of Health and Human Services, GA; 2014

[26] Spronk I, Kullen C, Burdon C, O'Connor H. Relationship between nutrition knowledge and dietary intake. Britain Journal of Nutrition. 2014;**111**:1713-1726

[27] Raaijmakers LG, Hamers FJ, Martens MK, Bagchus C, de Vries NK, Kremers SPJ. Perceived facilitators and barriers in diabetes care: A qualitative study among health care professionals in the Netherlands. BMC Family Practice. 2013;**14**(114):1-9

[28] Ajzen I, Joyce N, Sheikh S, et al. Knowledge and the prediction of behaviour: The role of information accuracy in the theory of planned behaviour. Basic and Applied Social Psychology. 2011;**33**(2):101-117

[29] Shrivastava SR, Shrivastava PS, Ramasamy J. Role of self-care in management of diabetes mellitus. Journal of Diabetes & Metabolic Disorders. 2013;**12**(1):1-14

[30] Breen C, Ryan M, Gibney MJ, O'Shea D. Diabetes-related nutrition

knowledge and dietary intake among adults with type 2 diabetes. British Journal of Nutrition. 2015;**114**:439-447

[31] Al-Sahouri A, Merrell J, Snelgrove S. Barriers to good glycemic control levels and adherence to diabetes management plan in adults with Type-2 diabetes in Jordan: A literature review. Patient Preference and Adherence. 2019;**3**(13):675-693. DOI: 10.2147/PPA.S198828

[32] Ralineba T, Netshikweta ML, Shilubane NH. Knowledge and practices associated with diabetes among patients with chronic diabetes mellitus in rural areas of Vhembe District, Limpopo Province, South Africa. Journal of Human Ecology. 2015;**51**(1-2):193-201. DOI: 10.1080/09709274.2015.11906912

[33] Mphasha MH, Mothiba TM, Skaal L. Assessment of diabetes dietary knowledge and its impact on intake of patients in Senwabarwana, Limpopo, South Africa. Journal of Endocrinology, Metabolism and Diabetes of South Africa. 2021;**26**(3):89-95. DOI: 10.1080/16089677.2021.1927584

[34] Fogelman Y, Goldfracht M, Karkabi K. Managing diabetes mellitus: A survey of attitudes and practices among family physicians. Journal of Community Health. 2015;**2015**(40):1002-1007

[35] Le Roux M, Walsh C, Reid M, Raubenheimer J. Diabetes-related knowledge, attitude and practices (KAP) of adult patients with type 2 diabetes mellitus in the Free State province, South Africa. South African Journal of Clinical Nutrition. 2018;**0**(0):1-8. DOI: 10.1080/16070658.2018.1468536

[36] Okonta HI, Ikombele JB, Ogunbanjo GA. Knowledge, attitude and practice regarding lifestyle modification in type 2 diabetic patients: Original research. African Primary Healthcare and Family Medicine. 2014;**6**(1):1-6

[37] Hood KK, Hilliard M, Piatt G, Ievers-Landis CE. Effective strategies for encouraging behavior change in people with diabetes. Diabetes Management (London). 2015;**5**(6):499-510

[38] International Diabetes Federation. IDF Diabetes Atlas. 8th ed. Brussels: IDF; 2017

[39] Karaoui LR, Deeb ME, Nasser L, Hallit S. Knowledge and practice of patients with diabetes mellitus in Lebanon: A cross-sectional study. BMC Public Health. 2018;**18**(525):1-9

[40] Umeh AE, Nkombua L. A study of the knowledge and practice of lifestyle modification in patients with type 2 diabetes mellitus in Middelburg sub-district of Mpumalanga. South African Family Practice. 2018;**60**(1):26-30

[41] Trikkalinou A, Papazafiropoulou AK, Melidonis A. Type 2 diabetes and quality of life. World Journal of Diabetes. 2017;**8**(4):120-129

[42] Pichon-Riviere A, Irazola V, Beratarrechea A, Alcaraz A, Carrara C. Quality of life in type 2 diabetes mellitus patients requiring insulin treatment in Buenos Aires, Argentina: A cross-sectional study. International Journal of Health Policy and Management. 2015;**4**(7):475-480. DOI: 10.15171/ijhpm.2015.80

[43] Daya R, Bayat Z, Raal FJ. Effects of diabetes mellitus on health-related quality of life at a tertiary hospital in South Africa: A cross-sectional study. South African Medical Journal. 2016;**106**(9):918-928. DOI: 10.7196/SAMJ. 2016.v106i9.9899

[44] Raghavendra N, Viveki RG, Gadgade A. An observational study to assess the health-related quality of life of type 2 diabetes mellitus patients attending a tertiary care hospital,

Belagavi. International Journal of Community Medicine Public Health. 2017;**4**:3347-3353

[45] Mohammadi S, Karim NA, Talib RA, Amani R. Evaluation of quality of life among type 2 diabetes patients. International Journal of Community Medicine Public Health. 2016;**3**:51-56

[46] Bulum T, Blaslov K, Duvnjak L. The use of anthropometric measurements of obesity in prediction of microvascular complications in obese type-2 diabetic patients. Acta Clinica Croatia. 2016;**55**:217-223

[47] Awasthi A, Rao CR, Hegde DS, Raon K. Association between type 2 diabetes mellitus and anthropometric measurements – a case control study in South India. Journal of Preventive Medicine and Hygiene. 2017;**58**:E56-E62

[48] Kamath A, Shivaprakash G, Adhikari P. Body mass index and waist circumference in type 2 diabetes mellitus patients attending a diabetes clinic. International Journal Of Biological and Medical Research. 2011;**2**:636-638

[49] Spollett GR. Diabetes: Treating the coming Tsunami. Diabetes Spectrum: A Publication of the American Diabetes Association. 2013;**26**:58-62. DOI: 10.2337/diaspect.26.1.58

[50] World Health Organization. Social Determinants of Healthhttps://doi.org/www.who.int

[51] Agardh E, Allebeck P, Hallqvist J, Moradi T, Sidorchuk A. Type 2 diabetes incidence and socio-economic position: A systematic review and meta-analysis. International Journal of Epidemiology. 2011;**40**(3):804-818. DOI: 10.1093/ije/dyr029

[52] Saydah S, Lochner K. Socioeconomic status and risk of diabetes-related mortality in the US. Public Health Reports. 2010;**125**(3):377-388

[53] Glazier RH, Bajcar J, Kennie N, Wilson K. A systematic review of interventions to improve diabetes care in socially disadvantaged populations. Diabetes Care. 2006;**29**(7):1675-1688. DOI: 10.2337/dc05-1942

[54] Mosley-Johnson E, Walker RJ, Thakkar M, et al. Relationship between housing insecurity, diabetes processes of care, and self-care behaviors. BMC Health Services Research. 2022;**22**(61):1-8. DOI: 10.1186/s12913-022-07468-7

[55] Keene DE, Guo M, Murillo S. "That wasn't really a place to worry about diabetes": Housing access and diabetes self-management among low-income adults. Social Science & Medicine. 2018;**197**:71-77. DOI: 10.1016/j.socscimed.2017.1

[56] Darin-Mattsson A, Fors S, Kåreholt I. Different indicators of socioeconomic status and their relative importance as determinants of health in old age. International Journal for Equity in Health. 2017;**16**:173. DOI: 10.1186/s12939-017-0670-3

[57] Mayberry LS, Osborn CY. Family support, medication adherence, and glycemic control among adults with type 2 diabetes. Diabetes Care. 2012;**35**:1239-1245

Chapter 14

Factors Contributing to the Academic Challenges Faced by South African Physiotherapy, Occupational Therapy and Biokinetics Students

Makwena Brink Ntjana, Yvonne Paul, Marine Burger and Terry Jeremy Ellapen

Abstract

Students of the Health Science professions of Physiotherapy, Occupational Therapy, and Biokinetics share mutual subjects detailing human bodily functions, as well as their pathology and subsequent rehabilitation, as such sharing similarly factors influencing academic success. Factors influencing students' academic success include matriculation scores, pedagogic techniques, successful integration into the university environment, self-efficacy, finances, and the language of instruction/teaching. While the three professions share similar prerequisite matriculation subjects, their university admission point scores vary, generating a degree of concern within a number of higher education institutions (HEIs). The global need to provide liberal access to HEIs has encouraged many tertiary institutions to adopt a policy of affirmative action that encompasses two fundamental strategies; the provision of financial support for deserving undergraduate students from previously disadvantaged communities, and the lowering of prerequisite admission scores. Despite these attempts at the creation of higher education equity, many students' academic performance is poor. The primary objective of this chapter is to review the factors, which influence the academic success rate of students engaged in a course of study geared at entry into the Physiotherapy, Occupational Therapy, or Biokinetics professions at a South African HEI. This paper chapter seeks to recommend potential strategies to improve student academic performance.

Keywords: university admission criteria, physiotherapy, occupational therapy, biokinetics, higher education, academic challenges

1. Introduction

"Higher Education Institutions" (HEIs) refers to tertiary educational institutions which provide and confer advanced credentials such as certificates, higher certificates, diplomas, advance diplomas, undergraduate/bachelor degrees, and post graduate degrees (honours, masters and doctoral degrees) in specific professions and/or disciplines [1]. The practice of equity and liberal access to HEIs is associated with the socialist philosophical ideology of justice and democracy. Mkude, Cooksey, and Levey suggested that equity and liberal access to HEIs contributes to the growth of a progressive society by encouraging social inclusiveness, thereby instilling national camaraderie [2].

South Africa is a nation composed of four primary ethnic groups: Black, Coloured, White, and Indian reflecting great socioeconomic diversity both within and across groups [3]. In 1999, Professor Kadar Asmal attempted to forge a democratic and liberal ethos among South African HEIs by convening a Council on Higher Education (CHE) in order to evaluate, recommend and subsequently transform national educational policies with the goal of promoting greater impartiality and providing improved opportunities for previously disadvantaged ethnic groups, making higher education more accessible to all South Africans. The primary findings of the CHE were that disparities and diversity between the great numbers of South African HEIs were "divisive" with regards to ethnicity, geography/location, finances, and resources; they furthermore shared dissimilar administrative structures which ultimately produced gross inequalities across the board [4]. The CHE guided the process of higher education transformation, aimed at addressing questions of accessibility and inequality [5].

HEIs embraced two fundamental strategies in order to address the concerns of inaccessibility and inequality: firstly, the provision of financial aid to deserving students from low socio-economic communities; secondly, the manipulation of admission and selection policies in an attempt to accommodate students with impoverished socio-economic backgrounds [6]. This approach is referred to as affirmative action, and has been met with mixed emotions [7]. Modisha reported that affirmative action instituted among South African HEIs was geared at the decolonisation of apartheid policies of inaccessibility and inequality [8]. Affirmative action further sought to create new policies of accessibility and equality, enhancing the educational and subsequent employment prospects of students from socio-economically disadvantaged communities, and thus improving their overall quality of life. The National Student Financial Aid Scheme (NSFAS) was founded in 1996 by the Department of Higher Education and Training, so as to financially support undergraduate students. The post millennium admission criteria of South African HEIs has been amended, following global trends of affirmative action, receiving mixed reactions from the 19 South African HEIs [9].

Regardless of these attempts to eliminate gatekeeping and create higher education impartiality, the academic success of many students remains poor. Factors influencing academic success include final school year academic performance, successful integration into the university environment, self-efficacy, finances, the language of instruction/teaching, and student organisational skills [10, 11]. The primary objective of this paper is to review the factors which influence the academic success rate of students engaged in a course of study geared at entry into the Physiotherapy, Occupational Therapy, or Biokinetics professions at a South African HEI. This paper further seeks to recommend potential strategies to improve student academic performance.

2. Methodology

2.1 Protocol

An electronic narrative literature surveillance adopting the Preferred Reporting Items for Systematic Reviews (PRISMA) benchmarks was followed.

2.2 Registration

This review protocol was not registered with the International Prospective Register of Systematic Reviews.

2.3 Search strategy and literature sources

The admission criteria for the disciplines of Physiotherapy, Occupational Therapy and Biokinetics at South African HEIs were surveyed through the examination of HEI online study prospectuses which are readily found via the Google search engine. Only HEIs offering four-year professional degrees in Physiotherapy, Occupational Therapy, and Biokinetics were considered. While 19 HEIs in South Africa offer advanced educational qualifications, not all of them offer professional four-year academic programmes. Eight HEIs offered degrees in Physiotherapy and Occupational Therapy, but only six offered degrees in Biokinetics; this chapter is thus concerned with the review of the prerequisite admission criteria of the latter sic institutions. The review of the prerequisite admission criteria reviewed 2020 HEIs admission criteria. The primary keywords in the literature search were: admission criteria, thereafter subsequent words such as Physiotherapy, Occupational Therapy, Biokinetics and South Africa were added. The selection criteria of literature was the prospectus of various South African Higher Education Institutes (HEI) that offer Physiotherapy, Occupational Therapy and Biokinetics four-year professional academic programmes.

A second electronic search was instituted to determine the academic success of Physiotherapy, Occupational Therapy and Biokinetics among South African HEIs in the search engine of Google.

2.4 Eligibility criteria

Participants were records pertaining to the admission criteria of various HEI Physiotherapy, Occupational Therapy and Biokinetics academic programmes. Pertinent themes which emerged: national senior certificate with bachelor degree endorsement, perquisite secondary schooling subjects, minimum admission point score (APS) and national benchmark test.

2.5 Research questions

The identified themes evolved research questions:

- What is the admission criteria of Physiotherapy programmes offered at South Africa Higher Education Institutions?

- What is the admission criteria of Occupational Therapy programme offered at South Africa Higher Education Institutions?

- What is the admission criteria of Biokinetics programme offered at South Africa Higher Education Institutions?

- What other factors influence Physiotherapy, Occupational Therapy and Biokinetics students' academic success at South Africa HEI?

2.6 Omitting criteria

Records preceding to 2020, non-South African HEI admission criteria of Physiotherapy, Occupational Therapy and Biokinetics, academic programmes besides Physiotherapy, Occupational Therapy and Biokinetics programmes, factors influencing the academic success of tertiary students registered for disciplines other than Physiotherapy, Occupational Therapy and Biokinetics, and, non-English papers.

3. Results

Table 1 reflects the prerequisite admission criteria employed by South African HEIs for the admission of prospective students in the aforementioned Health Science disciplines. Mathematics, Life Science, Physical Science, and English were common matriculation subjects identified as precursors for HEI admission. However, subject prerequisite scores at each institution varied: the matriculation prerequisite score for admission to Physiotherapy ranges from 28 to 39, while that for Occupational ranges from 25 to 36 and the prerequisite scores for admission to Biokinetics vary from 24 to 37. Furthermore, while the National Benchmark Test was a popular assessment for admissions to the disciplines of Physiotherapy and Occupational Therapy, this was not the case with admissions to Biokinetics.

University	National Senior Certificate with bachelor's degree endorsement	Prerequisite Secondary Schooling subject level				Minimum Admission Point Score	National Benchmark Test
		Mathematics	Life Science	Physical Science	English		
Physiotherapy							
Kwa-Zulu Natal	✓	4	4	4	4	30	X
Sefako Makgatho	✓	4	4	4	4	28	X
Witwatersrand	✓	5	5	5	5		✓
Western Cape	✓	4	4	4	4	39	X
Stellenbosh		4	4		4		X
Cape Town	✓	5	5	5	5	36	✓
Pretoria	✓	4		4	4	30	✓
Free State	✓	5	5	5	5	36	✓
Average	✓	4.4	4.4	4.4	4.4	33.5	✓
Occupational Therapy							
Kwa-Zulu Natal	✓	3	3	3	4	30	X
Sefako Makgatho	✓	4	4	4	4	25	X
Witwatersrand	✓	4	4	4	4		✓
Western Cape	✓	3	4		4	33	X
Stellenbosh	✓	3	4				✓
Cape Town	✓	5	5	5	5	34	✓
Pretoria	✓	4		4	4	30	✓

University	National Senior Certificate with bachelor's degree endorsement	Prerequisite Secondary Schooling subject level				Minimum Admission Point Score	National Benchmark Test
		Mathematics	Life Science	Physical Science	English		
Free State	✓	5	5	5		36	✓
Average	✓	3.9	4.1	4.1	4.1	31	✓
Biokinetics							
Venda	✓					34	X
Johannesburg	✓	4	5	5	5	30	X
North-West	✓	3	4	4		32	X
Nelson Mandela	✓	4	4			37	X
Tshwane	✓	4	4		4	24	X
Free State	✓	5	5	5		34	X
Mean	✓	4	4.4	4.7	4.5	31.8	X

** Post 2007 admission criteria was derived from 2020 prospectuses.*
** While a Biokinetics programme is offered by 12 universities, only the aforementioned six offer a four-year integrated professional degree.*

Table 1.
South African university admission requirements for physiotherapy, occupational therapy, and biokinetics as of 2020 [12].

Authors (year) (reference)	Findings
Grigorenko et al. (2009) [13]	This study describes the predicting index of secondary academic success relating to tertiary academic success
Govender et al. (2015)	First year students experienced personal stressors as being the most significant stressor while second, third and fourth students reported academic stressors to be significant.
Kuznekoff et al. (2015) [14]	This study demonstrated that sending and/or receiving mobile messages unrelated to class content negatively influences learning and note-taking.
Li et al. (2015) [15]	Individuals submitting too greater external locus of control experience a greater challenge to control the mobile phone use at inopportune times, which negative effects important cognitive tasks.
Gordon et al. (2020) [16]	University students spend more class time using their mobile phones (up to 20% of their classroom time) texting, emailing, surfing the web, checking social media, and even playing games, which negatively influence their academic performance.
Mabizela et al. (2020) [17]	Academic success is related to the NBT and Physical Sciences matriculation results. Clinical implications of this finding suggests that support programmes (supplementary tutorials and language supplementation programmes) in the first year of university study are required to augment student success
Henderson et al. (2021) [18]	Health science students experience stress due to academic tasks, interpersonal stress and clinical experiential learning stresses.

Table 2.
Factors influencing academic success of tertiary students.

Other factors influencing the success of Physiotherapy, Occupational Therapy and Biokinetics students studying among South African HEIs include lower academic matriculation scores, supportive social infra-structure (family and friends) and attentive listening challenging when students attend lectures (refer to **Table 2**).

4. Discussion

The discussion is focused on the following themes: commonality among the professions of Physiotherapy, Occupational Therapy, and Biokinetics; the influence of final school year academic performance on subsequent tertiary academic success; other factors influencing academic tertiary performance; and strategies for the improvement of tertiary academic success.

4.1 Commonality among the professions of physiotherapy, occupational therapy and biokinetics

The professions of Physiotherapy, Occupational Therapy, and Biokinetics are concerned with the rehabilitation of human pathology at various stages of healing, thus requiring the study of similar academic literature. These professions treat pathologies that range from neuro-musculoskeletal pathologies to non-communicable diseases, operating in both the pathogenic (illness) and fortogenic (apparently healthy) healthcare paradigms [12, 19]. Practitioners require a sound knowledge of human anatomy, physiology, kinesiology and biomechanics. In some South African HEIs Physiotherapy, Occupational Therapy, and Biokinetics students attend the same fundamental modules, underlining the commonality between the disciplines. Furthermore, the prerequisite academic modules are identical: English, Mathematics, Life Science, and Physical Science (**Table 1**). However, the admission scores varies (**Table 1**). Moreover, these professions follow similarly structured residency and work-integrated learning programmes which are synthesised by their respective HEIs.

4.2 The prerequisite matriculation subjects for admission to physiotherapy, occupational therapy, and biokinetics

Final school year academic performance is positively correlated with strong tertiary academic prowess in so far as the final school year is an essential foundation for subsequent education [13, 20, 21]. Good results enhance the admissions eligibility of prospective students enabling them to pursue studies in their chosen career-path at HEIs [21]. The aforementioned Health Science professions have identified the need for satisfactory mastery of Mathematics, Life Science, Physical Science, and English (**Table 1**), and these subject requirements are in line with international prerequisites for analogous professions [22].

i. McNaught and Hoyne have suggested that secondary schooling Mathematical prowess can be applied to many collegiate academic programmes that require critical analysis and problem solving, such as Health Sciences and Engineering [23]. However, many South African matric scholars experience challenges that adversely impact upon their Mathematics performance [24]. The 2019 results reflected a dip in Mathematics performance where the academic pass rate dropped by 4%, falling from 58% the previous year [24]. In 2018, 6763 scholars achieved distinctions in Mathematics, as compared to the 4415 Mathematics distinctions which were awarded to the 2019 class, yielding an average 2% decrease in performance [24]. The South African Mathematics class of 2019 was furthermore significantly (17.9%) smaller than the 2018 class, indicating that fewer students are pursuing secondary school Mathematics [24].

ii. The Physical Science prerequisite reflects a need for the comprehension of fundamental internal human biochemical reactions caused by injury, medication and/or physical rehabilitation. Physical Science is the cornerstone of modern technology and empowers students to comprehend various therapeutic technologies, as well as enabling them to ultimately develop new rehabilitation devices. As with the 2019 Mathematics matriculation results, Physical Science results have also declined with 24.5% of scholars failing the 2019 national senior certificate examination [25]. Comparing the 2019 results to those of the previous year, 3700 fewer scholars were able to secure pass marks in this subject [26].

iii. English proficiency is needed in so far as it is the predominant language of tuition among South African HEIs. English proficiency has been correlated with strong academic performance due to the fact that students are thus better able to comprehend the subject matter. While English is widely spoken, it is nevertheless not the first language of many South African students, a factor which limits their proficiency and places them at a disadvantage [8].

Academic performances in Mathematics, Life and Physical Sciences and English in the course of the final school year are strong predictors of the tertiary academic performance of prospective Health Science students [21, 22, 26]. Many South African scholars struggle to achieve strong grades in Mathematics, Physical Science, and English, which eventually adversely impact on their tertiary academic performance [24]. Many South African tertiary students studying Physiotherapy and Occupational Therapy experience academic challenges as evidenced by Govender *et al* who reported that Occupational Therapy students with lower academic matriculation admission scores took longer to complete their degrees as compared to students who possessed higher academic matriculation scores and maintained better grade average scores in the course of their studies [27]. Similarly Mabizela *et al* concur that secondary school competency strongly influences the academic success of Physiotherapy students [17].

4.3 The variation of the prerequisite matriculation scores allowing admittance into physiotherapy, occupational therapy and biokinetics

The minimum matriculation prerequisite admission scores allowing entry to the aforementioned South African HEIs for the study of Physiotherapy, Occupational Therapy, and Biokinetics vary (**Table 1**). While some South African HEIs have adopted a policy of lowering academic prerequisite scores in order to provide equitable access to tertiary education, this has not been favourably accepted by all HEIs [7, 9]. Varying prerequisite academic scores for admission have raised concerns regarding the integrity and the quality of the programmes offered at tertiary institutions who propose lower admission scores. This is especially relevant in so far as the various programmes share common prerequisite secondary school subjects, as well as common tertiary subjects (Human Anatomy, Physiology,

Kinesiology, Biomechanics, Clinical and Orthopaedic Pathology, and Principles of Rehabilitation). Unequal prerequisite admission scores for Physiotherapy, Occupational Therapy and Biokinetics among HEIs who ostensibly offer the same academic content, all of which is regulated and endorsed by the Health Professions of Council (HPCSA), show 9, 11, and 13 point variances [28]. The post millennium HEI policy of accessibility and equality has universally lowered prerequisite admission scores and is aimed at increasing overall student intake from socioeconomically disadvantaged communities. Further discrepancies among the already lowered prerequisite scores is therefore concerning. Rather than lowering their admissions criteria, South African HEIs should standardise their entry requirements, aligning the requirements to the mean score required for entry into the aforementioned vocations across the board, thereby accommodating previously disadvantaged students. This will serve to provide equity and liberal access to all eligible prospective students. However, not all HEIs are pleased to lower their prerequisite admission scores, in so far as they feel that it raises questions regarding the quality of the education provided by the university and consequently of the degree that is conferred upon the student [9]. Standardising entry requirements using mean scores effectively represents a compromise between the imperative to offer greater access and opportunities to students, and the maintenance of degree integrity and quality.

Another variation is the national benchmark test (NBT) that most HEIs offering Physiotherapy and Occupational Therapy require, and which is not required for entry into the study of Biokinetics. The NBT is a uniform South African test that all Grade 12 learners or any other prospective candidate intending to secure university admission have to complete, assessing Mathematical and Language Literacy together with overall readiness for tertiary-level education. This test measures the acumen of the candidate [29]. Given that Mathematics and English literacy are already prerequisites for admission to the aforementioned courses of study, the compulsory inclusion of the NBT will consolidate and standardise the prospective candidate's HEI application.

4.4 Other factors influencing academic tertiary performance

Academic success is further influenced by psychosocial factors including student self-efficacy and strong supportive social infrastructure (family and friends) [13]. Student self-efficacy is an intrinsic psychological motivation driving students to succeed academically with strong repercussions on tertiary academic accomplishment, lowering HEI drop-out rates. Strong academic success in the final year of schooling augments the confidence of prospective students thereby reinforcing their self-efficacy, engendering stronger tertiary academic success. Elements of self-efficacy include wisdom, intelligence and creative synthesis [13]. Additional factors influencing academic success include self-responsibility, regular class attendance, and attentive listening in class. Poor academic achievement is accomplished by students who attend class but rarely focus on what is said in class due to attentive listening challenges during lectures including students' preoccupation with their mobile phones [14–16]. Attentive listening is an essential soft skill imperative to problem solving, and which enables a person to become a strong leader and solid team member in so far as it improves their interpersonal communication skills. In the aforementioned professions, being able to attentively listen to a patient is imperative for successful rehabilitation. Kuznekoff *et al* and Gordon reported that the use of mobile phones to surf the internet, and to send and receive messages unconnected to the lecture at hand negatively impacted learning and note-taking [14, 16]. This is a worrisome concern.

4.5 Pedagogic strategies to augment academic success

The authors agree with concept of creating HEI equity and liberal access to all eligible prospective students. However, strategies aimed at overcoming the generally poor academic performances in South African HEIs need to be employed. South African HEIs should therefore enact strategies designed to augment their students' academic success. The following strategies have found success at other global HEIs, and these can serve as models for future pedagogic strategies adapted to specific institutional contexts:

i. Change from traditional teaching methods to more conventional approaches has proven to increase academic success [30, 31].

ii. Superficial learning of basic knowledge needs to be replaced with deeper understanding, which should be articulated through innovative pedagogic strategies. Educators have moved away from surface learning (the rote of memorization of knowledge) to deeper understanding, which is honed through active processes. Roehl et al. have recommended the idea of active learning through individual learning, paired groups, small informal groups, and larger co-operative student projects [31]. This approach encourages brain-storming, conceptual mapping, co-operative learning, and collaborative peer teaching. The student is no longer a spectator and becomes an active participant involved in the pedagogic process. During a single contact lecture, the students must be exposed to a traditional lecture format, coupled with individual problem solving, peer and group interaction, and learning which embraces the concept of active learning [31].

iii. The use of the flipped classroom model, whereby lecture content is assigned as homework, and which students are required to complete prior to the lecture, is also a recent and successful pedagogic strategy. This strategy allows students to familiarise themselves with the literature before attending class. Tucker contends that the adoption of the flipped classroom model allows the lecturer and students to use contact time for the discussion of advanced concepts, problem solving, and engagement in collaborative learning with colleagues. The flipped classroom model makes students active participants of the lecture [30].

iv. The luxury of readily available internet access is a common occurrence at most sites on HEIs campuses and should be readily adopted in so far as it allows for dynamic pedagogic strategic initiatives in order to encourage learning. Lecture notes, PowerPoint presentations and other materials should be uploaded onto the relevant teaching platforms so that each student is able to review the class material in their own time and at their own pace. This will ensure that teaching, and learning, can take place outside the classroom [31]. Classroom and lecture activities should include the use of smartphones and electronic tablets, thereby ensuring that student know how to use technology to supplement their learning. The use of mobile devices during the lecture for pedagogic purposes, will eliminate unwanted personal messaging.

v. The question of the translation of the primary language of instruction from English into one or many of the indigenous South African languages remains of concern. Many South Africans do not speak English as their first language and they furthermore lack proficiency in English (especially as regards the reading, writing and discussion of advanced academic topics), this consequently may limit their comprehension of both academic literature and of their lessons [32]. The translation of the language of instruction into their indigenous language will better facilitate comprehension of subject content as discussed in class [32]. At North-West University of South Africa the introduction of translators, who accompany the lecturer has proven successful. The lecturer is thus able to present the lecture in their preferred language, while the translator simultaneously provides students with an opportunity to garner a greater understanding of the matter in so far as the lecture is directly translated into their native language. Unfortunately, this service is available only for Sesotho and Afrikaans and there is a pressing need for the simultaneous translation of lectures into other indigenous South African languages in order to uniformly accommodate all students. Furthermore, while all theoretical tests and examinations should be translated into indigenous languages, the ever present question of the finances available for such initiatives means that certain languages will need to be prioritised over others. The authors recommend that the most commonly spoken indigenous language of each HEI should be identified. If a third or more of the student body speak the language as their first language, then this language should be identified and recognised as an indigenous language of the particular institution and attempts at establishing simultaneous translations of lectures should be considered. South African students should also realise that English is the primary global language and they should therefore also make a personal attempt to become proficient so as to enhance their educational outcomes.

vi. The use of student mentors in order to facilitate both the successful transition from secondary schooling to HEIs, as well as the progressive annual succession within each course of study has proven beneficial [11]. Lavhelani et al. have reported that the poor academic performance of many South African students is associated with the failure of academic support [33]. Vitali et al. reported that regular consultation with student mentors has assisted students in better organising their daily schedules, enabling them to balance their study and extra-curricular activities, positively impacting their academic performance [11]. Each semester, following the first round of assessments, all students should be strongly encouraged to consult the student mentor within their given discipline in order to seek advice regarding the way forward. This will help to identify students who are struggling to comply with study requirements. The earlier that student receive academic support, the greater their probability of success [34]. It is further recommended that NBT results should be reviewed at the beginning of the first semester in order to identify at risk students. This chapter concurs with the recommendations of Gultice et al. who state that new pedagogic criteria enabling the identification of at risk students should be invented [34].

5. Conclusion

Many factors influence tertiary academic performance; these include matriculation prerequisite results, the language of instruction, pedagogical methods and student mentoring. Physiotherapy, Occupational Therapy, and Biokinetics share communal matriculation subject prerequisites and professional subject content, but their university admission prerequisite scores differ. Consistent matriculation prerequisite admission scores are thus needed, given the overall similarity between the programmes. The authors recommend that the mean admission prerequisite score of the various HEIs be standardised across the board, allowing the aforementioned disciplines to satisfy both the need for HEI equity and maintaining educational quality. Furthermore, scholars interested in studying in these fields need to enhance their Mathematics and Physical Science marks as these serve as cornerstones of the aforementioned disciplines. The strategic use of predictive psychometric testing to identify the risk profile of prospective students is imperative for the provision of effective academic support programmes. Moreover, the need to prescribe and employ indigenous languages that students are familiar with is worth considering in an attempt to improve the overall quality of education.

Conflict of interest

None.

Author details

Makwena Brink Ntjana, Yvonne Paul, Marine Burger and Terry Jeremy Ellapen*
Faculty of Science, Department of Sport Rehabilitation and Dental Science, Tshwane University of Technology, Pretoria, South Africa

*Address all correspondence to: tellapen1@yahoo.com

References

[1] Benjamin KB, Dunrong B. Privatization of higher education in Tanzania. The Social Sciences. 2010;**5**(1):45-48. DOI: 10.3923/sscience.2010.45.48

[2] Mkude D, Cooksey B, Levey L. Higher education in Tanzania. The Journal of Modern African Studies. 2003;**43**(3):505-507

[3] Mzangwa ST. The effects of higher education policy on transformation in post-apartheid South Africa. Cogent Education. 2019;**6**(1):1592737. DOI: 10.1080/2331186X.2019.1592737

[4] CHE (council of Higher Education). National Plan For Higher Education in South Africa. 2000 dhet.gov.za

[5] Gibbon T, Kabaki J. Transformation in Higher Education: Global Pressures and Local Realities in South Africa. Dordrecht: Kluwer Academic Publishers; 2004. pp. 123-152

[6] Boulton G, Lucas G. What are universities for? Chinese Science Bulletin. 2011;**56**(23):2506-2517. DOI: 10.1007/s11434-011-4608-7

[7] Mkude D. Higher education as an instrument of social integration in Tanzania: Challenges and prospects. Research in Comparative and International Education. 2011;**6**(4):366. DOI: 10.2304/rcie.2011.6.4.366

[8] Modisha G. Employment equity: Can it produce a representative workforce? HSRC Review. 2007;**5**(4):14-15. Retrieved from: http://www.hsrc.ac.za/HSRC_Review_Article-69.phtml

[9] Villetee F. Mixed Reactions to Lowering of University Admission Requirements. Cape Town, South Africa: Cape Times; 2020

[10] Van Zyl G, Bezuidenhout J, Adefuye A. Factors affecting academic performance in anatomical sciences at a South African university: Students' perspective. Africa Education Review. 2020;**17**(3):52-73

[11] Vitali J, Blackmore C, Mortazavi S, Anderton R. Teritary anatomy and physiology: A barrier for student success. International Journal of Higher Education. 2020;**9**(2):289-296

[12] Ellapen TJ, Swanepoel M. The evolution of the profession of biokinetics. South African Journal of Research in Sport Physical Education Recreation. 2017;**39**(1):41-50

[13] Grigorenko EL, Jarvin L, Diffley R, Goodyear J, Shanahan EJ, Stemberg RJ. Are SSATS and GPA enough? A theory-based approach to predicting academic success in secondary school. Journal of Educational Psychology. 2009;**101**(4):964-981. DOI: 10.1037/a0015906

[14] Kuznekoff JH, Munz S, Titsworth S. Mobile phones in the classroom: Examining the effects of texting, twitter, and message content on student learning. Communication Education. 2015;**64**(3):344-365. DOI: 10.1080/03634523.2015.1038727

[15] Li J, Lepp A, Barkley JE. Locus of control and cell phone use: Implications for sleep quality, academic performance, and subjective well-being. Computers in Human Behavior. 2015;**52**:450-457

[16] Gordon S. How smartphones create distractions in classrooms. Very Well Family. 2020. Available from:

https://www.verywellfamily.com/how-smartphones-are-creating-distractions-in-the-classroom-4174646

[17] Mabizela SE, Roos R, Myezwa H, Potterton J. Predictors for the academic success of first-year physiotherapy students at a South African university. South African Journal of Physiotherapy. 2020;**76**(1):1-8. DOI: 10.4102/sajp.v76i1.1418

[18] Henderson RM, Chetty O, Gurayah T. Coping styles and sources of stress of undergraduate health science students: An integrative review. South African Journal of Occupational Therapy. 2021:**51**(2):29-38. Available from: http://www.scielo.org.za/scielo.php?script=sci_arttext&pid=S2310-38332021000200005&lng=en&nrm=iso

[19] Ellapen TJ, Paul Y, Swanepoel M, Strydom GL. Do biokineticists transgress on physiotherapists' scope of profession? Evidence-based analysis of two physical rehabilitation disciplines in South Africa. African Journal for Physical Activity and Health Science. 2018;**24**(3):316-331

[20] McKenise K, Schwetzer RD. Who succeeds at university? Factors predicting academic performance in first year Australian university students. Higher Education & Development. 2001:**20**(1):20-33

[21] Mills C, Heyworth J, Rosenwax L, Carr S, Rosenberg M. Factors associated with the academic success of first year health science students. Advances in Health Science Education. 2007;**14**(2):205-217 DOI: 10.1007/s10459-008-9103-9

[22] Anderton RS, Chivers PT. Predicting academic success of health science students for first-year anatomy and physiology. International Journal for Higher Education. 2016;**5**(1):250-260

[23] McNaught K, Hoyne G. Mathematics for first year success. In Proceedings of the 14th Pacific Rim First Year in Higher Education Conference, 29 June – 1 July, Fremantle, London, UK; 2011. Retrieved from http://fyhe.com.au/past_papers/papers11/FYHE-2011/content/pdf/4F.pdf

[24] Shay S. Why South Africa's Maths performance is worrying? SAST. 2020:**1**(1):1-4

[25] Head T. Matric results: Three subject areas facing alarming declines. Lifestyle. 2020;**1**(1):1-1

[26] Sadler PM, Tai RH. The two high-school pillars supporting college science. Science-New York Then Washington. 2007;**317**(5837):457-458

[27] Govendor P, Mkhabela S, Hlongwane M, Jetha CG. Occupational therapy Student's experience of stress and coping. South African Journal of Occupational Therapy. 2015;**45**(3):34-39. DOI: 10.17159/2310-3833/2015/v45n3/a7

[28] Health Professions Council of South Africa (HPCSA). No 1746: Regulations Defining the Scope of Practise for the Profession of Physiotherapy, Biokinetics and Occupational Therapy. 2020. Retrieved from http://www.hpcsa.ac.za

[29] Van der Merwe D, De Beer M. Challenges of students' selection: Predicting academic performance. South African Journal of Higher Education. 2006;**20**(4):547-562

[30] Tucker B. The flipped classroom. Education Next. 2012;**12**(1):82-83

[31] Roehl A, Reddy SL, Shannon GJ. The flipped classroom: An opportunity to engage millennial students through active learning strategies. FGCS. 2013;**105**(2):44-49

[32] Schreiber B, Yu D. Exploring student engagement practises at a South African university: Student engagement as reliable predictor of academic performance. South African Journal of Higher Education. 2016;**30**(5):157-175. DOI: 10.20853/30-5-593

[33] Lavhelani NP, Ndebele C, Ravhuhali F. Examining the efficacy of student academic support systems for 'At risk' first entering students at a historically disadvantaged South African university. Interchange. 2020;**51**:137-156

[34] Gultice A, Witham A, Kallmeyer R. Are students ready for anatomy and physiology? Developing tools for identifying students at risk for failure. Advances in Anatomy and Physiology. 2015;**39**(2):108-115

Chapter 15

In the Process of Being Left Behind: Rural-Urban Migration, Precarious Work Conditions, and the Health of Neglected Populations in Agbogbloshie, Accra, Ghana

Ransford Kwaku Afeadie, Mary Naana Essiaw, Susanna Adjei Arthur, Andrew Kweku Conduah, Dorothy Siaw-Marfo and Bridget Elikem Mensah

Abstract

Unlike international labour migration, there is a lack of substantive evidence of precarious work conditions and their associated poor health outcomes among rural-urban migrant labour workers. A lacuna that this paper attempts to fill in one of Ghana's urban slums, Agbogbloshie. We employed a sequential explanatory mixed methods design. In the absence of any sampling frame, simple random sampling was used to select 113 migrant household heads, while purposive sampling was used to select 12 in-depth interviews (IDI) and (8) key informant interviews (KII). The paper leans on the Harris-Todaro (1970) model and the ecological model. We found various precarious work activities, mostly dirty, demeaning, dangerous, and unrewarding. Logistic regression was performed on whether or not the type of work undertaken by the migrants resulted in ill-health. Using motor riders as reference, it indicates that electronic waste dealers' odds of ill-health (OR=1.0 [95%CI: 0.09–10.17]; P=1.0). Scraps dealers (OR=0.69[95%CI: 0.10–4.72]; P=0.71). Head porters (OR=0.25[95%CI: 0.22–6.97]; P=0.80. Street hawkers (OR= 0.5[95%CI: 0.03–7.45]; P=0.62). Truck pushers (0.83[95%CI: 0.05–13.63]; P=0.90). However, the association between precarious work and ill-health was insignificant across all work activities (P > 0.05). We found a slow pace in the government's response to addressing precarious work activities. We recommend work acceleration.

Keywords: rural-urban migration, precarious work, disease burdens, unfavourable informal workplace policy, slum

1. Introduction

In 2015, the number of international migrants reached 244 million [1]. However, a considerably higher number of migrants—740 million—moved within their countries, mainly from rural to urban areas or from one rural area to another [2]. This figure is expected to rise. The Department for International Development of the United Kingdom Government (DFID) estimates that in sub-Saharan Africa (SSA) 50%–80% of rural households include at least one migrant member [3]. The majority of the people who migrate are young individuals [4–13].

These young migrants are between the ages of fifteen and twenty-four and make up one-eighth of the migrant workers who are moving mainly in search of better opportunities [14]. As a number of young men and women lack sufficient access to quality education, job opportunities, and a decent standard of living in their rural areas, the expanding urban informal sector becomes attractive to most of these rural youths [15–17]. This situation is worsened by the fact that farming in some of rural areas is not very attractive, partly because of the lack of capital to acquire advanced farming implements that will help the farmers expand their business. Young people, therefore, see migration to the major cities as the only option to earn decent incomes that will make life comfortable for them [18, 19].

As a result of the lack of the necessary skills, they are unable to compete in the formal labor market at their destination. The same can also be said of the lack of sufficient economic assets, social capital, and cultural capital [20]. They normally end up living in informal settlements [21]. The consequence of this is that most of them are forced to accept low-income employment, precarious work, unemployment, or underemployment [20]. The term precarious work, as used in this study, means work that is uncertain, unstable, and insecure and in which employees are faced with work-related risks and receive limited social benefits and statutory protections [22–28].

What this also means is that the rise of precarious work in urban areas is of great importance not only for the work situations and career opportunities that workers can expect but additionally for large-scale social issues, including the role of the welfare state and the nature of economic policy [29]. Migration can lead to positive development results and eventually to achieving the objectives of the 2030 Agenda for Sustainable Development Goal 8, which talks about decent work for all. At the destination, migrants can provide labor where there are shortages and can also contribute to services, thereby increasing the government budget through the payment of taxes and social security contributions.

However, this does not mean that migration always achieves its full potential. For example, in their study on migration and sustainable cities, Lucci et al., [30] noted that vulnerable urban migrants often work in the informal sector, where the rewards of migration are unrewarding. In most of Ghana's urban areas, for instance, female head porters popularly referred to as "Kayayei", earn a living by carrying loads on their heads in market places and lorry stations. Though this indecent work serves as the main source of income for these female migrants, who are mostly from the northern parts of Ghana, the arduous tasks they perform on a daily basis create a number of health-related problems for them [31–33]. This indicates that migrants are also more likely to encounter work-related accidents and diseases [34, 35]. This situation is especially common among those working in the informal economy, who are also less likely to be protected through social-insurance schemes. Migrants may, therefore, lose extended periods of time to diseases. They may also end up with disabilities that limit their future earning potential or, in extreme cases, lose their lives. There is also the likelihood that if policies are not put in place to regularize the activities of controllers of the informal sector, most, if not all, of these migrants may return home with different health conditions, and the little money they might have earned will be used to treat these diseases. This can largely affect the migration intentions of many migrants, a situation that will make it difficult to achieve the 2030 Agenda for Sustainable Development Goal 8. It is important to note that the multi-faceted nature of the relationship between migration and development offers concrete and sector-specific policy entry points. For instance, the International Labor Organization (ILO) maintains that one factor that should always be considered in migration issues is the issue of decent work. Any decision to be taken as part of this agenda should consider the specific vulnerabilities of migrants in their various workplaces [30].

There is substantive evidence of precarious work conditions and their associated health outcomes, often connected to international migrant labor workers. For instance, Quandt et al., [36] note that these migrant labor workers are often engaged in what is known as 3-D jobs-dirty, dangerous, and demanding (sometimes degrading or demeaning), and these workers are often hidden from or invisible to the public eye and from public policy. They work for less pay, for long hours, and in worse conditions than non-migrants, and are often subject to human rights violations, abuse, human trafficking, and violence [37]. These conditions put immigrant workers at an increased risk of occupational fatalities and injuries when compared to native-born workers, even those doing the same job in the same industry [38].

However, anecdotal evidence suggests that similar precarious work activities are increasingly becoming common even among natives (internal migrants) of most developing countries who migrate from one part of the country to the cities in search of employment opportunities, and this phenomenon has escaped the research lens, a lacuna this paper attempts to fill. Therefore, this paper attempts to examine the precarious work conditions and health of rural-urban migrants living in the informal settlements of Agbogbloshie in Accra, Ghana. Specifically, the study seeks to ask the following questions: What are the precarious work activities often engaged in by these migrant workers living in the poor urban setting of Accra? How does the precarious work they undertake affect their health outcomes? What has been the government's response to address precarious work conditions among this subpopulation?

1.1 Theoretical underpinning

For the purpose of this study, we used the Harris–Todaro [19] model of migration and the ecological model of public health [39] to explain the study. The Harris–Todaro model of migration was utilized to explain why individuals engage in rural-urban migration in developing countries despite high joblessness rates in urban areas. Building on studies by early researchers, such as Ravenstein, Harris, and Todaro, view migration as an economic activity, which for the individual migrant could be a balanced choice in spite of the presence of urban unemployment [19]. They argued that migration is a result of urban-rural differences in expected income rather than actual earnings [19]. Potential migrants consider the various labor market opportunities available in both rural and urban areas and choose the one that augments their expected gains from migration. Although Harris–Todaro's model has been criticized as theoretically simplistic [40, 41], it can be credited with providing some explanations for why people migrate from rural to urban areas despite the lack of jobs. Migrants have no choice but to engage in any type of employment in the city, which is largely unregulated with accompanying health risks.

Our use of the ecological model [39] comes from the fact that it suggests structural changes better and highlights the enormous individual efforts of the migrants, which prevents them from working in activities that are hazardous in nature and ensures behavioral change. The ecological model is a framework widely employed in public health research and practice. It is also a framework of the processes and social conditions that facilitate health-promoting policy and environmental change. Ecological models are visual depictions of dynamic relationships among individuals, groups, and their environments. They derive from a systems orientation to human development in which individuals are understood to influence (and be influenced by) people and organizations with whom they interact, available resources and institutions, and societal norms and rules [39]. In the health promotion field, ecological models have been used to understand and identify targets for both general and specific health behavior interventions [42–48].

2. Research methodology

2.1 Study setting

The study focuses on Agbogloshie in Accra. Agbogbloshie is the nickname of a commercial district on the Korle Lagoon of the Odaw river, near the center of Accra, Ghana's capital city. Near the slum called "Old Fadama," the population of Agbogbloshie consists of economic migrants from northern and other rural parts of Ghana. To make a living, most Agbogbloshie residents engage in precarious economic activities [49]. For example, Ghana's e-waste dump site at Agbogbloshie is reportedly the biggest in sub-Saharan Africa, and this has attracted the attention of many international environmental groups, researchers, and journalists. The dump is currently a site for trading in products recovered from the waste stream [23, 50]. Migrant workers scavenge the waste, dismantling the scrap in open-air burning to recover precious components for sale, including gold, copper, silver, aluminum, iron, and brass [51]. Children who are able to attend school often spend every evening and weekend processing waste, and searching for metals [52]. Dwellings are wooden shacks that lack water and sanitation [53]. Besides, Agbogloshie also serves as an area for most migrants who work as head porters, locally referred to as "Kayayei," who are manual laborers and transport goods to and from the markets. Typically, these head porters carry their loads in a large pan placed on their heads, using a moistened coil of cloth as a buffer to make a living. This and many other precarious economic activities are what migrants are confronted with in their daily routine work for survival. As a result, Agbogbloshie serves as a prime location for this study (**Figure 1**).

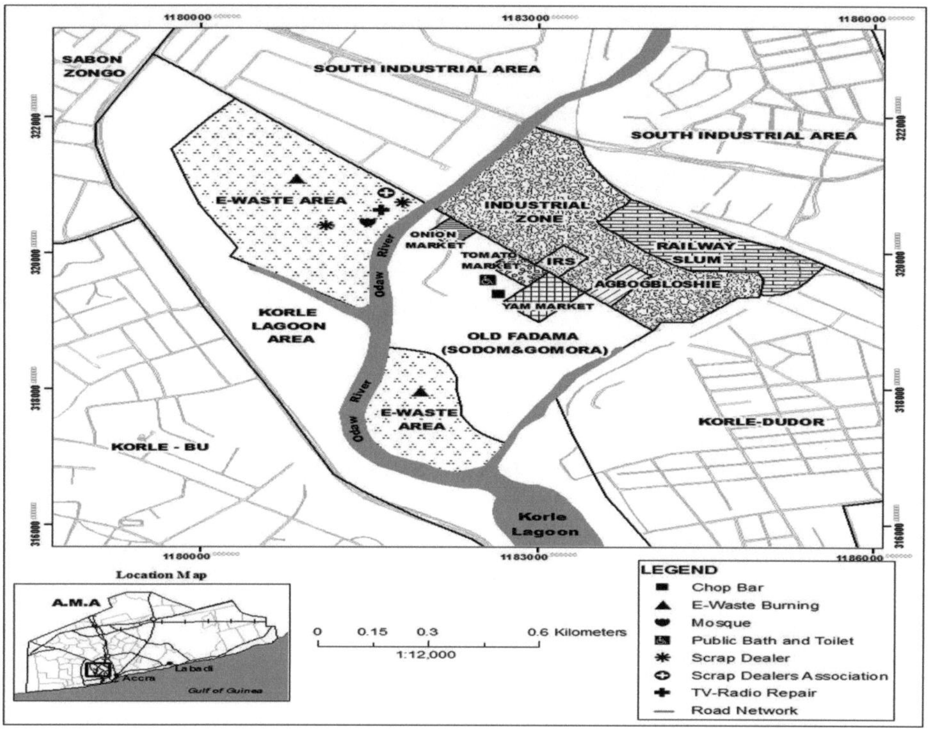

Figure 1.
Map of the study area.

2.2 Research design

We employed the mixed method approach of research investigation. The study further used the sequential explanatory mixed methods design. This approach is supported and accepted by the pragmatic paradigm [54]. This was to allow the initial quantitative data results to be explained further with the qualitative data. This triangulation of several methods provides the strengths and weaknesses of individual methods [55, 56]. We used questionnaire surveys and interview guides for primary data collection purposes. Secondary sources used included books, journals, articles, and some scholarly internet sites, such as jstor.org, database, and Google advanced search. The use of secondary data was to help us gain an initial insight into the research problem.

2.3 Study population and sample size

Migrant labor workers who are engaged in precarious work activities in the poor urban setting of Agbogbloshie served as the population for the study. An enumeration undertaken in 2009 shows that the area has a total population of 79,684, with a population density of 2,424 persons per hectare [57]. For the quantitative, an initial screening of rural-urban migrant slum households' heads or their representatives was conducted. In total, 119 of the respondents were identified to represent the total population of the respondents. The small sample size that was identified during the screening was a result of the fact that data were collected during the upsurge of COVID-19; hence, most of the migrants had gone back to their places of origin in order to avoid any threat posed by the virus. Yamane's formula was used to determine the sample size of 113. The formula is stated below:

$$n = \left[N/1 + N(e)2 \right]$$

Determination of sample size is based on the estimated population size (n = 119).
N - The sample size
N - The population size
e - The desired level of precision or level of acceptable error = 0.05)
Total sample size (n) = [119/(1+119(0.05)2] = [119/(1+119×0025)
= [119/1+0.05]
= [119/1.05]
=113

For the qualitative aspect, an estimated twenty-one (21) respondents were selected for the data collection. But due to saturation, a total of twelve (18) respondents were selected. Twelve (12) in-depth interviews (IDI) and eight (8) key informant interviews (KII) were held with the migrants. The use of the qualitative approach enabled us to select participants who were engaged in precarious work activities and were knowledgeable about the issue under investigation. It is also to allow the migrants to share their experiences about migration and precarious working conditions and how these have affected their health outcomes.

2.4 Sampling frame, sampling technique

In the absence of any existing reliable sampling frame, a household listing exercise was conducted in the migrant communities and a recording of the contacts of the household representatives (or heads) was made, to whom the questionnaires were administered. The simple random sampling technique was used to gather quantitative data. This was accomplished by labeling code numbers to the households, which were then placed in a box and shuffled. The labels were then picked randomly from the box to form the sample in a series of draws. The aim was to ensure that each household head had an equal chance of being selected [58].

For the qualitative study, the purposive sampling technique was used to select the respondents. Since the majority of the respondents did not understand English, the services of a translator were engaged to help with translation into the English language, and this served as the main mode of communication between the researcher and the migrants. To understand what the participants were saying, the translator used Dagbani and Mamprusi (i.e., their local dialects) to convey the information to the participants. Also, a key informant interview was conducted at the Ministry of Employment and Labor Relations, which is a government department. This was to enable us to understand the efforts being made by the government to address the precarious working conditions of migrant labor workers in Ghana.

2.5 Ethical consideration

We adhered to the national protocol on ethical issues in conducting research involving subjects. Permission was sought from the opinion leaders before entering the community by announcing the study. Also, written consent was obtained from the participants after carefully explaining the key issues to be considered before giving consent. Participants who did not want to participate or withdraw from the study could do so at any time.

While noting the caution in giving incentives to research participants, some incentives, such as soaps and the cost of transportation fare, were given at the end of every meeting.

2.6 Inclusion and exclusion criteria

For our inclusion criteria the following protocols were observed:

- Only rural-urban migrants residing in any of the informal settlements at Agbogbloshie.
- Participants should have resided in any of the slum communities for no less than 6 months.
- Participants should have demonstrated their willingness to participate in the study.
- Participants should have been engaged in precarious job activities.
- Participants should have been 18 years and older.

This means that the respondents who did not meet the above criteria were not allowed to participate in the study. Again, those who were unwilling to participate in the study were allowed to withdraw at any time.

2.7 Data collection instrument

Both structured and semi-structured instruments were used to collect data from the respondents in February 2021. The structured questionnaire was self-administered to the respondents. For the semi-structured interview, the researchers conducted the interview, which lasted for 20–30 minutes at each interview session. The questions were aligned with the objectives and the theories that were adopted for the study. Some of the questions that were asked included the types of precarious work activities engaged by the migrants; how the precarious work that was undertaken affected their health outcomes; and the attempts made by the government to address precarious work conditions among the migrants.

2.8 Pretesting

Pretesting of quantitative data was done at Madina with 40 questionnaires. The use of a 40-sample size for the pretest was due to the total migrant population available in the community at the time of pretesting of the data. This was because the upsurge of COVID-19 made most of the migrants go back to their places of origin. The aim of the pretesting was to allow for the restructuring of the questionnaire and the time needed to conduct each interview. Madina is a suburb of Accra in the La-Nkwantanang Madina municipality. The municipality has attracted and continues to attract, migrants from all over the country due to the major commercial activities that take place there. As a result, Madina has also become a home for a growing number of economic migrants [59].

2.9 Data analysis

The quantitative data gleaned from the study was coded and then analyzed with the use of SPSS software version 21. Chi-square tests were conducted to test whether there was a statistically significant relationship between the expected frequencies and observed frequencies in one or more categories of the study at the 0.05 level. Logistic regression was also performed on whether or not an association existed between work undertaken by the migrant and whether it resulted in a poor health outcome. Part of this report refers to findings from the qualitative results. For the qualitative analysis, data were transcribed and translated for uploading to NVIVO software. The data were done by identifying themes and sub-themes, coding those themes, and then interpreting the structure and content of the themes. Through this method, a codebook was developed, discussed, and accepted. Nodes were then created within NVivo using the codebook. Data triangulation were used to ensure that the findings were validated across different participants. The data were analyzed to understand the feelings and experiences of the migrants.

3. Results

3.1 Population characteristics and migration trajectory

As indicated in **Table 1**, most of the sampled population was female, which constituted (65.5%). The age group with the highest sample (61.9%) was between the ages of 18 and 25 (M = 1.52, SD = 0.84). A little over half (50.4%) of the respondents had had no education. Among the regions sampled, the northern region of Ghana had the highest proportion of respondents (93.8%) (see **Table 2**). The need to seek better employment opportunities (85.0%) accounted for most of the reasons for coming to the city of Accra. In an interview, it emerged that most of the migrants had come to Accra mainly to work to go back and trade. This was revealed in an interview:

> *I came to Accra to look for money to go and learn a trade [IDI, female migrant, Agbogloshie].*

Variables	Number	Percentage
Gender		
Male	39	34.5
Female	74	65.5
Total	**113**	**100**
Age		
18–25	70	61.9
26–33	30	26.5
34–41	8	7.1
42–49+	5	4.4
Total	**113**	**100**
Education		
No education	57	50.4
Primary	33	29.2
Middle/JSS	18	15.9
Voc/tech/SSS/O'level	5	4.4
Total	**113**	**100**

Table 1.
Population characteristics.

Variables	Number	Percentage
Region of origin		
Northern	106	93.8
Savanna	4	3.5
Upper East	1	0.9
Central	1	0.9
Bono East	1	0.9
Total	**113**	**100**
Reasons for migration		
Education	6	5.3
Seek employment	96	85.0
Others	9	8.0
Total	**113**	**100**

Table 2.
Migration history.

3.2 Precarious work activities among the migrants

More than half of the respondents (58.4%) were head porters, popularly referred to as "Kayayee." Scrap dealers came in second (20.4%). The least sampled occupation was truck driving, which had (3.5%) of its members. Long working hours were also reported by the majority of respondents; for example, exactly half (50.4%) reported working between 9 and 11 hours per day, while approximately 30.1% worked 12 to 14 hours per day (see **Table 3**). This observation was made in the course of an interview:

> *We do not intend to work for long hours...........but when you step out, sometimes you do not get customers. In that case, you have to extend your stay to cover the losses. In a nutshell, those of us who work long hours earn more than those who work less [IDI, Female migrant, Agbogbloshie].*

Analysis of the results of the chi-square test (see **Table 4**) has indicated that various health risk factors have been encountered by the respondents in their line of duty. For example, (84.6%) have been involved in motor accidents; (83.3%) have experienced burns/cults/explosions; approximately (80.0%) have experienced frequent falls; (78.3%) have received maltreatments/beatings from their masters; and 74.1% have faced the challenge of working in a dirty environment and its associated ill-health. Carrying heavy loads in the scorching sun was the least sampled health risk factor, accounting for 70.4%. Meanwhile, a statistical test shows an insignificant relationship between work activities and health risk factors ($\chi 2$ = 1.680, df =5, P =0.891).

The following was revealed in an interview:

> *We suffer here a lot. Sometimes while going about your duty, as in trying to cross the road with your load, you are knocked down by a car and the driver will not even stop. [KII, female migrant Agbogbloshie].*

Variables	Number	Percentage
Occupation		
Scrap dealers	23	20.4
Electronic waste dealer	7	6.2
Head porter	66	58.4
Motor cycle rider (Okada)	7	6.2
Hawkers (Yam & ice water)	6	5.3
Truck pusher	4	3.5
Total	**113**	**100**
Working hours		
1–2 hours	1	0.9
3–5 hours	3	2.7
6–8 hours	18	15.9
9–11 hours	57	50.4
Others	34	30.1
Total	**113**	**100**

Table 3.
Work activities.

Risk	Motor Accident N (%)	Heavy load/ sun N (%)	Burns/cuts/ explosions/ smoke N (%)	Falls N (%)	Mal-treat/ beatings N (%)	Dirty env't/ Sickness N (%)	Total N (%)	Chi-Square Test (χ^2)
Yes	11 (84.6)	19 (70.4)	15 (83.3)	4 (80.0)	18 (78.3)	20 (74.1)	87 (77.0)	χ^2 = 1.680,df = 5, P =0.891 (Insig)
No	2 (15.4)	8 (29.6)	3 (16.7)	1 (20.0)	5 (21.7)	7 (25.9)	26 (23.0)	
Total	13 (100)	27 (100)	18 (100)	5 (100)	23 (100)	27 (100)	113 (100)	

Table 4.
Assessment of precarious work and health risk factors.

> *Another respondent also noted that sometimes customers tell you to carry the load to that point, which is not far, but before you realize, they take you to a far place under the scorching sun, and in the end, they cheat you by paying you some small amount. It becomes more difficult while carrying a child behind you... As you can see, we are really suffering [IDI, Female Migrant, Agbogbloshie].*

Other respondents also expressed their views thus:

> *We have no work to do apart from scavenging just to feed ourselves and our families back home. Sometimes you inhale smoke from the burning site and it gives you a headache. But you cannot say you want to stop. You have to go to the burning site [KII, Male Migrant, Agbogbloshie].*

Another point was made: when attempting to break the metal, the hammer may strike your hand, causing severe bleeding. *So, if the bleeding does not want to stop, you go to the hospital. If not, there is no need to go to the hospital. You find a way of stopping the blood [IDI, Male Migrant, Agbogloshie].*

> *The loads we carry can be very heavy and they give us a lot of neck and sometimes severe body pains after you come from work... but you cannot say you would not go the next day. You will definitely go or else you will be hungry [IDI, Female Migrant, Agbogbloshie].*

3.3 Precarious work on health outcomes

Logistic regression was performed to investigate whether or not the type of work affects health outcomes. The results are presented in **Table 5**. Commercial motor riders, popularly known as "Okada," were taken as the reference group since they are mostly involved in accidents, whereas every other occupation was then compared in terms of the odds of suffering a poor health outcome. From the results, migrant workers who are engaged in electronic waste have 1.0 [95%CI: 0.09–10.17]; P = 1.0) sickness times the odds of those involved in Okada. However, there is no association between electronic waste dealers and Okada riders. When compared to Okada, people who work in scrap-yards have a lower risk of poor health outcomes by 0.69 [95% CI: 0.10–4.72]; P = 0.71]. The resulting p-value shows it is not significant. Similarly, people who are head porters have in excess of 25% increased odds of having experienced poor health of 0.25[95%CI: 0.22–6.97]: P = 0.80 when compared to motorcyclists, even though the p-value is not significant. Those who are engaged in street hawking, the sale of tubers of yams and sachets of water have 0.5[95%CI: 0.03–7.45]; P = 0.62] sickness times the odds when compared to Okada riders. However, the p-value is not significant. For the truck pushers, the odds of experiencing poor health outcomes are 0.83[95%CI: 0.05–13.63]; P = 0.90] when compared to the Okada riders. The resulting p-value shows it is not significant.

In the course of an interview, we made this observation:

> *As for sickness, we are always hit by headaches, body pains, joint pains, and several others, but you cannot complain to anyone. Sometimes you can experience these conditions 3–5 times a week [KII, female migrant Agbogbloshie].*

Logistic Regression		
Suffer health outcome	**OR (95%CI)**	**P-value**
Type of work		
Motorbike business (Okada)	Ref	
Electronic waste dealer	1.0 (0.09–10.17)	1.0
Scrap dealer	0.69 (0.10–4.72)	0.71
Head porter	0.25 (0.22–6.97)	0.80
Hawker (water and yam)	0.5 (0.03–7.45)	0.62
Truck pushers	0.83(0.05–13.63)	0.90

Table 5.
Assessment of precarious work and risk exposure.

In a related interview, this emerged:

> *What we suffer here mostly are injuries because of the metals we deal with. Accidents are common here. Sometimes, the heavy hammer we used to break the metal can hurt you. Sometimes, too, the metal plate can also cut you. But you cannot say anything [KII, Male migrant Agbogbloshie].*

3.4 Policy response

One of the strategies for reducing work-related precarity for migrant workers in the informal sector of the economy is the role played by the government in bringing an end to such occurrences.

The study showed that even though the government has unreliable accounts of labor migrants working in the informal sector of the economy; the government is yet to establish information on the indicated group of migrant workers. The Ministry further indicated that the National Labor Migration Policy, which was drafted in 2014, has been given cabinet approval, which is yet to be implemented, and once that is done, it would provide the framework. The framework would enable the government to address precarious work conditions among migrant workers in the informal sector.

The following came to light in one of the interviews:

> *The Ministry has anecdotal knowledge concerning labor migrants in the informal sector. The required monitoring and data collection exercise are yet to be done to acquire actionable information on the indicated group of migrant workers. However, the National Labor Migration Policy recently received cabinet approval and its implementation would provide the framework that would enable government and other relevant partners to address issues of workers in the informal sector, especially migrant workers [Ministry of youth and employment, KII].*

There are indications of efforts in revamping the country's employment centers and developing institutional capacities that will enable it to extend coverage to migrant workers due to the decent work deficits facing them as well as other workers in the informal sector. This was reported in one of the qualitative interviews:

> *The Ministry is aware of the decent work deficits facing workers in the informal sector. To that end, the Ministry, being responsible for the promotion of decent work for workers across all sectors, is revamping its public employment centers and developing institutional capacities that would enable it to extend coverage to informal workers, including migrant workers [Ministry of youth and employment, KII].*

Whereas the timely implementation of the responses in addressing precarious work conditions among this population is important not only to bring about hope to the migrant workers but also to meet SDG 8, our findings suggest otherwise. This was noted in our interview.

Meeting SDG 8, as well as most of the other goals of the 2030 Agenda, would be very difficult at the current rate of progress. World leaders and international and regional bodies all agree that efforts must be stepped up considerably if we are to achieve the targets set [Ministry of youth and employment, KII].

DOI: http://dx.doi.org/10.5772/intechopen.106907

4. Discussions

Our findings show that females accounted for the majority of the population sampled. The high number of females reported in the study indicates that the phenomenon of female migration has increased in recent times. Similar studies by Awumbila et al. [4] have also demonstrated that the migration of young females has become a common phenomenon due to the benefit of remittances from female members who work as head porters and domestic workers in the city.

The majority of those sampled for the study were young people. This is because most of the respondents at that stage of life want to explore the opportunities that migration can offer them. Similar findings from UNICEF [14] also note that the ages of most migrant workers often range from 15–24 years, accounting for one-eighth of the age groups that are often seen moving in search of better economic opportunities. One may be tempted to believe that migration in its widest sense is beneficial. However, certain age groups and categories of the population are particularly vulnerable to abuse, exploitation, discrimination, social exclusion, and violence. These have the tendency to expose them to poor health outcomes. Furthermore, the study found that most of the migrants had attained only a low level of education. It is not surprising, therefore, that most of them find themselves in low-paid work in the informal sector, with its associated long working hours. Such labor disparities do not only pose a health risk to them and their families but also contradict the ILO Constitution, which sets forth the principle that workers should be protected from sickness, disease, and injury arising from their employment [60].

Our finding also suggests that most of the migrants were from the three northern regions. The motivation behind the movement to Agbogbloshie was the need to seek better employment opportunities. This finding demonstrates the Harris–Todaro [19] model of migration, which explains why people move from rural areas to urban centers despite the high unemployment rates in the cities. Building on the works of early scholars, such as Ravenstein, Harris, and Todaro, see migration as an economic activity that for the individual migrant could be a rational decision despite the existence of urban unemployment. For most of the migrants that were sampled in this study, the unavailability of job opportunities in their places of origin forced them to seek better opportunities in the informal settlement of Agbogbloshie in the city of Accra. This makes migration to the city by many of the youth a gamble in seeking better opportunities [19].

We also found various precarious work activities ranging from scrap dealerships, electronic waste dealerships, head porterage, commercial motorbike riding, hawking on the main street of Accra, and pushing of trucks loaded with goods to be conveyed to their destinations, as well as long working hours and generally dirty, dangerous, and demeaning conditions under which this work is performed for a meager income. As noted by Piper et al. [61], this phenomenon is often common with migrants in search of better work and wages who often find themselves battling for jobs on the lowest rungs of the labor market. The work is often insecure, arbitrarily remunerated, and thinly regulated. This finding is consistent with Harris and Todaro's [19] model of migration, which further argues that migration occurs in response to rural-urban differences in expected income rather than actual earnings [19]. In the case of the migrants at Agbogbloshie, emigration to their current destination offers them employment opportunities despite the precarious nature of the work they find for themselves. As highlighted in the ecological models, individuals are understood to influence and be influenced by the people and organizations with whom they interact, available resources and institutions, and societal norms and rules [39]. Generally, efforts to address structural changes, such as equal geographic development, to address rural-urban migration and policies to regulate the activities in the informal sector of the economy can go a long way to address precarious work activity among migrants.

Results from the logistic regression that was performed on whether or not the type of work undertaken by the migrants resulted in poor health outcomes, using motor riders as a reference in the analysis, suggested that people who are engaged in electronic waste have the same odds of poor health outcomes when compared to motor riders (OR =1.0 [95%CI: 0.09–10.17]; P = 1.0). Scrap dealers have reduced the odds of falling sick when compared to motor riders. However, the reduced odds are not statistically significant (OR = 0.69 [95%CI: 0.10–4.72]; P = 0.71). Migrants who are head porters have in excess of 25% increased odds of falling sick when compared to motor riders even though the p-value is not significant (OR = 0.25 [95%CI: 0.22–6.97]; P = 0.80). The odds of street hawkers falling sick when compared to motor riders is (OR = 0.5 [95%CI: 0.03–7.45]; P = 0.62). However, the resulting p-value is insignificant.

Truck pushers have a reduced odds of experiencing sickness when they are compared to motor riders. The p-value is, however, insignificant (0.83[95%CI: 0.05–13.63]; P=0.90). In other studies, evidence of job insecurity and vulnerability have been shown to have significant adverse effects on self-reported physical and mental health. For example, results show that, relative to workers who remained in secure employment, self-reported morbidity was higher among workers reporting insecurity in their jobs [62]. As suggested by the ecological model, such behaviors that make migrants indulge in precarious work activities will need specific health behavior interventions in order to promote their health and wellbeing [42, 45, 47, 63–65].

While national legislation and policies determining migrant status play an active role in producing precarity for migrant workers, our study found that the government, through the Ministry of youth and employment, though in the process of fully addressing the issue of precarious work activity among migrant workers, work has been slow in achieving this goal. Such actions only exacerbate the plight of migrant labor workers, potentially delaying the achievement of SDG 8. According to Anderson, [66] and Lewis et al., [67], policies of national governments are very important not only for regulating the flow of migrants into a country but also for the types of migrant labor available to employers, that is, that can be paid minimal amounts and offered on highly flexible and insecure terms, and which needs to be regulated.

5. Conclusion and policy recommendation

This paper has, for the first time, contributed to our knowledge gap on precarious work conditions and the health of rural-urban migrant labor workers in the informal settlement of Agbogbloshie in Accra, Ghana. Precarious work conditions and their associated health outcomes have often been associated with international labor workers, leaving a huge gap in the area of internal migration. The study has found various precarious work conditions among rural-urban migrant workers, which have resulted in poor health outcomes. This paper is consistent with Harris and Todaro's [19] model of labor migration. This model has aided in explaining the causes of the migration of the youth to the informal settlement of Agbogloshie in Accra, despite the unavailability of job opportunities. Also, the paper's consistency with the ecological models [39] highlights the need for structural changes as well as individual migrants' efforts to engage in economic activities that promote their health and wellbeing. The study finally found a slow pace in which the government responds to addressing precarious work activities for the migrant labor workers in one of Ghana's urban slums, Accra. As a result, we proposed that structural changes can be implemented to address precarious work activities among migrants, as well as health promotion at the individual migrant level to address workplace-related health risk activities.

Competing interests

The authors have declared that no competing interests exist.

Author details

Ransford Kwaku Afeadie*, Mary Naana Essiaw, Susanna Adjei Arthur, Andrew Kweku Conduah, Dorothy Siaw-Marfo and Bridget Elikem Mensah
Institute of Work, Employment and Society, University of Professional Studies, Accra, Ghana

*Address all correspondence to: ransford.afeadie@upsamail.edu.gh

References

[1] United Nations Department of Economic and Social Affairs (UN DESA), 2015) International Migrant Stock: Revision. United Nations, New York. Available from: www.un.org/en/development/desa/population/migration/data/estimates2/estimates15.shtml

[2] United Nations Department of Economic and Social Affairs. (2013a). World population Prospects: the 2012 revision. New York, Population division, united nations (UN) online]. [Accessed 8 November 2015]. Available at:http://esa.un.org/unpd/wup/http://esa.un.org/wpp>/

[3] DFID. Migration and pro-poor policy in sub-Saharan Africa. Policy Briefing prepared by the Sussex Development Research Centre on Migration. 2004

[4] Awumbila M, Kofi Tehe J, Litchfield J, Boakye-Yiadom L, Deshingkar P, Quartey P. Are Migrant Households Better off Than Non-migrant Households? Evidence from Ghana. Ghana: Migration Out of Poverty; 2015

[5] Mitullah W. A Review of Street Trade in Africa. Cambridge: WIEGO; 2004

[6] Molini V, Pavelesku D, Ranzani M. Should I Stay or Should I Go? Internal Migration and Household Welfare in Ghana. Washington, D.C: World Bank; 2016

[7] Mosse D, Gupta S, Shah V. On the margins in the city: Adivasi seasonal labour migration in Western India. Economic and Political Weekly. 2005;**40**(28):3025-3038

[8] Mosley L, Singer DA. Migration, labor, and the international political economy. Annual Review of Political Science. 2015;**18**:282-301

[9] Msigwa ER. Determinants of internal migration in Tanzania. Journal of Economic & Sustainable Development. 2013;**4**(14):67-76

[10] Osei-Boateng C, Ampratwum E. The Informal Sector in Ghana. Accra: Friedrich Ebert Stiftung; 2011

[11] Picherit D. Migrant labourers' struggles between village and urban migration sites: Labour standards, rural development and politics in South India. Global Labour Journal. 2012;**3**(1):143-162

[12] Sabates-Wheeler R, Waite M. Migration and Social Protection: A Concept Paper. UK: University of Sussex; 2003

[13] Ginsburg C, Bocquier P, Afolabi S, Otiende M, Odhiambo F, Augusto O, et al. Determinants of internal migration in Africa: Does human capital necessarily end up in cities? Comparative analysis of health and demographic surveillance systems: Princeton University Paper; 2014

[14] UNICEF. Migration and youth: Challenges and opportunities. Edited by J. Cortina, P. Taran & A. Raphael on behalf of the GMG. 2014

[15] Deshingkar P, Grimm S. Internal migration and development: A global perspective. Geneva: IOM; 2005

[16] Deshingkar P. Internal migration, poverty and development in Asia: Including the excluded through partnerships and improved governance. In: Presented at the Promoting Growth, Ending Poverty – Asia 2015 Conference. 2006

[17] Deshingkar P, Grimm S. *Voluntary Internal Migration*: An Update.

September. London: Overseas Development Institute; 2004

[18] Hagen-Zanker J, Mosler Vidal E, Sturge G. Social Protection, Migration and the 2030 Agenda for Sustainable Development. London: Overseas Development Institute; 2017

[19] Harris JR, Todaro MP. Migration, unemployment and development: A two-sector analysis. American Economic Review. 1970;**60**(1):126-142

[20] WB. Migration and Poverty: Towards Better Opportunities for the Poor. Washington, DC; 2011

[21] McKay A, Deshingkar P. Internal Remittances and Poverty: Further Evidence from Africa and Asia, Migrating out of Poverty Working Paper 12. 2014. Available from: https://opendocs.ids.ac.uk/opendocs/handle/20.500.12413/14882

[22] Hewison K. Precarious work. In: Edgell S, Gottfried H, Granter E, editors. The Sage Handbook of the Sociology of Work and Employment. Thousand Oaks, CA: Sage; 2016. pp. 428-443

[23] Johnson NM, Afriyie-Gyawu E, Huebner H, et al. PAH exposure in a Ghanaian population at high risk for aflatoxicosis. Science Total Environment. 2009;**407**(6):1886

[24] Kalleberg AL, Hewison K. Precarious work and the challenge for Asia. American Behavioral Scientist. 2013;**57**(3):271-288

[25] Kalleberg AL. Nonstandard employment relations: Part-time, temporary, and contract work. Annual Review of Sociology. 2000;**26**:341-365

[26] Krejcie RV, Morgan DW. Determining sample size for research activities. Educational and Psychological Measurement. 1970;**30**:607-610

[27] Rodgers G, Rodgers J. Precarious Jobs in Labour Market Regulation: The Growth of Atypical Employment in Western Europe. Geneva: ILO; 1989

[28] Vosko L. Managing the Margins: Gender, Citizenship, and the International Regulation of Precarious Employment. Oxford: Oxford University Press; 2010

[29] Kalleberg AL, Vallas SP. Probing precarious work: Theory, research, and politics. Research in the Sociology of Work. 2018;**31**:1-30

[30] Lucci P, Mansour-Ille D, Easton-Calabria E, Cummings C. Sustainable Cities: Internal Migration, Jobs and the 2030 Agenda for Sustainable Development. London: ODI; 2016

[31] Agarwal S, Attah M, Apt N, Grieco M, Kwakye EA, Turner J. Bearing the Weight: The Kayayoo. Ghana: Centre for Social Policy Studies; 1997

[32] Tanle A. Perceptions of Returnee Migrants and Non – migrants to Female Migration: Case of Ghana. UMOJA Bulletin of the African and African American Studies Program. 2007;**2**(2):12-25 Retrieved from: www.ucweb.gvsu.edu

[33] Yeboah MA, Appiah-Yeboah K. An Examination of the Cultural and Socio-Economic Profiles of Porters in Accra Ghana. Nordic Journal of African Studies. 2009;**18**(1):1-21

[34] Belin A, Zamparutti T, Tull K, Hernandez G, Graveling R. Occupational Health and Safety Risks for the Most Vulnerable Workers. Brussels: Milieu Ltd; 2011

[35] ILO. Psychosocial Risks, Stress and Violence in the World of Work.

International Journal of Labour Research. 2017;**8**:1-2

[36] Quandt S, Kristen K, Courtney H, Klein BG, Langley R, Agnew M, et al. OccupationalHealthOutcomesforWorkers in the Agriculture, Forestry and Fishing Sector: Implications for Immigrant Workers in the Southeastern US. Wiley periodicals inc: American journal of industrial medicine; 2013

[37] ILO. The Right to Rest for Domestic Workers: Setting a Floor. Fact sheet. 2015

[38] Flynn MA. Safety and the diverse workforce. Prof. Saf. 2014;**59**(6):52-57

[39] Bronfenbrenner U. Ecological Systems Theory. London, England: Jessica Kingsley; 1992

[40] Lall SV, Selod H, Shalizi Z. Rural-Urban Migration in Developing Countries: A Survey of Theoretical Predictions and Empirical Findings. Policy Research Working Paper; No. 3915. Washington, DC: World Bank; 2006. Available from: https://openknowledge.worldbank.org/handle/10986/8669 41

[41] Lee ES. A theory of migration. Demography. 1966;**3**(1):47-57

[42] McLeroy KR, Bibeau D, Steckler A, Glanz K. An ecological perspective on health promotion programs. Health Education & Behavior. 1988;**15**:351-377

[43] Migration DRC. Place, Social Protection and Migration in Bangladesh: A Londoni Village in Biswanath. Sussex: University of Sussex; 2006

[44] Mitra A. Migration, livelihood and well-being: Evidence from Indian City Slums. Urban Studies. 2009;**47**:1371-1390

[45] Sallis JF, Owen N, Fisher EB. Ecological models of health behavior. Health Behavior and Health Education. 2008;**4**:465-485

[46] Sigerist H. Annual "Plans of Work". Bulletin of the History of Medicine. 1955;**71**:3

[47] Stokols D. Translating social ecological theory into guidelines for community health promotion. American Journal of Health Promotion. 1996;**10**:282-298

[48] Tacoli C, McGranahan G, Satterthwaite D. Urbanisation, Rural–urban Migration and Urban Poverty. London: International Institute for Environment and Development; 2015

[49] Safo A. End of the road fpr Sodom and Gomorrah squatters News from Africa. 2011. Archived from the original on 18 July 2011. Retrieved 15 March 2011

[50] Ghana e-waste Country Assessment. SBC e-waste Africa Project. GreenAd-Empa; 2011 [cited 2012 Jul 13]

[51] Gabel DA. E-waste dump in Africa contaminating community. Global Pollution. 2011;**2011**:2

[52] Claiborne R. E- waste in Africa, US trash is Ghana's problem ABC News. 2011.

[53] Afenah A. Reclaiming Citizenship Right in Accra. Ghana: DPH; 2011

[54] Creswell JW. Mapping the field of mixed methods research. Journal of Mixed Methods Research. 2009;**3**:95-108

[55] Creswell JW, Plano Clark VL, Gutmann ML, Hanson WE. Advanced mixed methods research designs. In: Tashakkori A, Teddlie C, editors. Handbook of Mixed Methods in Social and Behavioral Research. Thousand Oaks, CA: Sage; 2003. pp. 209-240

[56] Castro FG, Kellison JG, Boyd SJ, Kopak A. A methodology for conducting integrative mixed methods research and data analysis. Journal of Mixed Methods Research. 2010;**4**(4):342-360

[57] Housing the Masses. Community-led Enumeration of Old Fadama Community, Accra Ghana, People Dialogue on Human Settlement. 2010

[58] Brink HIL. Fundamentals of Research Methodology for Health Care Professionals. Kenwyn: Juta; 1996

[59] Ghana Statistical Service. Population and Housing Census: National Analytical Report. Accra: Ghana Statistical Service; 2010

[60] ILO. Social Protection for Domestic Workers: Key Policy Trends and Statistics. Social Protection Policy Papers. 2016; Papers No. 16

[61] Piper N, Rosewarne S, Withers M. Migrant precarity in Asia: Networks of labour activism for a rights-based governance of migration. Development and Change. 2017;**48**(5):1089-1110

[62] Marmot M. Income inequality, social environment, and inequalities in health. Journal of Policy Analysis and Management. 2001;**20**(1):156-159

[63] Tulloch O, Machingura F, Melamed C. Health, Migration and the 2030 Agenda for Sustainable Development. London: ODI; 2016

[64] World of Work Report. Developing with Jobs/International Labour Office. Geneva: ILO; 2014

[65] Yea S. The art of not being caught: Temporal strategies for disciplining unfree labour in Singapore's contract migration. Geoforum. 2017;**78**:179-188

[66] Anderson B. Migration, immigration controls and the fashioning of precarious worker. Work, Employment and Society. 2010;**24**(2):300-317

[67] Lewis H, Dwyer P, Hodkinson S, Waite L. Hyper-precarious lives: Migrants, work and forced labour in the Global North. Progress in Human Geography. 2015;**39**(5):580-600

Chapter 16

Perspective Chapter: Enhancing the Nurse-Initiated Management of Antiretroviral Therapy Training and Implementation – A Conceptual Framework

Sheillah Hlamalani Mboweni and Lufuno Makhado

Abstract

Task shifting of nurse-initiated management of antiretroviral therapy (NIMART) rather than doctors is crucial to meet the increasing demand for antiretroviral therapy (ART) in primary health care in low and middle-income countries with limited healthcare resources. This chapter will furnish cooperation between the NIMART conceptual framework, National Department of Health policies and guidelines, and empirical findings regarding the management of ART and tuberculosis (TB) in South Africa and globally through pre-service and in-service training and continuous professional development (CPD). It will also include regulations and WHO guidelines on task shifting, application in a healthcare setting, the HIV continuum of care use in identifying gaps, and the development of appropriate interventions to improve patients and population health outcomes. The training and health care systems or structural challenges or barriers and strategies or enablers to enhance effective training and implementation, including the role and responsibilities of NIMART nurses, will be explored and discussed in detail. The focus will mostly be on the primary health care (PHC) setting as the first level of care and entry into the healthcare system to decentralize healthcare services and facilitate access to HIV services by the community.

Keywords: nurse-initiated management of antiretroviral therapy training, HIV programme, NIMART-trained nurse, antiretroviral therapy, primary health care

1. Introduction

The dual burden of Human Immunodeficiency Virus (HIV) and tuberculosis (TB) are global public health of concern and demands integrated TB/HIV services collaboratively to manage and control the dual epidemic as well as Prevention of Mother to Child Transmission (PMTCT). According to WHO and UNAIDS [1], there were approximately 37.7 million people living with HIV (PLWH) worldwide in 2020, of which 19.3 million are women, 16.7 men above 15 years, 1.7 million children and adolescents less than 15 years old. Furthermore, an approximately 680,000 deaths from Acquired Immune Deficiency Syndrome (AIDS) have been reported from low and middle-income countries and reported a total of 190 million people who tested and receive results for HIV in 2018.

According to the UNAIDS [2] report, sub-Saharan Africa is the worst affected by HIV globally. It is home to the most significant number of PLWH, with an HIV prevalence of 6.7%, 730 00 new HIV infections, and 300,000 AIDS-related death. Young women, men who have sex with men, transgender people, sex workers, prisoners, and people who inject drugs are at an increased risk of acquiring HIV infection (UNAIDS, 2020). South Africa has the largest HIV population globally, with 8.2 million PLWH, HIV prevalence high at 20.4% in 2021, 200,000 new HIV infections, and 72,000 AIDS-related deaths. South Africa has the most extensive ART programme globally, with 3.4 million PLWH on ART because of the adoption of WHO task-shifting.

As a result, nurses rather than doctors initiate ART in the primary level of care, and it is crucial to train nurses in nurse-initiated management of ART (NIMART). Task shifting was adopted in South Africa, and training on NIMART was introduced in 2009 to improve access to ART. Therefore, it is crucial to enhance the NIMART training and implementation in South Africa by making all role players and stakeholders aware of the conceptual framework that can strengthen and optimize training and implementation to improve patient and HIV programme outcomes. The framework should cooperate with the national Department of Health policies and guidelines, including empirical studies on HIV management to enhance the quality of care, achieve the UNAIDS 95–95-95 target by 2030 and end the HIV and TB epidemic. The increasing number of PLWH in need of ART continues to exert excessive pressure on the health care system, which is already experiencing a dire shortage of resources and high staff turnover. This chapter will focus on the description of concepts related to enhancing NIMART training, education, and implementation, the objectives of NIMART training, the methodology of the conceptual framework, barriers and enablers of NIMART training and implementation, the HIV continuum of care, and the role and responsibilities of NIMART-trained nurses.

2. Definition of concepts

WHO defines education as the process of giving or acquiring knowledge, skills and developing attitudes and values at school or university, while training aims at improving the level of a trainee's competence in a specific area and may be defined as the process of developing, changing or strengthening the knowledge, skills, and attitudes of a target group [3].

NIMART training is a short course on essential HIV clinical management that tackles the fundamentals of HIV management and includes prevention, diagnosis, treatment initiation, management, control, referrals, monitoring and evaluation of treatment success. NIMART was developed in response to the call for action by the South African government to adopt WHO recommendations for task-shifting to strengthen the response to HIV and TB epidemics. It was specifically developed and aimed at professional nurses working in the primary health care (PHC) setting [4].

The NIMART-trained nurse is a professional nurse (PN) or midwife trained in nurse-initiated management of antiretroviral therapy or treatment and has undergone a clinical mentorship programme and assessed for competency in managing HIV and TB [4].

Clinical NIMART mentorship is an HIV programme that focuses on enhancing the skills, competencies, attitudes, and values of trained NIMART concerning HIV prevention, diagnosis, treatment initiation, and linkages to care and treatment, referrals, and monitoring of treatment success for children, adolescents, pregnant women, adults, co-infected with TB and the management of opportunistic infections. Upon completing the programme, the nurse is assessed and receives a competency certificate [5].

Pre-service training or pre-service education refers to any structured activity aiming at developing or reinforcing knowledge and skills before a health care professional joins service or takes up a job that requires specific training in addition to those of undergraduate courses either from the public health service or private practice, to provide competence needed to perform new services [3].

Continuous Inservice training refers to training provided to health care workers already employed in the public or private sector to acquire practical work experience and can be provided after one or two years of the theory are completed to enhance the performance of the health care workers or nurses [3].

Continuous professional development (CPD) is a term used to describe the learning activities in which healthcare professionals engage to develop and enhance their skills, knowledge, competencies, and abilities to perform their jobs [3].

According to WHO [3], *task-shifting* involves rational distribution or delegation of tasks among health workforce teams with a highly specialized or qualified workforce to less specialized health workers with shorter training and fewer qualifications to use valuable human resources for health efficiently. It is a great option or method to enhance efficiency in delivering health care services, especially HIV and TB services in low and middle-income countries with a high shortage of skilled human resources.

3. The objectives of NIMART training

The objectives of NIMART training are to upskill nurses' capacity in HIV and TB management. The training also seeks to cultivate positive attitudes among nurses dealing with PLWH and those affected by the diseases. NIMART training facilitates the decentralization of HIV services to the PHC level, thereby:

- increasing access to HIV and TB services to meet the growing demand for ART and improve the country's socioeconomic status through the provision of early ART initiation to PLWH,
- reducing complications and death related to HIV and TB,
- improving patient health outcomes, and increasing life expectancy,
- facilitating the optimal use of human resources for health,
- improving monitoring and evaluation of the HIV and TB programme,
- identifying strengths, gaps or weaknesses, or challenges and opportunities to guide policy and decision-makers on strategies to improve and end the HIV and TB epidemic [6].

4. Methodology of the conceptual framework

The conceptual framework (CF) was developed by conceptualizing the two stages of the study—The impact of NIMART training on HIV management and barriers to NIMART Training and Implementation. An explanatory sequential mixed method (QUAN-qual) was used [7]. Mixed methods refer to a research strategy in which a researcher combines qualitative and quantitative methods to comprehensively understand the phenomenon under study to produce a more complete and validated conclusion [8–10]. In order to develop a conceptual framework that will provide direction, strengthen NIMART training and implementation, and improve patient outcomes, a descriptive and explorative program evaluation design was used. Retrospective data were gathered from the District Health Information System (DHIS) and the three integrated electronic registers (TIER.NET), of the selected PHC facilities, including interviews with purposively selected NIMART-trained nurses and program managers directly involved in managing TB/HIV coinfection until data saturation was reached. Programme evaluation research refers "to an applied system scientific method used to measure or assess the implementation, conceptualization, design, utility and outcomes or impact of social programs for decision making purpose", and is very useful in mixed methods [11, 12].

The Donabedian structure-process-outcome (SPO) model and Dickoff, James, and Wiedenbach's practice-oriented theory were two models that were crucial in the creation of the theoretical lens through which this conceptual framework was developed. The Donabedian's SPO model gave the researcher a framework to assess and enhance the application of HIV management following NIMART training [13]. The structure of the fixed PHC facilities providing ART or health care system and the process of NIMART training to professional nurses greatly influence the achievement of the health outcomes. Furthermore, following the Preferred Reporting Items for Systematic Reviews and Meta-Analyses, a thorough review of the literature was conducted in studies conducted in Africa and around the world from January 2012 to February 2017 from various databases. The results were analyzed using the quality assessment research instrument created by the Joan Briggs Institute in 2014 to obtain a broader perspective of factors that can enable and those that can be a barrier to NIMART training and implementation and play a major role in the development of the conceptual framework. Studies consulted for the thorough literature review revealed positive and negative factors affecting NIMART training and implementation. These will be discussed in detail in section five as barriers and enablers to efficient NIMART training and implementation, together with study findings.

The final conceptual framework was developed following Dickoff et al.'s POT, with six elements presented as questions and integrated into Donabedian's SPO model [14], as presented in **Figure 1**. The six elements questions addressed include:

4.1 Who is expected to implement the NIMART conceptual framework? (the agent)

According to Dickoff et al. [14], the agent refers to the persons or things that implement the framework. According to Donabedian's SPO model, this refers to the structure that enables the implementation of the CF, including the recipient and the context [13]. The department of health provincial and district regional training centers (RTCs), Higher education institutions ((HEIs), partners supporting the department of health, the South African nursing council (SANC), Health and welfare Seta (HWSETA), and other stakeholders are regarded as the agents of the NIMART

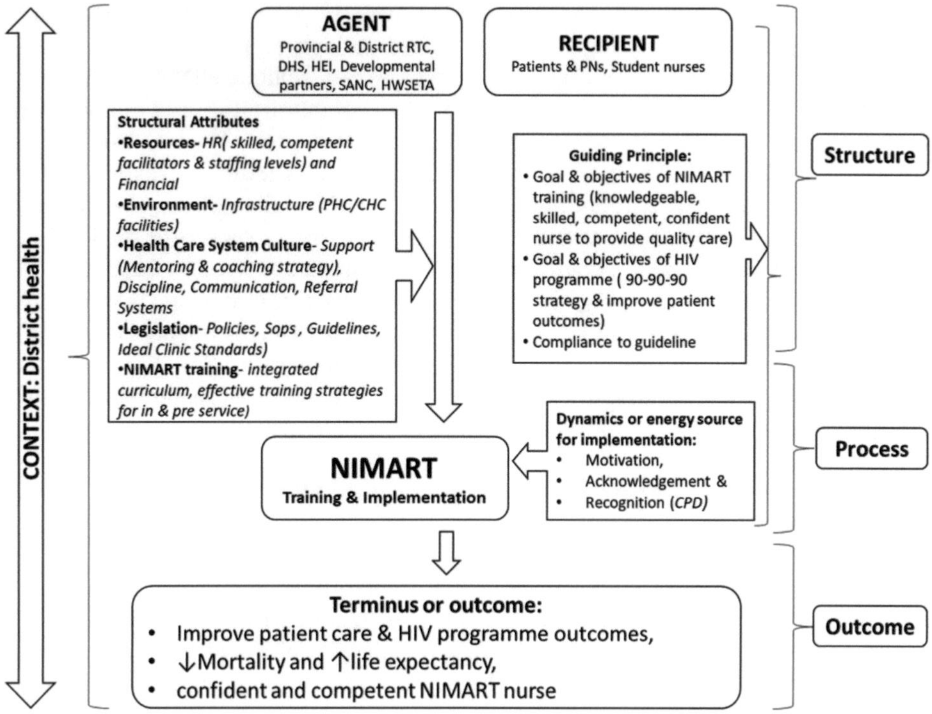

Figure 1.
Conceptual framework for strengthening NIMART training and HIV management implementation.

training process and has the responsibility to facilitate effective quality training to PNs and student nurses including patients that are receiving care from such nurses.

4.2 Who is the recipient of HIV management after NIMART training? The recipients

A recipient is a person or thing receiving action from the agent [14]. In this framework, the recipient is any health care worker receiving NIMART training. These can be PNs, facilitators, student nurses, nurse educators, or programme managers. The agent should provide comprehensive quality training to improve the skills, competence, and confidence of the NIMART nurse in providing quality care to the patients and facilitators and educators to transfer the skills to the students. In addition, the patients indirectly benefit from the NIMART training as they receive care from the NIMART nurse equally.

4.3 In what context is the NIMART training implemented? (the setting)

The context refers to resources, activities, and environments which enable or facilitate the implementation of the NIMART conceptual framework [14]. A combination of organizational resources and a conducive, safe and comfortable environment in the district primary health care system can facilitate implementation. Having adequate, independent, experienced, skilled human resources for health (HRH) with positive attitudes toward PLWH and HIV programmes facilitates robust implementation. Again, the development of a standard integrated NIMART curriculum and effective interactive strategies that stimulate critical thinking and facilitate the integration of theory and practice can influence implementation. Moreover, the provision of NIMART/HIV management pre-service training to student nurses, continuous professional development (CPD), and in-service training on HIV changes can facilitate NIMART implementation. This also includes the availability of good communication and relationship skills, compliance to HIV/TB and PHC policies, guidelines, protocols, and standard operating procedures (SOPs) to facilitate implementation. In addition, treating patients and nurses with respect and attending to their concerns or challenges can also facilitate implementation. Furthermore, maintaining the physical infrastructure of the PHC facilities, having enough space, re-organizing the facility in line with the ideal clinic integrated clinical services management (ICSM) standards, and reducing waiting times can facilitate implementation and quality. Prioritizing the PHC in budget planning is necessary to deal with the overt challenges influencing implementation. Provincial and district management team support, flexibility, coaching, and supervision are necessary to influence and facilitate discipline and meaningful implementation.

4.4 What are the support systems to strengthen NIMART training and implementation? (dynamics)

The dynamics refer to the sources of power or energy among the activities [14]. According to Donabedien [13], this refers to the process that facilitates the implementation of the CF, including the guiding principles. Provision of motivation, acknowledgement, and recognition of NIMART nurses for rendering services under difficult conditions substantially influences and facilitates implementation. Intrinsic and extrinsic recognition is necessary to motivate and enhance performance. This would invariably boost their self-esteem, build confidence, and improve their sense of responsibility and feeling worthy to the department. Again, the Department of Health should meet NIMART nurses' needs and deal with their frustrations. Furthermore, avoiding negative criticism and blame–punishment feedback would greatly influence successful implementation.

4.5 What are the guiding approaches, rules, or procedures to improve NIMART training and implementation? (the principle/s)

The guiding principle refers to the rule, technique, protocol, and routine governing the activities to achieve the terminus [14]. According to the Donabedian SPO model [13], the recipient, agent, and principles that guide NIMART training and implementation are referred to as the structure. Providing quality training, mentoring, support, and compliance to policies, guidelines, SOPs, and protocols are the guiding principles that facilitate achieving patient and framework outcomes. Again, monitoring, reporting, and evaluation facilitate the identification of gaps, signs of danger & success in arriving at the terminus. Another principle to facilitate and influence implementation is the involvement of all internal and external stakeholders, which includes district clinical specialist teams (DCST), facilitators, RTC managers, the province and district leadership, developmental partners, HEI, SANC, and HWSETA in implementation.

4.6 What is the outcome of the implementation of the NIMART training conceptual framework? (terminus)

Terminus refers to the outcomes or end results of the activity [14], while [13] describes a terminus as the end product or outcomes of the structure and process.

The outcomes of effective and efficient implementation of NIMART training facilitate the production of confident, competent, and skilled NIMART nurses who comply with policies and guidelines. This will also facilitate the improvement of patient health status by increasing linkages to ART, improving adherence and retention to care, reducing loss to follow-up (LTFU), enhancing viral suppression, and decanting of the stable patients, and relieving pressure on NIMART nurses. Furthermore, this reduces complications and death rates, thus increasing life expectancy. Dickoff et al.'s six elements questions and Donabedian's SPO described above were categorized and classified with the characteristics and activities from the study findings to develop a conceptual framework that can facilitate and influence the improvement of NIMART training and implementation in the district health system, thus improving patient and HIV programme outcomes as represented in **Figure 1**.

5. Barriers and enablers to effective NIMART training and implementation

A study conducted by Mboweni and Makhado [15] in South Africa revealed structural or health care system, environmental, patient, human resource, training, and mentoring factors as challenges influencing NIMART training and implementation and supported by various studies in Africa and globally. Such barriers should be dealt with decisively to enhance the effectiveness of NIMART training and implementation, improving the quality of care and HIV services.

5.1 Health care factors

Health care system or structural factors plays a significant role in the effectiveness and efficiency of delivering HIV services and health care services in general, including achieving universal health coverage (UHC). According to Mboweni and Makhado (2019), several challenges are influencing NIMART training and implementation in South Africa and other African countries, which includes:

- lack of NIMART training regulation,
- shortage of staff,
- poor work schedules and processes,
- inadequate systems for data management,
- drug stock-outs,
- poor integration of services,
- poor clinical supervision and management support,
- insufficient leadership role model,
- stigma and discrimination.

5.1.1 Poor leadership role model

The success of the HIV programme and ending the HIV and TB epidemic lies in the commitment of the district, provincial and national leadership with clear political will and leadership strategy. Therefore, poor leadership affects the implementation of the NIMART programme. All internal and external stakeholders should have clear roles and responsibilities to avoid duplication and overlapping of functions and facilitate the integration of HIV and non-communicable disease as they are both chronic diseases.

Supportive supervision by district and local management is key to dealing with gaps in training and implementation at facility levels, such as shortage of medication, equipment, and supplies as soon as possible. There is no district clinical mentorship programme; if available, it is mostly partner driven. Partners are HIV and TB communities or non-profit organizations mostly funded by donors. The United States President's Emergency Plan for AIDS Relief (PEPFAR) supports the government in preventing, controlling, and managing HIV and TB. Their existence is based on funding, meaning HIV management can collapse when they are unavailable and create dependency as most nurses working for government no longer render HIV services and rely on NIMART nurses from NGOs. Patient care is delayed as some patients are referred to another facility or have to wait for a partner NIMART-trained nurse.

5.1.2 Inadequate integration of service

The high shortage of skilled human resources for health requires better planning through integrating HIV, communicable and non-communicable services. Vertical integration might allow underutilized resources to remain and contribute to inefficient operations, excess capacity and duplication must be removed from the system. Health service integration is defined as the "managerial or operational changes to health systems to bring together inputs, delivery, management, and organization of particular service functions." Integration improves access, facilitates services, and addresses what has brought together inputs, delivery, management and organization of particular service functions." Integration improves access, encourages the use of services, and addresses what has been referred to as the four 'D's' – duplication, distortion, disruption, and distraction. A health facility should be a one-way stop where the patient can receive all services without moving from one consultation room to another. However, adequate staff allocation is key to ensuring quality, reducing long waiting hours, and improving patient satisfaction. Such staff needs to be provided with appropriate training to provide quality care and be integrated during NIMART training, where adult care 101 can be integrated and continued within the facility level during clinical mentorship support visits.

Integrating health services improves multiple healthcare outcomes among HIV-infected people who inject drugs. This can be relevant to managing other key population groups eye marked to reduce new HIV infections. A mind shift set from vertical programmes to context-specific equitable access to integrated services is crucial to achieving the 95–95-95 and 10–10-10 plus 90% targets by 2030 by dealing with issues related to:

- human rights,
- gender inequality,
- violence,

- preventing and addressing gender-based violence,
- intimate partner violence,
- stigma, discrimination,
- access to sexual reproductive health,
- mental health,
- communicable and non-communicable services,
- eliminate vertical transmission,
- stop criminalization and punitive laws and policies of key populations, especially people who inject drugs and sex workers.

All stakeholders should speak in one voice and put PLWH and communities at risk at the centre, with a non-judgmental attitude and embracing diversity [7]. Key populations in the HIV programme refer to a group of people who are vulnerable and disproportionately affected by HIV owing to risk behavior and marginalization and frequently lack access to health care services and include: lesbians, gays, bisexuals, transgender, sex workers, men who have sex with men, people who inject drugs, prisoners or inmates, and people in intergenerational relationships with older men or women groups and adolescents.

5.1.3 Inadequate information systems and processes

The healthcare process refers to interrelated or interacting healthcare activities transforming inputs into outputs. The processes and systems are essential in improving the quality and performance of the healthcare environment and can help providers with reliable, cost-effective, and sustained healthcare processes and enable them to achieve their goal of improving care delivery and enhancing patient outcomes. Therefore, inadequate information systems and the process can affect quality and decision-making.

5.1.3.1 Inadequate patient information systems and processes

There are inadequate information systems and processes for follow-ups and tracing of patients. It became difficult to provide continuous quality care to patients, especially those working in farming, mining, and industrial areas, as they are highly mobile and migrant workers. Facilities ended up with a high loss to follow-up and missed appointments, and systems and processes should be developed to address such. There should be one system nationally to track patients' movements as they visit other facilities using ID as a unique identifier.

5.1.3.2 Inadequate viral load management systems and processes

Viral load management is critical in managing and monitoring the effectiveness of treatment or treatment outcomes in HIV management. It is currently lacking or not implemented effectively in most health facilities. If no systems and processes are in place, it will affect patient outcomes. Most patients' blood for viral load is not collected per cohort. Either they are missed, or patients did not visit the facility, and there are no effective systems to identify such on time for tracing or tracking the patients. Viral load management is also crucial in monitoring the 95–95-95 UNAIDS target by 2030 to ensure that ART patients adhere to treatment and are virally suppressed. Quality improvement is key to identifying gaps and developing processes and systems that can be followed to improve VL monitoring in all health facilities. Patients, key populations, and the community should be educated on the slogan of undetectable equals untransmissible (U=U), to reduce new HIV infection through early ART initiation and adherence to lower the HIV viral load in the blood and by reaching that level where the transmission will be low and should be emphasized that this only applies to the transmission through sexual intercourse and not through other methods transmission; therefore they need to continue to implement relevant preventatives measures [16].

5.1.3.3 Poor data management systems and processes

Data management is collecting, keeping, and using data securely, efficiently, and cost-effectively. Managing digital data in an organization involves various tasks, policies, procedures, and practices. Data are critical to HIV programme management as it identifies gaps and monitors progress. Management should be data-driven to direct planning and allocation of resources. Therefore, the whole programme will lack direction if data are not managed well. The study revealed poor adherence to data management SOPs, incomplete clinical records, inconsistent clinical records quality audits, and lack of data verification. The facility manager's responsibility is to ensure that data are well managed in the facility. However, it is not happening in some facilities or is inadequate. Health care providers, including NIMART nurses, mostly do not accurately complete clinical records or registers. Such gaps make it difficult for the data team to capture quality data in the DHIS and TIER.NET. They also do not comply with the SOPs and HIV guidelines, compromising quality. Clinical records quality audits are not conducted consistently. Hence, gaps in clinical records are not attended to until data capturing. This is the responsibility of the clinical nurse mentor, HIV programme manager, and NIMART-trained nurse with the support of and under the leadership and guidance of the facility manager. The data team should ensure that the facility or institutional data is always verified, cleaned, timely, and ready to use. Access to timely and accurate facility data is vital for decision-making and planning. There should be a data collection system, processes, and equipment with a well-trained data or information team. A proper and highly effective ICT infrastructure is also necessary to collect real-time data from the facility or community level. The programme also needs well-trained staff to conduct data cleaning and verification process to ensure quality.

5.1.3.4 Stigma and discrimination

HIV was labeled as a gay disease from its beginning around the 1980s, which had the foundation of stigma and discrimination and has remained to the present. The failure of the HIV programme is owing to stigma and discrimination. Most PLWH are not accessing health services owing to stigma from community and health care workers. Stigma and discrimination become barriers that delay PLWH's early access to ART leading to complications and death. Suppose the world has to end the HIV epidemic. In that case, the focus will be on ending stigma and discrimination, especially among key populations such as adolescents, young women, LGBTQI–a common abbreviation for the lesbian, gay, bisexual, transgender, queer, and intersex community. Countries should end criminalization and punitive laws against LGBTQI and people who inject drugs and develop strategies to enhance access to health services. This will help deal with behavior that exposes them to HIV, reducing new HIV infections. Inequalities should be confronted to end the HIV epidemic [17].

5.2 Environmental factors

NIMART-trained nurses continuously reported poor infrastructure, that the health facilities are poorly maintained, small, and cannot accommodate the growing number of patients needing health services. They work in an overcrowded and congested environment, worsening infection during the COVID-19 pandemic. The consultation rooms are small and not well ventilated despite implementing ideal clinic initiative standards for quality care. Some patients have to wait outside for a long time and are exposed to heat or cold to implement infection control measures. Such small facilities do not have enough space for supplies, equipment, and medicines. Therefore, proper planning and budgeting is need to refurbish or extend the health facility.

5.3 Health care providers' factors

Health care providers can play a major role in ensuring that HIV services are accessible, efficient and effective. However, various factors must be considered to ensure quality, such as staff attitude, shortage, and scheduling.

5.3.1 Staff attitude

Some health care workers have negative staff attitudes toward patients and are a barrier to accessing health services, which has to change. Nurses must comply with their pledge and work according to SANC regulations and Batho Pele or customer care principles in line with the South African Constitution Act 108 of 1996 regarding human rights and patients' rights charter. Training should be provided to sensitize nurses on these legislations, including stigma and discrimination and key populations.

5.3.2 Shortage of skilled healthcare workers

Low- and middle-income countries like South Africa still experience a high shortage of skilled human resources for health, making those available staff overworked or overburdened and suffer from exhaustion and stress. This requires better planning, budgeting, and allocation of work schedules by the healthcare leadership. Some staff members resigned or transferred to work in other areas as they no longer cope with the workload, especially in rural provinces. Those left continue to be overworked, dissatisfied, and experience burnout, affecting the quality of HIV management and other programmes. Some form of intrinsic and extrinsic incentives is necessary to motivate nurses trained on NIMART. Despite task shifting, there is still high staff turnover, and more needs to be done. Nurses still perform non-clinical roles, and there is a need for task shifting in other roles like ordering and dispensing medication by assistant pharmacists rather than pharmacists, administrative work to administrators, and collecting specimens for phlebotomists or laboratory technicians as it delays actual management of patients. Nurses cannot become all-rounders as it compromises their clinical skills.

5.3.3 Confidence in HIV management

NIMART training should be aimed at providing knowledge and skills and building confidence and a positive attitude to manage PLWH. The districts should prioritize the establishment of the Department of Health district clinical mentorship teams and avoid reliance on partners to build the confidence of NIMART nurses at a facility level where patient care and management are taking place than at a classroom level where theory and simulation take place. On-job support to conduct the physical assessment, staging, interpretation of guidelines and results, selecting the correct regimen, drug interactions, and management of complications and opportunistic infections is key to improving the clinical competence of NIMART-trained nurses to the acceptable level of providing quality HIV management.

5.3.4 Clinical supervision and support by management

Management support is key to achieving the organizational goals and objectives, and once it is lacking, the HIV programme is not going to perform as expected. Management should manage by identifying gaps and be more proactive than reactive. Most challenges experienced by NIMART nurses and other health care providers might be minimized through the support of national, provincial, district, and local management. They will plan better and prioritize resources effectively where it is needed most.

5.4 Patient factors

Patients' social, psychological, physical, and financial factors need to be consider in HIV management. Failure to consider these factors might lead to poor clinical and virologic outcomes. Poor clinical outcome refers to a situation where the patient's condition is not improving despite taking antiretroviral treatment, while virologic outcomes refer to a situation where the viral load remains high or does not improve despite the patient starting on treatment.

5.4.1 Social factors

Patients need to modify their lifestyle, stop or reduce smoking, and alcohol consumption, eat a healthy diet, and exercise. Patients need treatment and scheduled appointments and avoid over-the-counter medication or traditional herbs that may interfere with treatment. Continuous patient self-care management education is key in every visit, including the importance of adherence to medication through health education and counseling. There is a need to modify a lifestyle that interferes with appointments and adherence to treatment because missing appointments interfere with the regular taking of medication, resulting in poor clinical and virologic outcomes. Some clients experience intimate partner violence (IPV) or gender-based violence (GBV), especially women when they have to disclose their HIV status and end up hiding and not taking medication as prescribed or missing their appointments.

5.4.2 Psychological factors

Stigma and discrimination also play a significant role in lack of disclosure, stress, anxiety, and depression, and loss of follow-up and should be dealt with decisively by NIMART nurses and the healthcare system. Factors leading to stigma and discrimination should be identified and addressed appropriately, including prevention. Sensitization of health care providers and the community about stigma and discrimination can be integrated into training and education and during community education and awareness campaigns. All stakeholders should be involved and sensitization, including PLWH, traditional and religious leaders, CBOs and NGOs. Mental health services should be provided to PLWH to reduce stress, anxiety, and depression. Enhanced adherence counseling (EAC) should be provided to all patients who missed appointments and did not adhere to treatment. Lack of support also results in poor adherence to treatment and lack of disclosure; patients need to identify a friend and family support and be referred to psychosocial counseling to help cope, accept the diseases, and move on with life. Community support groups can also be used to refer patients so that they have an opportunity to share their experiences with other people. Some do not have money to access health facilities monthly and can be registered for home or community medication distribution if they qualify or are assisted by community health workers. Some are physically disabled or very ill and need support with daily self-care management.

5.4.3 Financial or economic factor

Patients with financial difficulties or lack of support might miss appointments due to a lack of transport money to visit a health facility or pay for treatment in a private health facility or pharmacy. Some patients are unemployed without any government grant to support themselves, especially immigrants and those living with a disability or mental illness who need support. ART is available free of charge in South Africa's public health services. Stable patients on ART and the communities should be made aware of the minimum package of interventions to support linkage, adherence, and retention in care and differentiated models of care for stable chronic patients on treatment, which include repeat prescriptions (RPCs) collection strategies after six months on treatment through facility pick point (FAC-PUP), adherence clubs (AC) within the facility or community, external pick up points (EX-PUP) from the local shops, pharmacies or NGOs (National Department of Health AGL, 2021).

5.5 Inadequacy in NIMART training

South Africa has the largest and most high-profile ART programme globally, with 7.7 million initiated on treatment. However, quality is still a challenge and should be addressed through proper training, including standardization of the curriculum, use of strategies that can stimulate critical thinking, competency-based education, training and assessment, and application of the conceptual framework to enhance NIMART training and implementation.

5.5.1 Standardization of NIMART curriculum

The literature review and the study findings revealed that the NIMART curriculum was not standard and partner-driven, and recommendations were made to standardize the curriculum. The National Department of Health in South Africa did not have a standard curriculum to guide the country and train providers. The content covered and even the period offered differed. Some offer it in five days while others in ten days. The curriculum is a standards-based sequence of planned experiences where students practice and achieve proficiency in content and applied learning skills. The curriculum is the central guide for all educators as to what is essential for teaching and learning so that every student can access rigorous academic experiences. The disruption of onsite training by the COVID-19 pandemic has propelled the department to develop a standard training programme. It is now being attended to and offered online through the national knowledge and training hub and is accessible to all professional nurses either from m private or public sector and allocated CPD points. However, it is unclear which curriculum was followed in developing the training materials.

5.5.2 The use of strategies that stimulate critical thinking

Facilitators or educators should use interactive teaching strategies to stimulate critical thinking, including problem-based, reflective, case studies, and seminars. Health workers play a major role in learning and teaching by active participation based on their experience and knowledge of managing PLWH. Facilitators and educators should be adequately trained to facilitate NIMART and should be carefully selected during the recruitment process. Moreover, they should possess skills like nursing education or health sciences education with computer and good presentation skills, not just pick anyone to facilitate learning and teaching. In addition, experience in HIV and AIDS management is also necessary. They should do away or eliminate traditional strategies or didactics of the presentation without active participation or involvement of participants.

5.5.3 Use of competency-based education, training, and assessment model

Integrating theory with practice is key to improving health workers' competency levels and performance. Clinical mentoring and competency tools were developed to assess the competency of nurses after training and can be certified as competent than being presented with a certificate of attendance. All health workers trained should undergo a clinical mentoring process by allocating an experienced mentor for 6 to 12 months to support the trained health workers onsite or virtually through SMS, WhatsApp, and telephonically. Final assessments are conducted through OSCE or simulated case studies and onsite job assessments while managing the patients in the health facility to determine the competency of the trained health workers. NIMART-trained nurses should complete the logbook or portfolio of evidence with stipulated cases needed to manage children, men, women, ANC pregnant women, HIV/TB Co-infected cases, and adults. They need to show the integration of adult primary care in managing chronic diseases and integrated management of childhood illness when implementing NIMART or managing PLWH. Other education and training strategies that can improve NIMART implementation include pre-service, continuous in-service training, and CPD.

5.5.3.1 Pre-service training

Introduction or strengthening of NIMART as pre-service training to nursing students can help facilitate capacity building of new nurses before they can enter or join the health care system and prepare them to work effectively and efficiently in providing quality services to the community and PLWH. According to WHO (2014), **pre-service education** or **pre-service training is used interchangeably** and refers to any structured activity aiming to develop or reinforce knowledge and skills before a health care professional enters public health service or private practice. "Pre-service" refers to activities before a person takes up a job requiring specific training, i.e. before a person 'enters service. This also includes courses for graduates and undergraduates, which are 'pre-service courses' if they provide the competence needed to perform new services. *Pre-service training* is the *training* nurses receive before they begin managing patients in a health facility after completing formal training. This stage is vitally important as it lays the foundations for motivation and ensures that new nurses are competent before entering the consultation room.

Pre-service coordination is meant to increase efficiency for patients and office staff. Patients know upfront what their service will cost before they arrive, and they have the opportunity to pay for that service in full, in part, or to make payment arrangements. Nurses should be exposed to HIV and non-communicable and communicable disease guidelines, policies, and protocols before they start working as part of induction and orientation to their new roles in health facilities to provide integrated, comprehensive quality care to their clients or patients. This will also reduce time spent orientating the new nurses and be used effectively for patient clinical management. Again, training will reduce stress and anxiety as the new nurses will be familiar with such guidelines and confidently manage the patient. Unnecessary referral to other professionals or facilities will be reduced, facilitating access to services in the first or primary level of care. This can be designed through stakeholder coordination by the national, regional, or district training centres together with higher education institutions offering training and education to nurses and partners supporting the Department of Health, and can be offered through staggering the content every academic year or allocating weeks specifically for NIMART and Adult Primary care (APC) 101 like how Integrated Management of Childhood Illness (IMCI) is being integrated into HEIs learning and teaching programmes. Adult Primary Care (APC) is the new name for Primary Care 101 (PC 101). APC is a symptom-based integrated clinical management tool using a series of algorithms and checklists to guide the management of common symptoms and chronic conditions.

In adults, a clinical tool is a comprehensive approach to the adult's primary care for 18 years or older. APC has been developed using approved clinical policies and guidelines issued by the national Department of Health and is intended for use by all healthcare practitioners working at the primary care level in South Africa as a clinical decision-making tool. This tool accompanies a training package consisting of short onsite sessions using simulated case scenarios. APC is being implemented as part of the Integrated Clinical Services Management (ICSM), a key focus within the Ideal Clinic Realization and Maintenance (ICRM) initiative to improve the quality of care delivered and is complemented by the health for all health promotion tool to promote healthy lifestyles and health education. Therefore, APC 101 is a step-by-step training provided to health workers for the integrated management of communicable, and non-communicable diseases in the primary level of care with limited resources and facilitates the provision of integrated management of NCDs and communicable diseases, including HIV.

5.5.3.2 Continuous in-service training

Providing continuous or ongoing in-service training is key to keeping health workers updated on the current development and changes in national HIV policies, guidelines, and protocols to provide appropriate services to the community and PLWH. According to WHO, in-service training refers to training persons already employed, e.g. health providers working in the public or private sector.

In-service training refers to practical work experience during studies and usually, after one or two years of the theory are completed. In-service nurse training enhances the performance of a nurse. A nurse feels enriched with additions of ideas, concepts, and activities. In-service training improves the overall personality of a nurse. Sometimes it is called in-service education and training (INSET), and it improves various aspects of the overall performance of a nurse. This has to be planned periodically and facilitated within the facility to access all staff members and encourage discussion of real cases within the facility. Online nursing is a dynamic profession subject to rapid changes, like the HIV programme hence the need for in-service training for nurses. In-service training can be described as training that has been systematically planned, is carried out by a trainer within an institution, and takes place during normal working hours. Nurses are essential in transforming healthcare and health systems. Being educated to degree-level ensures nurses are well equipped to provide high-quality care. It also prepares them to take the lead, inform and design health services delivery, decision making, and policy development.

5.5.3.3 Continuous professional development

CPD is the term used to describe the learning activities professionals engage in to develop and enhance their skills. Health workers are expected to keep themselves abreast of the current trends and development in research to provide quality services. NIMART should be registered and accredited as one of the CPD programmes with SANC or HWSETA that must attend annually to accumulate points. CPD enables learning to become conscious and proactive rather than passive and reactive. Furthermore, CPD is professionals' holistic commitment to enhancing personal skills and proficiency throughout their careers. CPD combines different methodologies for learning, such as training workshops, conferences and events, e-learning programmes, best practice techniques, and ideas sharing, all focused on helping an individual to improve and have effective professional development. This can be managed by professional bodies such as SANC and HWSETA.

5.5.4 NIMART training and implementation regulation

NIMART training is not yet registered and accredited as a formal pre-service or CPD programme. It is not recognized as an expert in government even though it is recognized by non-governmental organizations (NGOs) supporting the government with HIV management. There are no incentives for providing an additional expert role as a NIMART nurse or clinical mentor, which demoralizes NIMART nurses. This delays the implementation of WHO recommendations for task shifting of creating an enabling regulatory environment for implementation, sustainability, and quality care. This requires all stakeholders, guideline developers, decision, and policymakers to fast-track engagements to register and apply for accreditation of the NIMART training with all relevant education and training quality assurance bodies such as SANC, HWSETA, and Department of Higher Education and Training as vocational training and consider as expert skills with additional remuneration for scarce skills or other forms of incentives can be implemented to motivate nurses.

5.5.5 Development of a conceptual framework to strengthen NIMART training and implementation

According to Mboweni and Makhado (2020), there was no conceptual framework to guide the training and implementation of NIMART, and this study developed a framework that needs to be implemented and reviewed before adoption. A further study can be conducted to upgrade the framework into a model that can be tested and approved for use. A framework is a particular set of rules, ideas, or beliefs that you use to deal with problems or decide what to do, and it can guide how to conduct training and implementation of NIMART. According to Adom and Hussein (2018), a *conceptual framework* is a structure that the researcher believes can best explain the natural progression of the phenomenon to be studied. The application of NIMART training and implementation was discussed in section five of this chapter.

6. The HIV continuum of care

The HIV continuum of care is a public health model that indicates steps or stages people living with HIV take from diagnosis until they achieve and sustain viral load suppression. The stages include diagnosis of HIV infection, linkage to treatment or ART, management of a patient on ART, retention to care and achievement, and maintenance of viral suppression, as illustrated in **Figure 2** [18].

The HIV care continuum is useful as both an individual and population-level tool or framework to assess care outcomes, and analyzing the proportion of PLWH in a given community, helps policymakers to plan and make a decision about the allocation of resources, and service providers can identify gaps in service delivery and develop interventions to improve the quality of care to PLWH to achieve the treatment goal of viral suppression. Achieving viral suppression has health and prevention benefits. Health benefits to PLWH as the viral load becomes low and can live healthy and longer, increasing life expectancy. The prevention benefit is that PLWH who take treatment as prescribed and have undetectable viral load have no risk of transmitting HIV to their HIV-negative sexual partners. However, these patients need continuous

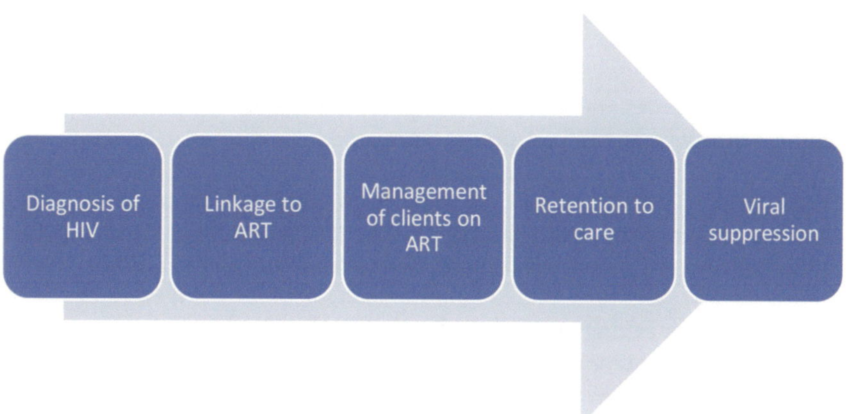

Figure 2.
HIV continuum of care.

engagement in HIV care with support, and knowing where the problem helps develop targeted intervention to break the cycle of HIV transmission. Therefore, it requires the involvement and collaboration of all stakeholders such as local health departments, community-based organizations, traditional and religious leaders, traditional healers, health care providers, public health officials, and PLWH to develop and implement quality improvement systems to support all PLWH to navigate the continuum and achieve and maintain viral suppression successfully. NIMART nurses play a major role throughout this continuum.

Diagnosed HIV infection can measure the percentage of the total number of PLWH whose infection has been diagnosed and measures prevalence, and NIMART nurses achieve this by conducting provider-initiated counseling and testing (PICT) to all patients coming to their care and confirming those without documented HIV status. This ensures that no one is left behind. Linkage of people who tested HIV positive to quality care is one of the crucial roles of NIMART nurses as clinicians and continues to ensure that PLWH receives effective and efficient care through follow-up, management of OIs, complications and provide adherence counseling messages, thereby keeping PLWH in care until they are viral suppressed, which indicates treatment or failure if the viral load is high while on treatment. It is very easy to lose PLWH if this continuum is not implemented properly. A combination of preventive interventions is also very important in reducing new HIV infections.

7. The role and responsibilities of NIMART nurses

The NIMART nurse plays an expert role and responsibilities in managing HIV and TB and includes the following [19, 20]:

Promote universal prevention and control of infection

- Prevention of Transmission of Communicable infections across all age groups and key populations, including from mother to child (HIV, Hepatitis, Listeriosis, Malaria, Syphilis, COVID-19, and TB) through education, community awareness, and campaigns and provide combined preventions strategies or refer clients for Voluntary Medical Male circumcision (VMMC), Pre- Exposure Prophylaxis (PrEP), Post Exposure Prophylaxis (PEP), including condom distribution.

- Strengthening antenatal and postnatal care for both HIV-negative and positive mothers through the PMTCT programme.

- Confirm the HIV test for those without documented HIV status and conduct provider-initiated counseling and testing for all clients under their care, including HIV index and recency testing services for partners and children.

- Conduct History taking and physical examination: To identify potential risk, baseline assessment, and identify conditions that need urgent attention and referral, the physical examination also helps to identify contradictions, OIs, and staging of the patients, which helps to understand the severity of the client's clinical condition, associated risks of mortality and determine the urgency and timing of ART initiation.

Conduct Screening of the following

- Conduct screening for TB to identify clients with a positive TB screen who requires further investigations such GeneXpert, and identify those with negative TB screen who may be eligible for TPT.
- Symptoms for meningitis to diagnose and treat clients with cryptococcal and other forms of meningitis and reduce associated morbidity and mortality.
- Mental health: Active depression and other mental health issues such as psychosis and substance abuse to identify potential adherence risks and side effects.
- Non-communicable Diseases (NCDs) such as hypertension, diabetes, and epilepsy to identify and manage major chronic diseases or co-morbidity and prevent drug interactions or contraindications.
- Pregnancy: Ask if not pregnant or planning to conceive for early referral to ANC, and measures to prevent mother-to-child transmission, assess fertility and contraceptive needs if not pregnant, and assess eligibility for ART regimens.
- Screen STIs, especially in sexual active clients, to identify and to provide early treatment.
- Neurodevelopmental screening among children for early referral and follow-ups.
- Cervical screening to identify women with cervical lesions and manage them appropriately.
- Nutritional assessment – to identify recent weight loss that may indicate active opportunistic infections or other conditions, also identify under/overweight clients that require nutritional and lifestyle support. Promoting breastfeeding and counseling the mother on feeding options is key to improving and maintaining the nutritional status of infants and children exposed to HIV, as it strengthens the immune system.
- Facilitate the collection of baselines clinical specimens- CD4 cell count to identify eligibility for CPT, cryptococcal antigen screening, to identify asymptomatic clients that need pre-emptive fluconazole treatment, Creatinine and Estimated glomerular filtration rate (eGFR) to assess renal sufficiency, HB to identify and manage anemia and eligibility for some ART where necessary such as Zidovudine (AZT), Hepatitis B, to identify those co-infected with hepatitis.

Interpretation of National Health Laboratory Services (NHLS) results and reports and develop appropriate interventions.

7.1 ART initiation and managing clients on ART

Fast track linkage to ART initiation, determine eligibility criteria and reason to defer ART, select the correct regimen, and provide key adherence messages for adults, children, and adolescents, including lifestyle modification.

- Re-initiating ART in clients who have interrupted treatment.

- Managing clients with TB/HIV coinfection.

- Switching stable clients on ART between first-line regimens and clients not responding well to the first-line regimen with confirmed virologic failure to a second-line regimen.

- Early referral of complicated cases for expert management.

- Management of opportunistic infection and complications related to HIV and TB.

- Provide routine integrated care to other conditions, including sexual reproductive health such as contraceptive and mental health services, identify and address stigma and discrimination, intimate partner violence, and gender-based violence.

- Care for HIV-exposed infants and children.

Identify eligibility for prophylaxis such as TB preventive therapy (TPT), and cotrimoxazole preventive therapy for infections (CPT).

Monitoring clients on ART.

Quality care at the follow-up visits promotes adherence, achieves and sustains viral suppression, minimizes side effects and toxicities, and promotes quality of life.

Viral load monitoring and management – to determine clinical, virologic, and immunological response to ART, management of viral load results in infants, children, adolescents, ANC pregnant women, and adults and conduct routine viral load monitoring.

Implement interventions to suppress viral load, including enhanced adherence support.

Provide clinical support to staff – experienced NIMART nurses in the health facility are expected to provide support to pre-service trained nurses, those newly trained, and staff on interpretation of guidelines, results, and ART initiation, and interventions and can be trained as clinical nurse mentors through the district clinical mentorship programme to transfer skill, knowledge to newly trained nurses thus improve clinical competence in the management of PLWH. They can also provide in-service training to keep staff and NIMART-trained nurses up-to-date with current development and research.

Data management and quality improvement – NIMART nurses are responsible for documentation of clinical findings, results, and interventions, and this should be legible, signed, and dated as per record management policy. Data management requires systems and processes, including clinical records audits to identify gaps and develop a quality improvement plan and projects to improve such gaps.

8. Conclusion

Enhancing NIMART training and implementation is key in HIV management to improve the quality of care and achieve the goal of ending new HIV infections and ending the HIV epidemic in low and middle-income countries through proper training, clinical mentorship, leadership, and management support, and dealing with structural challenges influencing the implementation of NIMART in healthcare services. The HIV continuum should continue to provide direction on managing the programme and identify individual and population gaps that require appropriate action by policy, decision-makers, health care providers, PLWH, community, and other stakeholders to end the HIV epidemic.

Acknowledgements

The authors also want to acknowledge the Department of Health in North West Province, South Africa, Regional Training Centre, and NIMART trained nurses for participating in the study.

Conflict of interest

The authors declare no conflict of interest.

Author details

Sheillah Hlamalani Mboweni[1] and Lufuno Makhado[2]*

1 University of South Africa, Pretoria, South Africa

2 University of Venda, Thohoyandou, South Africa

*Address all correspondence to: lufuno.makhado@univen.ac.za

References

[1] World Health Organization, UNAIDS & United Nations Children's Fund (UNICEF). Global HIV/AIDS response: Epidemic update and health sector progress towards universal access: Progress report 2011. World Health Organization. 2011. Available from: https://apps.who.int/iris/handle/10665/44787

[2] W. H. O. N. Diseases in Emergencies. G. Switzerland: WHO; 2019 No Title

[3] WHO. Task Shifting. Global Recommendations and Guidelines. World Health Organization; 2008. pp. 1-88. DOI: 10.1080/17441692.2011.552067. Available from: https://apps.who.int/iris/bitstream/handle/10665/43821/9789241596312_eng.pdf

[4] Mboweni SH, Makhado L. Conceptual framework for strengthening nurse-initiated management of antiretroviral therapy training and implementation in northwest province. Health SA Gesondheid. 2020;**25**:1-10. DOI: 10.4102/hsag.v25i0.1285

[5] Mboweni SH, Makhado L. Impact of NIMART training on HIV management in Ngaka Modiri Molema District, northwest province. International Journal of Africa Nursing Science. 2019;**11**(January):100170. DOI: 10.1016/j.ijans.2019.100170

[6] South Africa National Department of Health. South Africa National Department of Health ART Clinical Guidelines. Pretoria: South Africa National Department of Health; 2019

[7] Creswell JW, Creswell JD. Research Design: Qualitative, Quantitative, and Mixed Methods Approach. 5th ed. Los Angeles: Sage Publications Inc.; 2018

[8] Gray JR, Grove SK, Sutherland S. The Practice of Nursing Research. 8th ed. China: Elsevier; 2018

[9] Brink H, van der Walt C, van Rensburg G. Fundamentals of Research Methodology for Healthcare Professionals. 4th ed. Cape Town: Juta; 2018

[10] Babbie E, Mouton J. In: Vorster P, Prozesky B, editors. The Practice of Social Research. Cape Town: Oxford University Press; 2011

[11] Polit DF, Beck CT. Nursing Research. Generating and Assessing Evidence for Nursing Practice. 9th ed. W & W. Lippincott; 2017

[12] Donabedian A. Evaluating the quality of medical care. 1966. The Milbank Quarterly. 2005;**83**(4):691-729. DOI: 10.1111/j.1468-0009.2005.00397.x. Available from: https://pubmed.ncbi.nlm.nih.gov/16279964/. PMID: 16279964; PMCID: PMC2690293

[13] Dickoff J, James P, Wiedenbach E. Theory in the practice discipline. Part 1. Practice-oriented theory. 1968;**17**(5):415-434 Nursing research

[14] Mboweni SH, Makhado L. Challenges influencing nurse-initiated management of antiretroviral therapy training and implementation in Ngaka Modiri Molema district, northwest province. Heal. SA Gesondheid. 2020;**25**(January):1-11. DOI: 10.4102/hsag.v25i0.1174

[15] Chan M. Ten Years in Public Health. WHO report; 2017

[16] UNAIDS. The Need for Routine Viral Load Testing. UNAIDS 2016 Ref.; 2016. pp. 1-12. Available from: https://www.unaids.org/en/resources/documents/2016/JC2845

[17] UNAIDS. Confronting Inequalities. 2021. Available from: https://www.unaids.org/en/resources/documents/2021/2021-global-aids-update

[18] Hogg RS. Understanding the HIV care continuum. Lancet HIV. 2018;**5**(6):e269-e270. DOI: 10.1016/S2352-3018(18)30102-4

[19] South African National Department of Health. 2019 PMTCT Clinical Guidelines. South African National Department of Health; 2019

[20] Wessels J, Sherman G, Bamford L, Makua M, Ntloana M, Nuttall J, et al. The updated South African National Guideline for the Prevention of Mother to Child Transmission of Communicable Infections (2019). Southern African: Journal of HIV Medicine. 2020;**21**. DOI: 10.4102/sajhivmed.v21i1.1079. Available from: https://www.researchgate.net/publication/342791700_The_updated_South_African_National_Guideline_for_the_Prevention_of_Mother_to_Child_Transmission_of_Communicable_Infections_2019/citation/download